Methadone:
Experiences and Issues

DRUG ABUSE SERIES
Sheldon R. Roen, Ph.D., Series Editor

The Yearbook of Drug Abuse
    Edited by Leon Brill, M.S.S. and
    Ernest Harms, Ph.D.

Major Modalities in the Treatment of Drug Abuse
    Edited by Leon Brill, M.S.S. and
    Louis Lieberman, M.A.

Methadone
    Edited by Carl D. Chambers, Ph.D. and
    Leon Brill, M.S.S.

METHADONE: EXPERIENCES AND ISSUES

Edited by

Carl D. Chambers, Ph.D.
Co-Director and Assistant Professor
Addiction Sciences Division
Department of Psychiatry
University of Miami School of Medicine
Leon Brill, M.S.S.
Associate Professor of Psychiatry
Addiction Sciences Division
University of Miami
School of Medicine

Behavioral Publications   New York City
1973

Library of Congress Catalog Card Number 72-6122
Standard Book Number 87705-072-4
Copyright ©1973 by Behavioral Publications

BEHAVIORAL PUBLICATIONS, 2852 Broadway—Morningside Heights,
New York, New York 10025

Printed in the United States of America

Library of Congress Cataloging in Publication Data

Chambers, Carl D
  Methadone.

111438

  Bibliography: p.
  1. Methadone. I. Brill, Leon, joint author.
II. Title. [DNLM: 1. Drug Abuse. 2. Drug Addiction
--Drug therapy. 3. Methadone--Therapeutic use. WM270
C444m 1972]
RC568.M4C48   616.8'63   72-6122
ISBN 0-87705-072-4

To
Vincent P. Dole
and
Marie E. Nyswander

In recognition of their outstanding pioneering efforts and continuing contributions to the field of methadone treatment.

CONTENTS

PART 3. DETOXIFICATION THERAPY: RECENT EXPERIENCES AND ISSUES

FOREWORD

METHADONE:
EXPERIENCE AND ISSUES

Dr. Stanley F. Yolles,
Professor and Chairman,
Department of Psychiatry,
State University of New York at Stony Brook

Formerly Director
National Institute of Mental Health

The American public, aghast at the notion that a narcotic such as heroin has any significant relationship to the life style of the population, is now turning to another narcotic—methadone—to solve the problem of heroin addiction. The proliferation of methadone maintenance programs in efforts to treat heroin addiction now poses questions related to the safety and efficacy of a treatment which substitutes one addiction for another, as the lesser of two evils.

Methadone is an experimental drug, but if the public considers it to be a universal panacea to the heroin problem, its experimental prescription will be perverted, the caveats to be considered will instead be ignored and it is possible that the entire problem of narcotic addiction will be compounded by a hasty and cavalier effort to find an easy way out of the dilemmas surrounding the abuse of heroin.

For these reasons, publication of this volume *at this time* is extremely important both to professionals and the public whose concerns in providing effective

1

treatment for heroin addiction are genuine. The editors and authors of this book have attempted to assemble and analyze the experiences gained and the issues raised as components of what can best be termed "the methadone controversy." They have presented a thoughtful commentary which comes as close to being a definitive presentation both of the problem and the state of the art as is currently available. It is now the task of those persons responsible for the operation of methadone maintenance programs to evaluate the effectiveness of their work as it proceeds. This is a difficult assignment at best and the conditions under which methadone is being prescribed today make such ongoing evaluation as necessary as it is difficult.

Under Federal regulations set forth in 1971, Methadone may be used in drug maintenance programs on an experimental basis under closely supervised conditions. The use of methadone is seen by the Food and Drug Administration and the National Institute of Mental Health as part of a total rehabilitation program including counseling, occupational training and appropriate psychotherapy. As an investigational drug, it is available to community clinics for "controlled, scientific programs designed to rehabilitate drug addicts."

There is little doubt that methadone programs, when operated under strictly controlled conditions, will help in the collection of data relating to the selection of subjects, to treatment, recordkeeping and the evaluation of results. However, it will probably not be easy to achieve effective conditions for control of prescription of methadone since the distribution of any narcotic carries with it the potential for abuse.

It is in the full awareness of these problems that the authors of this volume present their discussions of past and current experience, since, for better or worse, the prescription of methadone has already become an important treatment modality. It is the authors' contention, as well as my own, that the approach to methadone programs has already become too uniform and too rigid. Any hope for success within the program must be based on the adaptation of a methadone therapy to each indi-

vidual's needs, and this will of necessity call for rehabilitative follow-up far beyond that which is presently provided. Only in the provision of such long-term continuity
of care will it be possible to assess the potential and
known undesirable effects, as well as the desirable actions attributable to the effects of the drug itself, within
a wider treatment approach.

The authors, in assembling the content of this book as
it relates to methadone, have also included current data
on research and utilization of narcotic antagonists, in an
effort to present for the reader's consideration the relative values of treatment of narcotic addiction by substitution therapy and by blockade therapy which antagonizes
the effects of opiates. It is suggested that strategy for
further development of the usefulness of each chemotherapeutic approach involves extensive experimentation.

As the editors point out, to have any pragmatic value
for the treatment of addiction to morphine-like drugs, the
ideal-typical medication employed, whether it be a drug
substitute or a drug antagonist, must: eliminate the euphoric appeal of heroin; preclude abstinence symptoms;
produce no toxic of dysphoric effects; be orally effective;
have long duration; be medically safe; be of moderate
cost; and be compatible with normal social roles.

Obviously, no such comprehensive treatment modality
has as yet been evolved. The content of this volume, however, is a significant contribution of information and
analysis of value to those who continue the search.

PART ONE

Early Experiences and Issues

Chapter 1
Introductory Overview—
Historic Background

Leon Brill

The use of methadone maintenance as a treatment approach can best be understood if examined against a broad legal and historical perspective, covering the international and American backgrounds. The American context would need to include such areas as: *a*) the Harrison Act and subsequent Supreme Court decisions interpreting treatment of the addict; *b*) discussion of the 44 ambulatory clinics for dispensing drugs established between 1919 and 1923; *c*) the "British System" of managing addicts; *d*) early forerunner plans to methadone treatment; and *e)* current regulations governing methadone programming.

LEGAL BACKGROUND

Federal Legislation

Congress does not have the power to legislate to restrain the purchase of opiates and other drugs. Its ability to enact Federal legislation regulating all phases of the production, manufacture, sale and use of narcotic drugs derives rather from the commerce and tax clause of the United States Constitution. Under the commerce power, it can forbid the importation of drugs and make violation of the statute a criminal offense. Under its taxing power, Congress may prohibit all purchase or sale of narcotics except in or from the original stamped package.

5

With these constitutional bases, Federal legislation enabling the Convention to bring about legal control of narcotics, with restriction of their sale and use, is contained in a series of statutes. Congress adopted a law entitled "An Act to Prohibit the Importation and Use of Opium for Other Than Medicinal Purposes" in 1909. Five years later, in fulfillment of the obligations of the United States under the Hague Convention of 1912, this law was amended to prohibit the export of narcotic drugs except to a country which regulated their entry.[1]

That same year, to implement the Hague Convention further, this country enacted its basic narcotic law, the Harrison Narcotic Act, as a revenue measure and exercise of Federal power to tax. By imposing penalties for illegal manufacture and distribution, the effect of its provisions was to regulate the production, manufacture and distribution of narcotics, and to limit the availability of narcotic drugs to medical and scientific use. Thus, in an effort to minimize the spread of narcotic addiction, the Harrison Narcotic Act was applied as a measure to control the domestic narcotic traffic.

Because there was need for tighter control over the import and export of narcotic drugs than provided by the Act of 1909 as amended in 1914, a revised form of this older statute was reenacted by Congress in 1922 as the Narcotic Drugs Import and Export Act. The importation of only such quantities of opium and cocoa leaves as the then Federal Narcotics Control Board found necessary to meet medical needs was authorized. With this legitimate exception, importation of any form of narcotic drug was prohibited. Under the special amendment to this statute in 1924, the legal manufacture of heroin in the United States ended.

With the growing abuse of marijuana, Congress enacted the Marijuana Tax Act of 1937, which requires the registration and payment of a tax by persons who produce, import, manufacture, sell, or transfer marijuana. When growing of the opium poppy, ostensibly for seed yield, sprang up as the result of a shortage of imported poppy seed during World War II, Congress en-

acted the Opium Poppy Control Act of 1942, which prohibited the growth of the opium poppy in the United
States except under a special license issued only upon a
demonstrated need for domestic production of the opium
poppy to supply opium derivatives for medical and scientific uses.

Because the Harrison Narcotic Act has been used to
control the domestic trade in narcotics, its constititution-
ality has been debated and subjected to court tests. Several cases have arisen testing the constitutionality of the
Act on grounds that it is not really a tax measure, but
rather an indirect method of invading the police powers
of the states; that it undertakes to regulate matters
within the exclusive control of the state, and that the penalties amount to a denial of due process of law. The point
at issue concerns the constitutionality of these statutes
and the extension of indirect control by the Federal government over objects which it is forbidden to regulate directly. The Harrison Narcotic Act has twice been
declared constitutional by the Supreme Court, solely as a
revenue measure and as an exercise of the Federal power
to tax. (*Ibid.*)

The Federal Bureau of Narcotics

Congress in 1930 established the Bureau of Narcotics
in the Treasury Department. To this Bureau were
transferred all functions and duties of control over narcotic drug imports and exports and enforcement of the
narcotic law previously exercised by the Federal Narcotics Control Board and the Bureau of Internal Revenue respectively. The policy of the new Bureau was to cut off
the supply of the illicit drug traffic at the source. Recently, in the President's Reorganization Plan effective
April 8, 1968, the Federal Bureau of Narcotics, and the
Bureau of Drug Abuse Control were combined and
transferred to the Department of Justice as the Bureau of
Narcotics and Dangerous Drugs. The "BNADD" thus ex-
ercises all control over heroin and the dangerous drugs.
(*Ibid.*)

The Law and Rehabilitation—the Two Federal
Public Health Service Hospitals

The Federal government has attempted to provide rehabilitation of the addicts through hospitalization in two Federal institutions. These hospitals in Fort Worth, Texas, and Lexington, Kentucky, cared for 1) those who, on conviction, were sentenced to confinement in such institutions; 2) those who were ordered to submit to such treatment as a condition of probation; and 3) patients who applied voluntarily for treatment. The pronouncement laid down in the Federal Regulations regarding the treatment of addicts is interesting:—"It is well established that the ordinary case of addiction yields to proper treatment, and that addicts will remain permanently cured when drug taking is stopped and they are otherwise physically restored to health and strengthened in will power." Actual treatment begins with gradual withdrawal of the drug "in a drug-free environment" in order to break the addict's physical dependence on it. The concept of the drug-free environment in an institutional setting as the *sine qua non* of all treatment long held sway, and has only recently been questioned and modified. [2,3]

COURT DECISIONS AND SUBSEQUENT LEGISLATION

In 1919, a special Treasury Department Committee reported that one million persons in the U.S. had become addicted to narcotics, which aroused the country and kept public concern at a high pitch. The Treasury Department, supported by medical leaders, began an intensive campaign against physicians who prescribed narcotics to addicted individuals.

In the Supreme Court that same year, in the case of *Webb vs. U.S.*, the Government sought an authoritative ruling on what constituted the legal and proper practice of medicine with addicts. The phrasing of the question posed by the Government influenced the decision: if a practicing and registered physician issues an order for morphine to an habitual user thereof, the order not being issued by him in the course of professional treatment in the attempted cure of the habit, but being issued for the purpose of providing the user with morphine sufficient to keep him comfortably by maintaining his customary use, is such order a physician's prescription under exception b) of Section (2) of the Harrison Act?

In this first Supreme Court decision on the case of a doctor who had prescribed large quantities of narcotics to an addict, it was ruled that drugs prescribed indiscriminately for an addict "not in the course of professional treatment in the attempted cure of the habit, but being issued for the purpose of providing the user with morphine sufficient to keep him comfortable by maintaining his customary use" did not fall within the exemption provision of the law. With this opinion, it became possible for the narcotics authorities to warn physicians against prescribing drugs for the purpose of avoiding withdrawal distress or keeping them comfortable.[4]

In the Jim Fuey Moy case in 1920, the Court decided that a doctor could not legitimately prescribe drugs "to cater to the appetite or satisfy the craving of one addicted to the use of the drug." But in 1922, the Behrman decision decreed that such prescriptions were illegal *regardless of the doctor's purpose*. The addict was forced to turn to illegal channels to obtain his drugs, and thus his involvement with the criminal world and the addiction system was confirmed—"a self-fulfilling prophecy".

The Supreme Court nevertheless displayed, in this opinion, a beginning realization that it had encroached on the medical profession by defining what a physician could or could not do for an addict patient in his medical capacity. The Court suggested that the physician might not have been subject to conviction if he had prescribed a smaller dose of narcotics. This was reflected in the subsequent *Linder decision* in 1925. Dr. Linder was accused of having sold a female addict with withdrawal symptoms one tablet of morphine and three tablets of cocaine for self-administration; she was an informer and he was arrested. The ruling stated that the Harrison Act

" . . . says nothing of addicts and does not undertake to prescribe methods for their medical treatment. *They are*

> *diseased and proper subjects for such treatment, and we cannot possibly conclude that a physician acted improperly or unwisely or for other than medical purposes solely because he has dispensed to one of them, in the ordinary course and in good faith, four small tablets of morphine or cocaine for relief of conditions incident to addiction. What constitutes bona fide medical practice must be determined upon consideration of evidence and attending circumstances."*

Further, the Court stated that

> "the direct control of medical practice in the states is beyond the power of the Federal Government and that an incidental regulation of such practice by Congress through a taxing act cannot extend to matters plainly inappropriate and unnecessary to reasonable enforcement of a revenue measure."

Thus, within 7 years after Webb, in *Linder vs. U.S.* and then *Boyd vs. U.S.,* the Supreme Court significantly clarified the rights of physicians under federal law to dispense and prescribe narcotic drugs. The subsequent interpretation was that a doctor who dispenses drugs in good faith for a medical purpose has not violated the Act. (*Ibid.*) Despite this clear holding, the Bureau of Narcotics regulations, based on language in Webb which Linder and Boyd repudiate, has never itself been appropriately modified.

Although the Supreme Court had recognized that addiction is a disease and the addict a proper subject for medical treatment, the physician could never know in advance whether he might be arrested and subjected to a "consideration of evidence and attending circumstances." The successful prosecution of so many doctors for a decade in the late teens and early twenties led them to realize that treating addicts entailed enormous professional risks. Dr. Linder's exoneration cost him $30,000 and his medical license for 2 years—and few private physicians were willing to expose themselves to these risks.[4]

Linder and Boyd are nevertheless important decisions, confirming the medical profession's right to deal with addict patients. A physician, *acting in good faith and adher-*

ing to accepted standards of medical practice, could prescribe moderate amounts of a narcotic for an addict in order to relieve conditions incident to his addiction. Unfortunately, this did not end the problems of physicians. Dr. Kolb has reported that, during the period 1931-1935, 10 years after the Linder decision, 757 physicians were convicted and 1347 were reported to State Boards for revocation of licenses on grounds of narcotics violations. From the year of the Harrison Act to 1938, it is estimated that 25,000 physicians were arraigned and 3,000 served penitentiary sentences on narcotics charges. About 20,000 were said to have made a financial settlement. Even now, about 50 per cent of revocations of medical licenses are for narcotics violations. It is probable that some of these physicians may themselves have been addicted.[4]

In the later *Robinson vs. California* case, (1962) the Court held that to convict a drug addict criminally for being an addict was a violation of the Eighth and Fourteenth Amendments. The majority held that the State has very broad powers to regulate the narcotic drug traffic within its borders and can punish for unauthorized manufacture, prescriptions, sale, purchase or possession of drugs. The State can even establish compulsory civil-commitment treatment programs for drug addicts to discourage violations of law or to protect the health and welfare of its citizens. But it cannot convict a man for his status alone without proof that a specific violation of the narcotic laws took place. In a dissenting opinion, Justice White wondered why, if it is cruel and unusual punishment to convict an addict for being an addict, he can be convicted for ministering to his addiction (or illness) by procuring the necessary supplies. In subsequent decisions related to alcoholics (*Driver vs. Hinnant, The Easter Case*) a chronic alcoholic was defined as a person powerless to stop drinking. To punish him for this is a violation of the Eighth Amendment. The court leaned on the Robinson case in the *Driver vs. Hinnant* decision, using the concept of *"mens rea"* so that the addict could avoid legal responsibility because he was not responsible for his actions.

RECENT FEDERAL NARCOTIC ENACTMENTS

Although there has been no Federal judicial redefinition of the Harrison Act since 1925, there have been legislative amendments concerned with the imposition of harsher penalties for violations. The Harrison Act provided for a maximum prison sentence of 10 years, the particular penalty to be determined by the judge before whom the case was tried.

In July 1965, the Drug Abuse Control Amendments of 1965 were added to the Federal Food, Drug, and Cosmetic Act, to be effective in February 1966. The new law requires that record-keeping be increased in the manufacture and distribution of stimulant and depressant drugs other than narcotics and marijuana, which are covered by the Harrison Act, and gives the Food and Drug Administration investigatory powers somewhat similar to those currently held by the Bureau of Narcotics. Agents are authorized to seize stimulant and depressant drugs being manufactured or distributed illegally and to arrest persons engaged in illegal activities.

Precisely which "dangerous drugs" (barbituates, amphetamines, tranquilizers) are covered by the new legislation is not specified, such classification having been made the administrative province of the Secretary of Health, Education and Welfare, who is to act on the advice of a committee of non-government experts. Prescriptions for drugs to which the new law becomes applicable will not be valid for more than 6 months, nor may they be filled more than five times without reauthorization from the prescribing physician. Persons over 18 who sell or give these drugs to anyone under 21 are subject to imprisonment for 2 years and a fine of up to $5,000 for a first offense. Imprisonment of up to 6 years and fines of up to $15,000 may be imposed for subsequent violations.

THE PRIVATE PHYSICIAN

Under the Harrison Act, which was enacted for revenue purposes, the medical and allied professions are charged with the responsibility of prescribing narcotics under restrictions. These restrictions are specifically set forth in the Federal regulations:

" . . . This Bureau has never sanctioned or approved the so-called reductive ambulatory treatment of addiction, however, for the reason that where the addict controls the dosage he will not be benefitted or cured. The Bureau cannot under any circumstances sanction the treatment of mere addiction where the drugs are placed in the addict's possession, nor can it sanction the use of narcotics to cover a period of excess of thirty days, when personally administered by the physician to a patient either in a proper institution or unconfined. If a physician, pursuant to the so-called reductive ambulatory treatment, places narcotic drugs in the possession of the addict who is not confinced, such action will be regarded as showing lack of good faith in the treatment of addiction and that the drugs were furnished to satisfy the cravings of the addict."[4]

NARCOTIC CLINICS 1919-1923

Efforts were made between 1919 and 1923 to deal with the fact that addicts exist and require treatment. At that time, there were virtually no inpatient hospital facilities available to the drug user. Even these began refusing to admit them altogether due partly to the discouraging rate of "cure" and partly to sensational publicity given episodes in which addicts either bribed or forced hospital attendants to give them quantities of drugs as well as reports of overprescribing by some doctors. Consequently, 44 outpatient narcotic clinics were opened throughout the country.[5]

The following AMA account of the clinics must, therefore, be read in light of the deficiencies of the material on which it is based.* The narcotic dispensaries were oper-

---

* With some small modifications or interpolations, the following discussion of the Ambulatory Clinics follows that of the AMA Committee on Mental Health under Dr. Leo Bartemeier Chairman, in their ABA Report.

ated by states and municipalities to meet a purported emergency created by the Supreme Court decision which held that dispensing narcotics to an addict merely to gratify his addiction was not proper professional practice and was therefore, illegal under the Harrison Narcotic Law. Many of the physicians who had prescribed for addiction stopped doing so, and addicts in some states and municipalities therefore applied to Boards of Health for relief. Some clinics were established at the suggestion of the Treasury Department agents. Of the 44 clinics or dispensaries established in various cities, some continued only a few weeks, others as long as four years. On the whole, the clinics seem to have had no purpose other than dispensing drugs to addicts in order to prevent their exploitation by drug peddlers. In some instances, the clinics dispensed cocaine as well as opiates. The directors of some clinics stated that they were not attempting to cure the patients of their addiction, i.e. their goal was detoxification. In all instances, it was eventually found necessary to give drugs to addicts for self-administration (Ibid).

Apparently, there were some exceptions to the general lack of direction and purpose in the clinics. The clinic in Shreveport, Louisiana, is reported to have required addicts to register in the clinic and obtain employment before drugs were dispensed. The New Orleans clinic did not register its addicts and the director states that drugs were dispensed with no idea of the addicts' being cured, but, rather to prevent exploitation of the addict. The clinic operated in New York City by the New York Board of Health deserves special comment. It served as a means of bringing the addict into the open, supplying him with drugs so that he could obtain employment, begin rehabilitation, and reduce the extent of his use, preparatory to hospitalization in the institution operated on North Brothers Island in New York City (later known as the Riverside Hospital for Adolescent Addicts in the 50's). Seventeen hundred of the 7,400 addicts registered in the New York City clinic finally went to the island for withdrawal, although the clinic was operated for a period of only 10 months. (Ibid.)

Actual reasons for closing the clinics remain obscure. Dr. Charles Terry and Mildred Pellens of the USPHS imply in the "Opium Problem (1928)" that the clinics were forced to close because of pressure from law enforcement officers before they had a chance to develop more definitive programs. Law enforcement officers, on the other hand, claim that the clinics were closed as a result of local public pressure, including those from the medical profession. Terry and Pellens believe that the medical profession did indeed play a decisive role in shutting down the clinics.[6]

Apparently as a result of the experience of the New York City clinics, a resolution at the meeting of the New York State Medical Association in 1920 condemning ambulatory treatment of addiction by private physicians and by clinics was adopted. At the meeting of the House of Delegates of the American Medical Association in New Orleans in 1920, the American Medical Association's Committee on the Narcotic Drug Situation in the United States recommended the following: "That ambulatory treatment of drug addiction, as far as it relates to prescribing and dispensing of nartocic drugs to addicts for self administration at their convenience, be emphatically condemned."

In 1920 and 1921, the Committee on Narcotic Drugs of the Council on Health and Public Instructions of the American Medical Association pursued its investigations, and in June 1921, made a recommendation which appears to have been extremely influential in molding medical opinion. This recommendation read that "any method of treatment for narcotic drug addiction . . . which permits the addicted person to dose himself with the habit-forming narcotic drugs placed in his hands for self-administration, is an unsatisfactory treatment of addiction . . . . Therefore, your Committee recommends that the American Medical Association urge both federal and state governments to exert their full powers and authority to put an end to all manner of so-called ambulatory methods of treatment of narcotic drug addiction, whether practiced by the private physician or by the so-called 'narcotic clinic' or 'dispensary.' " At the meeting of the American Medical Association of 1924, this resolution was adopted by the House of Delegates and, therefore, became the official policy of the American Medical Association.[5]

In spite of the Treasury Department's contention, based primarily on the failure of the New York Clinic, that the clinics were all disastrous failures, contradictory evidence is offered by Terry and Pellens. The resolution adopted by the House of Delegates in 1924, which condemns any system of treatment that places opiates in the hands of addicts for self-administration nevertheless remained the official policy of the American Medical Association for a number of decades.[6] Many of the arguments used against ambulatory treatment and clinics were revived when the issue arose again in the 50's and 60's.

THE "BRITISH SYSTEM"

The storm of controversy about narcotics clinics has often focused upon the pros and cons of the so-called "British System" for managing the addiction problem in England.[8] The differences between the incidence of the problem in the United States and Great Britain were attributed to a difference in regulations regarding prescriptions for opiates in the two countries though their Dangerous Drugs Act is similar to our Harrison Act. In 1963, Schur reported before the Presidential Advisory Commission in the U.S. that British narcotics policy approached the problem from a primarily medical orientation rather than stringent law enforcement standpoint. The guiding principle concerning prescription of drugs for addicts continued to be that set forth in the Departmental Committee on Morphine and Heroin Addiction in 1926:

" . . . morphine or heroin may properly be administered to addicts in the following circumstances, namely: *a)* Where patients are under treatment by the gradual withdrawal method with a view to cure, *b)* Where it has been demonstrated, after a prolonged attempt at cure, that the use of the drug cannot be safely discontinued entirely, on account of the severity of the withdrawal symptoms produced, c) where it has been similarly demonstrated that the patient, while capable of leading a useful and relatively normal life when a certain minimum dose is regularly administered, becomes incapable of this when the drug is entirely discontinued.[7]

It was not a criminal offense in Britain to be an addict or to possess or use narcotics that were properly prescribed. In connection with his use of drugs, the addict committed an offense only if he obtained illicit supplies, forged a prescription, or obtained drugs fraudulently from more than one doctor at a time. There were, however, no specialized addiction treatment facilities and no compulsory withdrawal treatment for addicts. The medical profession had a high degree of autonomy in the treatment of addiction. *(Ibid.)*

Under this policy the prevalence of addiction remained remarkably low (around 500 or so addicts estimated for the whole country at that time). Addicts were mostly native-born white Britons, over 30 years of age, of middle-class background and position—and about as often female as male. A disproportionately high number of these addicts were reported for the medical and allied occupations, but no other special occupational concentration was noted. A definite separation existed between addiction on the one hand, and the personnel and activities of the criminal underworld on the other.

Brill & Larimore British-On-Site Reports

Because of the great interest in the British management of the addiction problem especially as it related to ambulatory treatment, Brill and Larimore in 1959 and later again in 1965, undertook to study the "British System."[9,10] The first report was based on a brief visit to Britain and the Continent and contained the conclusion that there had never been a significant narcotic addiction problem in Britain. Particularly, it was noted that what was called a "British System" was no system at all, but merely a collection of administrative practices and information developed over a period of years in a situation so mild as to call for virtually no effort at control beyond some persuasive activities with respect to physicians who were careless.[9]

The *Second Report (1967)* noted there had been a significant change for the worse in the British narcotics situation in the seven years which elapsed since their site visit in 1959. The following points were of particular importance to understand the nature of the change and the direction countermeasures were taking:

1. The number of heroin addicts jumped from 56 in 1958 to over 300; the total for all opiate addicts from 300–700, with unknowns perhaps estimated at 1500–3000.

2. Type of addicts which accounts for the increase corresponds to the American "street addict." Cases were young, mostly men concentrated in the London metropolitan area. A prior step is amphetamines and barbituates. In studying the "British System," one of Larimore and Brill's objectives was to ascertain whether the British experience actually provided support for the clinic plan. They concluded: "The British experience to date does not provide support for the adoption of the "clinic plan" in this country. Their second objective was to determine whether all or part of the British system might be applied in this country. Their conclusion was that they found compelling reasons not to introduce the British system in this country.[10]

Schur questioned these findings, stating that the authors failed to document any of their conclusions; and there was no real evidence to support their belief that the British system was the result of the favorable British situation and not the cause of it. The British system was sharply divergent from ours in its humane handling of the addict.

Recent Enactments in Britain

Griffith Edwards in 1969 further summarized recent revisions in approach in England. Dr. Edwards reports that the legal context within which the doctor takes on the treatment of this patient is clear. Deriving from the Dangerous Drugs Acts of 1965 and 1967, the Dangerous Drugs (Notification of Addicts) Regulations of 1968, which came into operation on Feb. 22, 1968, and the Supply to Addicts Regulations, which came into force on April 16, 1968, in essence lay down between them the following rules:

1. Heroin and cocaine "unless given for the relief of pain due to organic disease or injury" may be prescribed only by doctors specially licensed by the Home Secretary. It is not proposed to issue licenses to general practitioners.

2. The Government is empowered at any time to limit prescribing of other dangerous drugs in similar manner. "This, of course, does not include the amphetamines or barbiturates."

3. A license is valid for prescribing only at a named hospital which, in London at least, largely means the new special centers located in teaching hospitals.

4. Any doctor seeing a patient he has reason to suppose is addicted must, within 7 days, furnish in writing certain particulars to the Home Office. This is a statuatory requirement and is not dependent on the patient's consenting to such notification.

The regulations mean that the addict in Britain is still, as ever, to be treated as a sick person, and it is the medical profession which is required by society to accept responsibility for the addict's care. There is no abrupt departure from the fundamental ethic of the "British system," but the way in which the system now operates is certainly a break with the past. Until 1968, any doctor who so wished could supply any narcotic in any amount (provided he kept proper records) to anyone he chose, charge fees for such prescribing, and was under no official obligation to notify. Intemperate prescribing by a handful of doctors under this old dispensation was thought by the second Brain Committee to have been responsible for the great increase in heroin addiction which has occurred during recent years.[11]

FORERUNNER PLANS TO METHADONE MAINTENANCE AND RELATED LEGISLATION

Over the years, the claim has frequently been made that some individuals could lead socially productive lives if maintained on moderate doses of an opiate. The Rolliston Committee in England appeared to have this view when it recommended to the Government in 1926 that physicians have the right to decide whether or not a patient should receive a continuous supply of opiates. The Scientific Study Group on Treatment of Addiction of the WHO in 1957 recommended a "perfunctory phase of treatment" before withdrawal though the eventual goal was abstinence.[12]

The Berger & Eggston Plan

An early proposal was for use of "depot morphine," which presumably would prevent withdrawal signs for 24 hours. This preparation would not be given the addict for self-administration, but would be administered once daily in the clinics established. At a meeting of the American Medical Association in San Francisco in June, 1954, Dr. Eggston submitted a resolution which proposed that the American Medical Association favor the legalization of distribution of narcotics to addicts under suitable safeguards.

The Kolb Plan

Dr. Lawrence Kolb, Sr. also proposed that narcotics be dispensed to addicts under certain safeguards. He requested "an increase in treatment facilities and recognition that some opiate addicts, . . . should be given opiates for their condition. Medical societies or health departments would appoint physicians to decide which patients should be carried on an opiate while being prepared for treatment and which ones should be given opiates indefinitely. Dr. Kolb's plan specified that opiates be prescribed by the addict's individual physician rather than by clinics.[13,14]

Academy of Medicine Plan

In 1965, the Committee on Public Health of the New York Academy of Medicine recommended that a procedure be instituted to "bring all addicts under medical supervision because they are sick people." The report also noted that "because of the psychological element in addiction and the high frequency of recurrence, the addict should not be removed from narcotics until another salutary crutch is provided"; that "maintenance therapy on a narcotic . . . should be restricted to highly selected subjects. . . . The academy does not favor indiscriminate dispensing of narcotics but . . . would not object to a demonstration project."[15]

REGULATIONS CONCERNING USE OF METHADONE MAINTENANCE

Gewirtz, in a cogent article in the *Yale Law Journal,* discusses the many legal questions surrounding the use of methadone maintenance. He states that because of the recency of methadone as used by Dole and because of its addictive qualities, potential restrictions on its use arise under both the Federal Food, Drug, and Cosmetics Act and the Harrison Act.

1. Under the Federal Food, Drug, and Cosmetics Act, the use of methadone maintenance presents unusual problems since the Act establishes procedures to assure that "new drugs" will not be introduced into interstate commerce until their safety and effectiveness have been proven. Before a "new drug" is marketed across state lines, the Food and Drug Administration must approve a new drug application (NDA), where there is not sufficient proof that a new drug is safe and effective. An alternative procedure permits the drug's manufacturer or sponsor to claim an investigational new drug exemption (IND) and send the drug into interstate commerce for testing only.

The first question concerning methadone maintenance under the FD&C Act is whether the "new drug" provisions are applicable. Methadone is not a "new" drug in the customary sense: the use of methadone as a painkiller has been confirmed and its use as the drug of choice during withdrawal from opiates, or for a brief period prior to withdrawal on a maintenance basis is widely accepted. However, an accepted drug like methadone would require new drug approval if it were marketed in interstate commerce for a new use "not generally recognized as safe and effective."[16]

Manufacturers of methadone have remained clear of the controversy, making no labelling changes or new claims for the drug, and they have not been required to file a new drug application.

2. Under the Harrison Act, according to the Bureau of Narcotics, any doctor who used methadone maintenance as treatment for heroin addicts violated federal law. The basis for the Bureau's position was the Harrison Act, which required the registration of narcotics dispensers, and imposes an excise tax on narcotics.

3. Analysis of case law and administrative history indicates that the Bureau's interpretation of the Harrison Act is improper, and that its current approach to methadone maintenance should be modified to protect the many physicians who believe that methadone maintenance is a sound form of treatment. The Bureau has further confused the issue by permitting methadone maintenance when it is a "research undertaking," but not allowing a widespread therapeutically-oriented program. (*Ibid.*)

4. Outpatient Treatment—In February 1962, the Medical Society of the County of New York stated its position that "physicians who participate in a properly controlled and supervised clinical research project for addicts on a non-institutional basis be deemed to be practicing ethical medicine." This research was to include the prescribing of narcotics. Several institution-based programs involved with the administration of narcotic drugs to addicted persons were soon in operation, and in New York State were specifically authorized by a 1965 law. The current most extensive maintenance research program is directed by Drs. Vincent Dole and Marie Nyswander at Manhattan's Bernstein Institute of the Beth Israel Medical Center. Governor Rockefeller, in

1970, recommended the appropriation through the NYS Narcotic Addiction Control Commission, of $15,000,000 to fund private and State Commission methadone programs; and this is currently being implemented throughout the State. Methadone programs are further spreading to other parts of the United States and abroad.

NEW FDA & BNADD REGULATIONS RE: USE OF METHADONE IN MAINTENANCE PROGRAMS

In a press release dated June 11, 1970, the Department of Justice announced its plan to promulgate new rules governing the distribution and use of methadone in community drug addiction programs. The new regulations, which apply only to "experimental use" of the drug in methadone maintenance programs, were publicized in the Federal Register in the summer of 1970 to invite reactions. The announced division of function between the two agencies was for the FDA to review applications for use of the drug for scientific validity and for the BNDD to consider the safeguards against diversion into illicit channels and other possible abuses of the drug.

The new regulations required advance approval of methadone rehabilitation projects from both agencies. The aim of this new regulation is "to clarify the ambiguous position of methadone today under current laws, to establish responsible medical-legal guidelines for its use and to facilitate controlled scientific research into methadone problems. Currently, methadone is viewed as a narcotic drug much like morphine. Its use is controlled by various federal drug laws. Possession and use are generally prohibited. However, it may be prescribed by physicians in the course of legitimate medical practice, and it may be used in drug maintenance programs on an experimental basis under closely supervised conditions."

A further statement by Charles C. Edwards, Commissioner of the FDA follows:

"The Food and Drug Administration takes the position that Methadone alone is not a cure for heroin addiction. It has not even been proved to be a satisfactory treatment. It may prove to be useful. If it does, we believe it will be as part of a total rehabilitation program, which may include counseling, occupational training, and in some cases, psychotherapy. FDA considers methadone to be an *investigational* drug subject to special regulations when used in maintenance therapy for narcotic addiction. On this basis, the Food and Drug Administration today has approved regulations which will make the drug available to the community clinics for controlled, scientific programs designed to rehabilitate heroin addicts. The regulations will aid community groups to set up programs to study the best methods of rehabilitation and make sure that the drug is used under strictly controlled conditions to provide safety and efficacy data. This plan was worked out with the National Institute of Mental Health and has their approval. FDA regulations include a recommended protocol or plan for such an investigation which outlines the method of selection of subjects, treatment regimen, record-keeping, and evaluation of results. FDA requires scientific evidence to establish the long-term safety and effectiveness of any drug for a particular purpose before the drug can be released for that particular use. The new regulations will facilitate the collection of that data. The Eli Lilly Co. of Indianapolis, working closely with FDA's Bureau of Drugs, has developed an oral dosage diskette form of methadone to minimize the possibility of abuse.[17]

TITLE 21—FOOD AND DRUGS

CHAPTER I—FOOD AND DRUG ADMINIS-TRATION, DEPARTMENT OF HEALTH, EDUCATION, AND WELFARE SUBCHAPTER C—DRUGS

PART 130—NEW DRUGS

CONDITIONS FOR INVESTIGATIONAL USE OF GRAMS FOR NARCOTIC ADDICTS

A notice was published in the Federal Register of June 11, 1970 (35 F.R. 9014), proposing establishment (21

CFR 130.44) of acceptable guidelines for programs for the investigation of methadone in the maintenance treatment of narcotic addicts. The guidelines of the Bureau of Narcotics and Dangerous Drugs, Department of Justice, were also proposed June 11, 1970 (35 F.R. 9015).

In response, a substantial number of comments were received from the medical community through the American Medical Association, Student American Medical Association, American Psychiatric Association, National Academy of Sciences-National Research Council, known authorities in the treatment of drug addiction, and from individuals and municipalities currently operating methadone maintenance programs.

The majority of the comments are in the form of objections to provisions of the protocol and the regulation, as follows:

1. The criteria in the protocol for the exclusion of subjects from the studies: Pregnancy, psychosis, serious physical diseases, and persons less than 18 years of age.

2. The requirement in the protocol that no more than a 3-day supply be given to a subject at one time.

3. The necessity for making records available to the Food and Drug Administration and to the Bureau of Narcotics and Dangerous Drugs and the lack of a guarantee of confidentiality of patient records.

4. The requirement that one of the objectives of the studies be a return to the drug-free state.

5. The requirement that the dosage level be limited to 160 milligrams per day.

6. The necessity of obtaining prior approval from the Bureau of Narcotics and Dangerous Drugs.

7. The requirements for weekly urine analysis and other laboratory tests and examinations.

8. The classification of the use of methadone in the maintenance treatment of narcotic addicts as an investigational use.

9. The regulation being overly restrictive and not in the best interest of the public.

The Commissioner of Food and Drugs, having considered the comments and having met with representatives of interested groups, associations, and individuals for further discussion, finds that:

1. The majority of the comments are a result of interested persons interpreting the proposal as restricting investigators to the suggested protocol. This is a misinterpretation since the protocol is intended only as a guide to assist the profession, municipalities, organizations, and other groups who are interested in sponsoring programs for the investigation of methadone in the maintenance treatment of narcotic addicts. It is not intended that every methadone program be confined to the limits of this protocol. Modification of the protocol and completely different protocols will be accepted, provided they can be justified by the sponsor. Modifications and completely different protocols consistent with public welfare and safety will be approved.

2. Since the suggested protocol is intended as an aid to those who wish to sponsor the programs for the investigation of methadone in the maintenance treatment of narcotic addicts. It is recognized that it would be to the benefit of the Food and Drug Administration, the Bureau of Narcotics and Dangerous Drugs, and the sponsors of the investigations to have a suggested protocol that would be acceptable to the majority of sponsors while satisfying the requirements of the two aforementioned agencies. Accordingly, the following revisions have been made in the regulation as adopted below:

a. The provision of the protocol "Criteria for exclusion from the program" has been changed to "Patients requiring special consideration." Pregnancy, psychosis, serious physical disease, and being less than 18 years of age are not reasons for automatic eliminations from a program but are conditions that merit special considerations which are detailed.

b. A provision has been added to the protocol to permit the investigator to exceed the dosage of 160 milligrams per day when the investigator finds it essential to do so and describes the considerations leading to such dosage levels in his protocol.

c. The requirement for laboratory examinations at 6-month intervals has been changed to 1-year intervals.

d. The objectives of the study have been clarified.

3. The remaining comments concerning the protocol

and not mentioned above deal primarily with problems that can be met by submission of a modified protocol to be judged on individual merit.

4. Regarding the objection that the record-keeping requirements and the necessity for making records available to the Food and Drug Administration and the Bureau of Narcotics and Dangerous Drugs could violate the confidential relationship between the patient and the physician: The Federal Food, Drug, and Cosmetic Act provides for promulgating regulations that require the sponsor of the drug investigations to maintain adequate records and that these records be made available to authorized personnel of the Food and Drug Administration. These records must be adequate in the event that follow-up on adverse reaction information requires identification of the patient. The Bureau of Narcotics and Dangerous Drugs is authorized to have access to these records under the Harrison Narcotic Act.

5. Methadone used in the maintenance treatment of narcotic addicts is an investigational use drug because, despite recent research gains, there remains inadequate evidence of long-term safety and of long-term effectiveness for this use to permit general marketability of methadone for maintenance treatment under the Federal Food, Drug, and Cosmetic Act standards for new drugs.

6. It is necessary that prior approval for methadone maintenance programs be obtained from the Bureau of Narcotics and Dangerous Drugs as well as the Food and Drug Administration because of this drug's potential for abuse. The Bureau of Narcotics and Dangerous Drugs' approval will be based on the existence of adequate control procedures to prevent diversion of the drug into illicit channels. Since the applications will be submitted only to the Food and Drug Administration and reviewed simultaneously by the two agencies, the inconvenience to the sponsor and the delay of approval will be minimal.

Therefore, pursuant to provisions of the Federal Food, Drug, and Cosmetic Act [secs. 505, 701(a), 52 Stat. 1052-53, as amended, 1055; 21 U.S.C. 355, 371(a)] and under authority delegated to the Commissioner (21 CFR 2,120), the following new section is added to Part 130:

§ 130.41 Conditions for investigational use of methadone for maintenance programs for narcotic addicts.

(a) There is widespread interest in the use of methadone for the maintenance treatment of narcotic addicts. Though methadone is a marketed drug approved through the new-drug procedures for specific indications, its use in the maintenance treatment of narcotic addicts is an investigational use for which substantial evidence of long-term safety and effectiveness is not yet available under the Federal Food, Drug, and Cosmetic Act standards for the general marketability of new drugs. In addition, methadone is a controlled narcotic subject to the provisions of the Harrison Narcotic Act and has been shown to have significant potential for abuse. In order to assure that the public interest is adequately protected, and in view of the uniqueness of this method of treatment, it is necessary that a methadone maintenance program be closely monitored to prevent diversion of the drug into illicit channels and to assure the development of scientifically useful data. Accordingly, the Food and Drug Administration and the Bureau of Narcotic and Dangerous Drugs conclude that prior to the use of methadone in the maintenance treatment of narcotic addicts, advance approval of both agencies is required. The approval will be based on a review of a Notice of Claimed Investigational Exemption for a New Drug submitted to the Food and Drug Administration and reviewed concurrently by the Food and Drug Administration for scientific merit and by the Bureau of Narcotics and Dangerous Drugs for drug control requirements.

(b) No person may sell, deliver, or otherwise dispose of methadone for use in the maintenance treatment of narcotic addicts until a study providing for such use has had the advance approval of the Commissioner of Food and Drugs on the basis of a Notice of Claimed Investigational Exemption for a New Drug justifying such studies.

(c) An abbreviated Notice of Claimed Investigational Exemption for a New Drug shall be submitted in four copies to the U. S. Food and Drug Administration, 5600

Fishers Lane, Rockville, Md. 20852. Forms entitled "Notice of Claimed Investigational Exemption for Methadone for Use in the Maintenance Treatment of Narcotic Addicts," suitable for such a submission may be obtained from the above address. The submission should be signed by the person in charge of the maintenance program who will be regarded as the responsible party and sponsor for the exemption. (If the sponsor is a manufacturer or distributor of the drug, the regulations as outlined in § 130.3 should be followed, except where the guidelines set forth below in this section are appropriate.) The notice shall contain the following:

(1) Name of sponsor, address, and date and the name of the investigational drug, which is methadone.

(2) A description of the form in which the drug is purchased (for example, bulk powder or tablet or other oral dosage form), the name and address of the manufacturer or supplier, and a statement that the drug meets the requirements of the United States Pharmacopeia or the National Formulary if recognized therein. If it is in an oral form designed to minimize its potential for abuse, and is not recognized in the U.S.P. or N.F., assurance that the drug meets adequate specifications for its intended use should be provided. This information may be obtained from the manufacturer. If bulk powder is used, a statement detailing how it is to be formulated, the name and qualifications of the person formulating the dosage form, and the address of where the formulating will take place if it is to take place at any location other than the principal address of the sponsor.

(3) The name, address, and a summary of the scientific training and experience of each investigator, and all other professional personnel having major responsibility in the research and rehabilitative effort, and individuals charged with monitoring the progress of the investigation and evaluating the safety and effectiveness of the drug if the monitor is other than a physician-sponsor. An investigator, other than a physician-sponsor (and investigators immediately responsible to a physician-sponsor and named in his submission) who has signed a form FD-1571 or the form entitled "Notice of Claimed Investiga-

tional Exemption for Methadone for Use in Maintenance Treatment of Narcotic Addicts," is required to sign a form FD-1573, obtainable from the Food and Drug Administration.

(4) A description of the facilities available to the sponsor to perform the required tests including the name of any hospital, institution, or clinical laboratory facility to be employed in connection with the investigation.

(5) A statement regarding the number of subjects to be included in the program.

(6) A statement of the protocol. The following is an acceptable protocol; however, it is not to be construed that this protocol must be adhered to in order to obtain clearance by the Food and Drug Administration and the Bureau of Narcotics and Dangerous Drugs. This protocol is intended primarily as a guide for investigators who wish guidance in what said agencies consider acceptable. Investigators who wish to do so may submit modifications of this protocol or other protocols; these will be judged on their merits.

Protocol

A. *Objectives*. 1. To evaluate the safety of long-term methadone administration at varying dosage.

2. To evaluate the efficacy of oral methadone per se in decreasing the craving for other narcotic drugs and in minimizing their euphoriant effect.

3. To evaluate the efficacy of methadone as a pharmacological moitié in facilitating social rehabilitation of narcotic addicts.

4. To determine which addicts are capable of returning to an enduring drug-free state.

B. *Admission criteria*. 1. Documented history of physiological dependence on one or more opiate drugs, the duration of which is to be stated.

2. Confirmed history of one or more failures of treatment for their physiological dependence on opiates.

3. Evidence of current physiological dependence on opiates.

An exception to the third criterion (current physiological dependence on opiates) is allowable in exceptional circumstances for certain subjects for whom methadone maintenance may be initiated a short time prior to or upon release from an institution. This procedure should be justified on the basis of a history of previous relapses. In these circumstances, appropriate descriptions of the facilities, procedures, and qualifications of the personnel of the institution are to be included in the application filed by the sponsor.

Subjects who wish to do so may be transferred from one approved program to another.

C. *Patients requiring special consideration*—1. *Pregnant patients*. Safe use of methadone in pregnancy has not been established. There is limited documented clinical experience with pregnant patients treated with methadone, and animal reproduction studies have not been done. It is therefore preferable that pregnant patients be hospitalized and withdrawn from narcotics. If such a course is not feasible, pregnant patients may be included provided the patient is informed of the possible hazard. To minimize the risk of physiological dependence of the new born, or other complications, pregnant women should be maintained on minimal dosage. The investigator should promptly report to the Food and Drug Administration the condition of each infant born to a mother in a methadone maintenance program.

2. *Patients with serious physical illness*. Patients with serious concomitant physical illness are to be included in methadone maintenance program only when comprehensive medical care is available. Such patients require careful observation for any adverse effects of methadone and interactions with other medications. The investigator should promptly report adverse effects and evidence of interactions to the Food and Drug Administration.

3. *Psychotic patients*. Psychotic patients may be included in methadone maintenance programs when adequate psychiatric consultation and care is available. Administration of concomitant psychotrophic agents requires careful observation for possible drug interaction. Such occurrences should be promptly reported.

Investigators who intend to include in their programs patients in categories 1, 2, and or 3 above should so state in their protocols and should give assurance of appropriate precautions.

4. *Patients less than 18 years of age.* It is imperative that adolescents be afforded the benefit of other treatment modalities whenever possible and that those with minimal histories of physiological dependence be excluded from methadone maintenance programs. Investigators who wish to include adolescents in the program are therefore required to submit special protocols for this purpose. These protocols should state in detail the number of such patients to be treated, the alternative treatment methods available, the criteria for selection, the screening procedures, and the anciliary procedures to be employed.

D. *Admission evaluation.* 1. Recorded history to include age, sex, history of arrests and convictions, educational level, employment history, and past and present history of drug abuse of all types.

2. Medical history of significant illnesses.

3. History of prior psychiatric evaluation and/or treatment.

4. Assessment of the degree of physical dependence on and psychic craving for narcotics and other drugs, and evaluation of the attitudes toward and motivations for participation in the program.

5. Formal psychiatric examination in subjects with a prior history of psychiatric treatment and in those in whom there is a question of psychosis and/or competence to give informed consent.

6. Physical examination.

7. Chest X-ray.

8. Laboratory examinations to include complete blood count, routine urinalysis, liver function studies (including SGOT, alkaline phosphatase, and total protein and albumin globulin ratio) blood urea nitrogen, and scrologic test for syphilis.

E. *Procedure*—1. *Dosage and administration.* The methadone is to be administered in an oral form so formulated as to minimize misuse by parenteral injection. The initial dosage is to be low for example, 20 milligrams per day. Subsequently, the dosage is to be adjusted individually, as tolerated and as required, up to 160 milligrams per day. In exceptional cases, investigators may find it essential to exceed this dosage to obtain the intended effect. If such cases are encountered, the initial protocol or an amended protocol should include the maximum dosage to be administered, the number of patients for whom such dosage is required, and a description of the considerations leading to such dosage levels. The methadone is to be administered under the close supervision of the investigator or responsible persons designated by him. Initially, the subject is to receive the medication under observation each day. After demonstrating adherence to the program, the subject may be permitted twice weekly observed medication intake with no more than a 3-day supply routinely allowed in his possession. Additional medication may be provided in exceptional circumstances, such as illness, family crisis, or necessary travel, where hardship would result from requiring the customary observed medication intake for the specific period in question.

2. *Urinalysis.* Urine collection is to be supervised; urine specimens are to be analyzed for methadone, morphine, quinine, cocaine, barbiturates, and amphetamines; urine specimens are to be pooled or selected randomly for analysis at intervals not exceeding 1 week.

3. *Rehabilitative measures.* Rehabilitative measures as indicated may include individual and/or group psychotherapy, counseling, vocational guidance, and job and educational placement.

4. *Abnormalities.* There shall be adequate investigation and appropriate management (including necessary referral and consultation) of any abnormalities detected on the basis of history, physical examination, or laboratory examination at the time of admission to the program or subsequently, including evaluation and treatment of intercurrent physical illness with observation for complications which might result from methadone.

5. *Repeated examinations.* Physical examination,

chest X-ray, and laboratory examinations conducted at the time of admission are to be repeated annually.

6. *Discontinuation and followup.* Consideration is to be given to discontinuing the drug for participants who have maintained satisfactory adjustment over an extended period of time. In such cases, followup evaluation is to be obtained periodically.

7. *Records.* Adequate records are to be kept for each participant on each aspect of the treatment program, including adverse reactions and the treatment thereof.

F. *Other special procedures.* Within the limitations of personnel, facilities, and funding available and in the interest of increasing knowledge of the safety and efficacy of the drug itself, the following procedures are suggested as worthwhile, to be carried out at baseline and periodically in randomly selected subjects: EKG, EEG, measures of respiratory, cardiovascular, and renal function, psychological test battery, and simulated driving performance.

G. *Voluntary and involuntary terminations.* Subjects who have demonstrated continued frequent abuse of narcotics or other drugs, alcoholism, criminal activity or persistent failure to adhere to the requirements of the program are ordinarily to be terminated and their records should reflect that they are treatment failures. If they are continued indefinitely in the program, the reasons for so doing should be stated in the protocol.

H. *Results.* 1. Evaluation of the safety of the drug administered over prolonged periods of time is to be based on results of physical examination, laboratory examinations, adverse reactions, and results of special procedures when these have been carried out.

2. Evaluation of effectiveness or rehabilitation is to be based on such criteria as:

a. Arrest records.

b. Extent of alcohol abuse.

c. Extent of drug abuse.

d. Occupational adjustment verified by employers or records of earnings.

e. Social adjustment verified whenever possible by family members or other reliable persons.

f. Withdrawal from methadone and achievement of an enduring drug-free status.

3. Evaluations are to be recorded at predetermined intervals; for example, monthly for the first 3 months, at 6 months, and at 6-month intervals thereafter.

I. *Evaluation group.* Whenever possible, a locally oriented independent evaluation committee of professionally trained and qualified persons not directly involved in the project nor organized by the sponsor will inspect facilities, interview personnel and selected patients, and review individuals' records and the periodic analysis of the data.

(d) The sponsor shall assure that adequate and accurate records are kept of all observations and other data pertinent to the investigation on each individual treated. The sponsor shall make the records available for inspection by authorized agents of the Food and Drug Administration. The Bureau of Narcotics and Dangerous Drugs is also authorized to inspect these records under the Harrison Narcotic Act.

(e) The sponsor is required to maintain adequate records showing the dates, quantity, and batch or code marks of the drug used. These records must be retained for the duration of the investigation.

(f) The sponsor shall monitor the progress of the investigations and evaluate the evidence relating to the safety and effectiveness of the drug. Accurate progress reports of the investigation and significant findings shall be submitted to the Food and Drug Administration at intervals not exceeding periods of 1 year. All reports of the investigation shall be retained for the duration of the investigation.

(g) The sponsor shall promptly notify the Food and Drug Administration of any findings associated with the use of the drug that may suggest significant hazards, contraindications, side effects, and precautions pertinent to the safety of the drug.

(h) The physician-sponsor or individual investigators

in admitting addicts to the investigational treatment program are required to give to the addict an accurate description of the limitations as well as the possible benefits which the addict may derive from the program.

(i) The physician-sponsor or each individual investigator of this program shall certify that the drug will be used and administered only to subjects under his personal supervision or under the supervision of personnel directly responsible to him; a statement to this effect shall be included in the notice. The signing of the form "Notice of Claimed Investigational Exemption for Methadone for Use in the Maintenance Treatment of Narcotics Addicts" by a physician-sponsor or the form FD-1573 by an investigator will satisfy this requirement.

(j) The physician-sponsor or each individual investigator shall certify that all participants will be informed that drugs are being used for investigational purposes, and will obtain the informed consent of the subjects and shall include a statement to this effect in the notice. The signing of the forms as indicated in paragraph (i) of this section will satisfy this requirement.

(k) Failure to conform to the protocol for which approval has been received from the Food and Drug Administration and the Bureau of Narcotics and Dangerous Drugs will be a basis for termination of the claimed investigational exemption.

(l) The sponsor of a "Notice of Claimed Investigational Exempttion for a New Drug" already on file with the Food and Drug Administration should review and amend his submission to bring it into accord with the acceptable protocol where appropriate within 60 days after the effective date of this section. All differences in his protocol from the suggested protocol should be justified.

(m) Provisions under the Harrison Narcotic Act enforced by the Department of Justice are applicable to this use of methadone.

Effective date. This order is effective upon publication in the Federal Register (4-2-71).

[Secs. 505, 701(a), 52 Stat. 1052-53, as amended, 1055; 21 U.S.C. 355, 371(a)]

Dated: March 25, 1971.

Charles C. Edwards,
Commissioner of Food and Drugs,
[FR Doc. 71-4553 Filed 4-1-71; 8:46 am]

TITLE 26—INTERNAL REVENUE
CHAPTER I

INTERNAL REVENUE SERVICE
DEPARTMENT OF THE TREASURY
[TREASURY DECISION 7076]
PART 151—REGULATORY TAXES ON
NARCOTIC DRUGS
ADMINISTERING AND DISPENSING
REQUIREMENTS

On June 11, 1970, there was published in the Federal Register, 35 F.R. 9015, 9016, a notice of proposed rule making amending § 151.411 of Title 26 of the Code of Federal Regulations in order to make clear the conditions upon which practitioners may administer or dispense narcotic drugs in the course of conducting clinical investigations in the development of methadone maintenance rehabilitation programs. Essentially, the proposal would require that practitioners obtain approval prior to the initiation of such an investigation by submission of a Notice of Claimed Investigational Exemption for a New Drug to the Food and Drug Administration which would then be reviewed concurrently by that agency for scientific merit and by the Bureau of Narcotics and Dangerous Drugs for drug control requirements.

This proposal was published in conjunction with a notice of proposed rule making published by the Commissioner of Food and Drugs for addition of a new section to Part 130 of Title 21 of the Code of Federal Regulations. Among other matters this notice contained acceptable criteria and guidelines agreed upon by the Food and Drug Administration and the Bureau of Narcotics and

Dangerous Drugs for the conduct of clinical investigations of this nature. Since the original publication of both of these notices, two extensions of 30 days each have been granted for the receipt of additional written comments. After extensive review of the written comments received, both agencies have agreed upon certain alterations in the proposed criteria and guidelines which are designed to facilitate further research and to accommodate the diverse needs and interests of the scientific community. These changes have been effected by appropriate modification of the new section to be added to Part 130 of Title 21 of the Code of Federal Regulations published elsewhere in this issue of the Federal Register. Inasmuch as the bulk of comments received concern the criteria and guidelines appearing originally in that proposal, no modifications of the proposed amendment to § 151.411 of Title 26 of the Code of Federal Regulations as published on June 11, 1970, have been undertaken.

As previously set forth, it is recognized that the investigational use of methadone, a class "A" narcotic drug requiring the prolonged maintenance of narcotic dependence as part of a total rehabilitation effort, has shown promise in the management and rehabilitation of selected narcotic addicts. In addition, it is a drug which has been shown to have a significant potential for abuse. The amendment which follows is designed to clarify the conditions under which it may be used for the specific investigational purpose indicated until such time as the results of present and future clinical investigations may indicate the necessity for reevaluation of current uses and control mechanisms. It does not authorize the prescribing of narcotic drugs for any such purpose, see 26 CFR 151.392. Moreover, it does not affect any other uses of narcotic drugs, or waive any requirements concerning the control, security, use, transfer, or distribution of narcotic drugs imposed by other Federal narcotic laws or regulations. The amendment shall become effective as of the date of this publication; however, those practitioners currently engaged in the operation of a bona fide clinical investigation shall have a period of 60 days in which to submit or resubmit a Notice of Claimed Investigational Exemption for approval.

Accordingly, under the authority previously cited in the notice of proposed rule making published in the Federal Register on June 11, 1970, 35 F.R. 9015, 9016, the word "Dispensing" preceding § 151.411 of Part 151 of Title 26 of the Code of Federal Regulations is hereby deleted and § 151.411 is amended to read as follows:

§ 151.411   Administering and dispensing.

(a) Practitioners may administer or dispense narcotic drugs to bona fide patients pursuant to the legitimate practice of their profession without prescriptions or order forms.

(b) The administering or dispensing of narcotic drugs to narcotic drug dependent persons for the purpose of continuing their dependence upon such drugs in the course of conducting an authorized clinical investigation in the development of a narcotic addict rehabilitation program shall be deemed to fall within the meaning of the term "in the course of professional practice" in sections 4704(b)(2) and 4705(c)(1) of title 26 of the United States Code: *Provided,* That approval is obtained prior to the initiation of such a program by submission of a Notice of Claimed Investigational Exemption for a New Drug to the Food and Drug Administration which will be reviewed concurrently by the Food and Drug Administration for scientific merit and by the Bureau of Narcotics and Dangerous Drugs for drug control requirements; and provided further that the clinical investigation thereafter accords with such approval; see 21 CFR 130.44. The prescribing of narcotic drugs is not authorized for any such purposes.

Effective date. This Treasury decision shall be effective when published in the Federal Register (4-2-71).

Dated: March 25, 1971.

John E. Ingersoll,
Director, Bureau of Narcotics and Dangerous Drugs, Department of Justice.

Randolph W. Thrower,
*Commissioner, Internal Revenue Service,
Department of the Treasury.*
Approved: March 25, 1971.

Edwin S. Cohen,
Assistant Secretary of the Treasury.
[FR Doc. 71-4554 Filed 4-1-71; 8:46 am]

REFERENCES

1. New York Academy of Medicine, Subcommittee on Drug Addiction: *Report on Drug Addiction,* 1955.
2. Wieland and Chambers: Two methods of utilizing methadone in the outpatient treatment of narcotic addicts, 1970.
3. Brill and Jaffe: The relevancy of some newer American treatment approaches for England, 1967.
4. New York Academy of Medicine, Subcommittee on Drug Addiction: Report on Drug Addiction, II, 1963.
5. American Medical Association, Council on Mental Health: Report on Narcotic Addiction, 1957.
6. Terry and Pellens: The Opium Problem, 1928.
7. White House Conference on Narcotic and Drug Abuse: Proceedings, 1963.
8. Schur: Narcotic addiction in Britain and America, 1962.
9. Brill and Larimore: The British narcotic system. Report to Governor Rockefeller, 1960.
10. Brill and Larimore: Second on-site study of the British narcotic system. Report to Governor Rockfeller, Reprinted, New York State Narcotic Addicition Control Commission, 1967.
11. Edwards: The British approach to the treatment of heroin addicts, 1969.
12. Eddy: Methadone maintenance for the management of persons with drug dependence of morphine type, 1969.
13. Kolb: Drug addiction: a medical problem, 1962.
14. Kolb: Drug addiction. Statement before Committee of United States Senate, published in *Bulletin of New York Academy of Medicine,* 2nd series, 1965.
15. New York Academy of Medicine, Committee on Public Health, Subcommittee on Drug Addiction: Report on Drug Addiction, 1965.
16. Gewirtz: Notes and Comments—methadone maintenance for heroin addicts, 1969.
17. Bennett: Development of a newly-formulated tablet for methadone maintenance program, 1970.

Chapter 2.

The Addiction Liability of Methadone (Amidone, Dolophine, 10820) and its use in the Treatment of the Morphine Abstinence Syndrome*

Harris Isbell
Victor H. Vogel

The discovery of any potent analgesic drug always raises the question of the danger of addiction to the drug. The idea that the drugs of the phenanthrene series (morphine and related compounds) were the only analgesics which possessed addiction liability had to be modified when Himmelsbach[1] showed that Demerol was an addicting drug. Accordingly, when methadone (which has also been called 10820, amidone, and dolophine) was shown to be a potent analgesic which possessed many of the pharmacologic actions of morphine[2], a study of its addiction liability became necessary. The studies, which are reported here, were carried out under the auspices of the Drug Addiction Committee of the National Research Council, and were conducted at the U. S. Public Health Service Hospital, Lexington, Kentucky.

In these studies particular attention was paid to the qualities which Himmelsbach[3] has regarded as characteristic of addiction to the opiate drugs: tolerance, physical dependence, and habituation, or emotional or

* This article was reprinted with permission from the *American Journal of Psychiatry,* **105,** 909-914, 1949.

psychic dependence. *Tolerance* is defined as the gradual decrease in the effect produced on repeated administration of the same dose of the drug. *Physical dependence* refers to an altered physiological state brought about by the repeated administration of a drug which necessitates continued use of the drug to prevent the appearance of a characteristic withdrawal illness (the abstinence syndrome). *Habituation* means emotional or psychic dependence upon the use of a drug. Of these three qualities, habituation is now regarded at Lexington as the most important and should be given the greatest weight in assessing the addiction liability of a drug.

After tolerance and physical dependence to methadone had been established experimentally in animals[4] studies on the administration of methadone to man were started at the Lexington hospital. When single doses of 5-10 mgm. of methadone were given to former morphine addicts, there was no evidence of euphoria. However, administration of doses of 20 mgm. or more of methadone subcutaneously to former morphine addicts regularly produced unmistakable euphoria. The patients began to talk more freely with each other and with the attendants; became boastful; compared the effects of the drug favorably with those of morphine; asked how it could be obtained, etc. The euphoria was slower in onset than that after the administration of morphine and persisted for as long as 48 hours after doses of 30-60 mgm. Intravenous administration of 20-30 mgm. of methadone produced particularly striking effects. The addicts would writhe in joy, and comment as follows: "O boy! that's a fine shot of dope. Can we get it outside? Who makes it? Will it be put under the Harrison Law?" The subjects were unable to distinguish the effects of methadone from those of heroin or dilaudid when the drug was given intravenously. Methadone became the favorite drug of many of the patients who received it intravenously, and they requested methadone in preference to morphine, heroin, or dilaudid when called for further experiments.

DIRECT ADDICTION IN MAN

Fifteen former morphine addicts, who volunteered for

the experiments, were given 4 doses of methadone subcutaneously daily for periods varying from 28 to 186 days.
The dosage was increased, as tolerance permitted, from
an initial level of 5-10 mgm. per dose to as high as 100
mgm. per dose in 3 of the cases who received the drug for
the longest period of time.

When the men were receiving only 5 mgm. of
methadone per dose, no evidence of euphoria or sedation
could be detected and the men complained that the drug
did not produce the pleasurable sensations they desired.
When the dosage was elevated to 10-15 mgm. 4 times
daily definite evidence of sedation and euphoria
appeared, and the patients began to express satisfaction
with the effects of the drug. These effects did not become
manifest until the third or fourth injection of the
increased dosage. Apparently, these actions of methadone
are cumulative. The behavior of the men then became
strikingly similar to that seen during addiction to
morphine. They ceased nearly all productive activity and
spent most of their time in bed in a dreamy semisomno-
lent state, which they termed being "on the nod," or
"coasting." This semisomnolence is regarded as a highly
desirable state by addicts. The patients neglected their
persons and their quarters.

Psychological tests[4] showed changes similar to those
seen in morphine addiction. As measured by the Otis
test, there was a loss of 6.8 IQ points in the week prior to
withdrawal as compared with the week prior to addiction. The arithmetic test was performed at almost the
same rate of speed, but there were more errors. Visual-motor coordination and perseveration tests were performed
at somewhat higher rates of speed, but with considerably more errors. The greater rapidity of visual-motor response and the increased fluidity of shift appear to be
vitiated by greater inaccuracy. A decrease in the efficiency of intellectual functioning is indicated.

The subjects used in this study appear to be diverse in
personality structure as measured by the Rorschach
methods. However, in every case there were changes between the test administered prior to addiction and that
administered during addiction. These changes may be

said to fall into two general categories. Those subjects whose primary difficulty appeared to involve inhibition conflicts in relation to the expression of their instinctual drives showed, during addiction, a decrease in the guilt and anxiety associated with these conflicts, accompanied either by increased sensuality, immaturity, and egocentricity or by decreased accessibility to affective stimulation. Where records of the same subjects were compared while on morphine sulfate and on methadone, the first result occurred most often with methadone, while the second most often accompanied the use of morphine. A second group, whose original records suggested that they were relatively free from anxiety, but were egocentric, self-centered, and emotionally withdrawn, revealed a greater accessibility to affective stimulation during addiction. When subjects in this group were compared while on morphine sulphate and on methadone results were quite similar for both drugs.

As the experiment proceeded, partial tolerance to the sedative actions of the drug became evident. The men, if maintained on a given dosage level, ceased to stay in bed, began to play cards, etc. When the dosage was elevated the men became somnolent, and, after they had remained on the new dosage level for a varying period of time, tolerance to the sedative effects again developed.

Definite tolerance to the pain threshold elevating action of methadone appeared during the experiment and is shown in Fig. 1.

No serious toxic effects appeared during addiction, even though some of the men received as much as 400 mgm. of the drug daily. Pulse and respiratory rates and systolic blood pressures were depressed throughout addiction. Five of the men developed a mild normochronic, normocytic anemia after the third month. The anemia, however, did not progress. All the subjects developed severe inflammation and induration of the skin over the injection sites.

WITHDRAWAL OF METHADONE

When the drug was abruptly withdrawn very little evidence of an abstinence syndrome was observed in 3 subjects who had received the drug for only 28 days. Definite evidence of physical dependence was, however, detected in all 12 subjects who received the drug for 56 days or more. The abstinence syndrome which developed was slower in onset, milder, and perhaps more prolonged than abstinence from morphine. The men had no complaints for the first 2 days. Thereafter, they complained of weakness, anxiety, anorexia, insomnia, and tinnitus. These symptoms persisted for as long as 6 to 8 weeks. Very few signs of disturbances in autonomic function (yawning, lacrimation, rhinorrhea, etc.) were seen. Vomiting and diarrhea were seldom observed. All subjects developed fever, elevated respiratory rates, elevated blood pressure, and tachycardia. Fig. 2 shows the intensity of abstinence from methadone as compared to abstinence from morphine.

The intensity of abstinence was estimated according to the point-scoring system of Himmelsbach. In this system arbitrary values are assigned to the various signs of physical dependence—1 point for lacrimation, 3 points for mydriasis, 5 points for a bout of vomiting, and so on. The scores are totalled and one thus obtains a semiquantitative estimate of the intensity of abstinence. The scoring system has been carefully calibrated on men with strong physical dependence to morphine. Such cases usually score 50 to 60 points in the second and third days of abstinence. Scores of less than 15 are regarded as nonsignificant, scores between 15 and 20 as very mild, and scores of 20 to 35 as fairly mild. The curve obtained on 5 men who received the drug for 142 to 186 days illustrates very well the slow development of the syndrome of abstinence from methadone as well as its mildness as compared to the course of abstinence from morphine.

USE OF METHADONE
IN THE TREATMENT
OF ABSTINENCE FROM MORPHINE

Methadone has now been administered to 17 men who

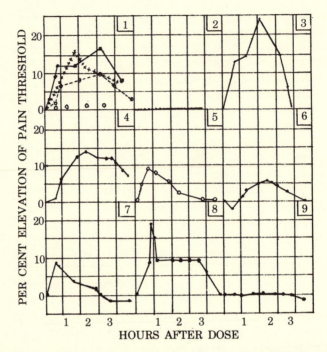

FIG. 1. Development of tolerance to the pain threshold-elevating action of methadone in Subject No. 729. *Curve 1.* Solid circles: greatest response to a 5 mgm. dose of methadone prior to addiction. Open circles: smallest response to a 5 mgm. dose. Crosses: average response to a 5 mgm. dose. Open circles with dots: control after injection of distilled water. *Curve 2.* Response to a 5 mgm. dose after 7 days of addiction. *Curve 3.* Response to a 15 mgm. dose on the 8th day of addiction. *Curve 4.* Response to a 15 mgm. dose after 14 days of addiction. *Curve 5.* Response to a 15 mgm. dose after 21 days of addiction. *Curve 6.* Response to a 25 mgm. dose after 28 days of addiction. *Curve 7.* Response to a 30 mgm. dose after 35 days of addiction. *Curve 8.* Response to a 45 mgm. dose after 42 days of addiction. *Curve 9.* Response to a 45 mgm. dose after 56 days of addiction.

were showing signs of abstinence from morphine. In all cases the intensity of abstinence has been greatly reduced or abolished (Fig. 3).

Methadone has been substituted for morphine in 12 subjects who were strongly addicted to morphine. Fig. 4 shows the average intensity of abstinence following preliminary withdrawal of these men from morphine. This preliminary withdrawal was carried out to prove and to assess the degree of physical dependence to morphine. The men were then returned to morphine and after 7 days methadone was abruptly substituted for the morphine at an average ratio of 1 mgm. of methadone for each 4 mgm. of morphine. The substitution was completely smooth. No signs of physical dependence appeared and the men did not notice the change. When the methadone was abruptly withdrawn a mild abstinence syndrome ensued which was quite similar to, but even milder than, that seen after direct addiction to methadone. This fact forms the basis for our present method of withdrawing morphine from addicts in the clinical section of the hospital. Methadone is substituted for morphine and the dosage of methadone is rapidly reduced over the course of 7 to 10 days. It is the most satisfactory method of withdrawal we have used. It is, however, necessary to emphasize that, 'though physical depen-

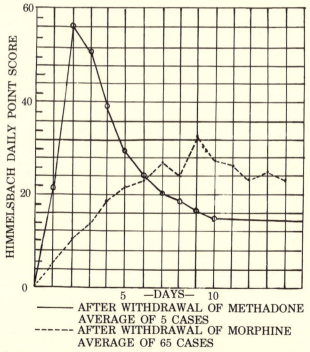

FIG. 2. Intensity of abstinence after administration of methadone for 4½ to 6 months.

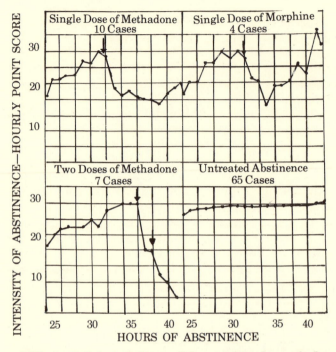

FIG. 3. Relief of abstinence from morphine by methadone. The intensity of abstinence is expressed in hourly points (31). *Upper left:* Average point scores of 10 subjects who received 21 mgm. of methadon at the 32nd hour of abstinence. Arrows indicate injection of drugs. Note prompt decline in the intensity of abstinence and prolonged effect. *Upper right:* Average point scores of 4 of the same subjects who received 30 mgm. of morphine at the 32nd hour of a subsequent abstinence. Note decline in the intensity of abstinence followed by a return to the original level about the 7th hour after the injections. *Lower Left:* Average point scores of 7 subjects who received methadon at the 36th and 38th hour of abstinence. Note almost complete abolition of abstinence 4 hours after the second dose. *Lower right:* Course of untreated abstinence from morphine based on 65 control cases of Himmelsbach.

dence can be handled nicely with this technique, the emotional factors in withdrawal remain and that loss of emotional control occurs just as frequently following substitution and withdrawal of methadone as it does after withdrawal of morphine. It should be emphasized that withdrawal is only the first and least important step in the treatment of narcotic addiction.

Methadone is an optically active substance and the

dextro- and levorotatory isomers have been resolved and studied separately. The levorotatory isomer accounts for all the analgesic effect of the racemic form and also for all the addiction liability. Levomethadone relieves and suppresses abstinence from morphine, whereas dextromethadone is totally inactive in this respect.[5] Racemic isomethadone, a structural isomer of methadone, is only one-fourth as potent as racemic methadone in relieving or suppressing abstinence from morphine. Following withdrawal of isomethadone from post-addicts who had been experimentally addicted to isomethadon for 56 days, an abstinence syndrome came on very rapidly. Abstinence from isomethadone was, qualitatively, very similar to abstinence from morphine. All the

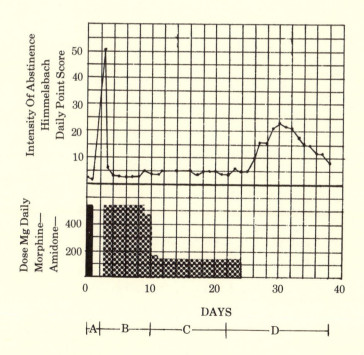

FIG. 4. Substitution of methadone (amidone) for morphine, average of 12 cases. A, preliminary withdrawal from morphine. B, restabilization on morphine. C, substitution of methadone. D, withdrawal of methadone.

signs of disturbances in autonomic function which are so characteristic of abstinence from morphine were noted. Quantitatively, abstinence from isomethadone was more severe than abstinence from methadone, but less severe than abstinence from morphine.[5] Both levomethadone and isomethadone must be regarded as addicting drugs.

DISCUSSION

The results leave absolutely no doubt that methadone is a dangerous addicting drug. Tolerance has been shown to develop to many actions of the drug in both animals and in man. Physical dependence to methadone has been shown to occur in dogs, and a real, however mild, physical dependence occurred in man after prolonged administration of larger doses. The drug in sufficient dosage produces a type of euphoria which is even more pleasant to some morphine addicts than is the euphoria produced by morphine. The similarity of the behavior of the subjects addicted to methadone to the behavior of men addicted to morphine; the similarity of the psychological changes; the requests for increases in dosage during addiction—all point to the development of strong habituation to the drug. Unless the use and manufacture of methadone are controlled, people with neurotic and psychopathic personalities will abuse it. Following our recommendation methadone has been brought under control of the Harrison Narcotic Law.

Morphine addicts like methadone because it produces a long sustained type of euphoria and because it will suppress signs of physical dependence when substituted for morphine. These qualities make methadone a particularly dangerous drug. The veteran morphine addict is skilled in ways of obtaining drugs illegally and has few scruples about introducing nonaddicts to the use of the drug. It requires some time for a person who becomes addicted for the first time to acquire the education and contacts necesary for illegal trafficking in narcotics. Addiction to a drug which is popular with morphine addicts is likely to spread much more rapidly than addiction to a drug which is liked only by people who have never been addicted to morphine.

The view that the addiction liability of methadone is slight because physical dependence to the drug is mild in man is very dangerous. Addicts are unwilling to bear even mild discomfort and would continue to use methadone despite the low grade of physical dependence to the drug. A mild grade of physical dependence might actually encourage addicts to use the drug, since the penalty (from the viewpoint of physical suffering) would be less if they were forcibly interrupted. Furthermore, addicts repeatedly relapse to the use of morphine long after withdrawal, not because they are suffering with any physical distress, but because they desire the euphoria produced by the drug or the relief from psychic and emotional discomfort which it gives. This is simply another way of saying that habituation is more important in addiction than in physical dependence.

It is hoped that the addiction liability of methadone will be clearly understood and accurately reported by all who write professionally and for the public press, thus avoiding unnecessary addiction such as occurred with demerol. It was disquieting to read in the American Weekly, a syndicated Sunday supplement magazine, for October 19, 1947, under the headline "New Drug for Breaking the Dope Habit" that ". . . . methadone does not produce the euphoria, the feeling of exaltation which comes to the addict from cocaine or other narcotics," and ". . . . it is the safest narcotic drug yet produced."

What is the danger of addiction to methadone in ordinary, legitimate medical usage? It is probably equal to the danger of addiction to morphine in the same circumstances—that is to say, slight. Mild signs, possibly indicative of developing physical dependence, have been seen in only 2 of 19 cases on temporary abrupt withdrawal of methadone after its administration for pain relief in cancer for from 35 to 180 days.[6] As long as the dosage of either morphine or methadone is held to the minimum required for pain relief, there is very little likelihood of addiction to either drug. The danger of "medical" addiction is great only when physicians mistakenly believe that a drug is not addicting and are careless in its use.

REFERENCES

1. Himmelsbach: Studies of the addiction liability of demerol (D-140), 1942.

2. Scott and Chen: The action of 1, 1 diphenyl-1 (dimethylamino-isopropyl)-butanone-3, a potent analgesic agent, 1945.

3. Himmelsbach and Small: Clinical studies of drug addiction II "Rossium" treatment of drug addiction, 1937.

4. Wikler and Frank: Tolerance and physical dependence in intact and chronic spinal dogs during addiction to 10820 (4-4 diphenyl-6-dimethylamino-heptatone-3) (Abstract), 1947.

5. Isbell and Eisenman: The addiction liability of some drugs of the methadone series.

6. Isbell, et.al.: Tolerance and addiction liability of 4-4-diphenyl-6-dimethylamino-heptatone-3 (amidone), 1947.

Chapter 3.

A Medical Treatment for Diacetylmorphine (Heroin) Addiction: A Clinical Trial with Methadone Hydrochloride*

Vincent P. Dole
Marie E. Nyswander

The question of "maintenance treatment" of addicts is one that is often argued but seldom clearly defined. If this procedure is conceived as no more than an unsupervised distribution of narcotic drugs to addicts for self-administration of doses and at times of their choosing, then few physicians could accept it as proper medical practice. An uncontrolled supply of drugs would trap confirmed addicts in a closed world of drug taking, and tend to spread addiction. This procedure certainly would not qualify as "maintenance" in a medical sense. Uncontrolled distribution is mentioned here only to reject it, and to emphasize the distinction between distribution and medical prescription. The question at issue in the present study was whether a narcotic medicine, prescribed by physicians as part of a treatment program, could help in the return of addict patients to normal society.

No definitive study of medical maintenance has yet been reported. The Council on Mental Health of the American Medical Association, after a thorough review of evidence available in 1957, concluded that "The advisability of establishing clinics or some equivalent

* This article was reprinted with permission from the *Journal of the American Medical Association,* **193**(8), 80-84, 1965.

system to dispense opiates to addicts cannot be settled on the basis of objective facts. Any position taken is necessarily based in part on opinion, and on this question opinions are divided." With respect to previous trials of maintenance treatment, the Council found that "Assessment of the operations of the narcotic dispensaries between 1919 and 1923 is difficult because of the paucity of published material. Much of the small amount of data that is available is not sufficiently objective to be of great value in formulating any clear-cut opinion of the purpose of the clinics, the way in which they operated, or the results attained." No new studies bearing on the question of maintenance treatment have appeared in the eight years since this report was published. Meanwhile, various medical and legal committees have called for additional research.

The present study, conducted under the auspices of the departments of health and hospitals, New York City, has yielded encouraging results; patients who before treatment appeared hopelessly addicted are now engaged in useful occupations and are not using diacetylmorphine (heroin). As measured by social performance, these patients have ceased to be addicts. It must be emphasized that this paper is only a progress report, based on treatment of 22 patients for periods of 1 to 15 months. Such limited study obviously does not establish a new treatment for general application. The results, however, appear sufficiently promising to justify further trial of the procedure on a larger scale.

PROCEDURE

The patients admitted to the program to date were men, aged 19 to 37, "mainline" diacetylmorphine users for several years with history of failures of withdrawal treatment. They have reported no substantial addictions to other agents (although most of them had used barbiturates or tranquilizers when narcotic drugs were unavailable). and they were not psychotic. Patients came from the streets, from drug withdrawal units, from referrals by social agencies and physicians who had heard of the program, and from recruitment of addicted friends by

Table 1
Incidence of Drug Abuse Among 65 Detoxification Patients

Daily Methadone Dose	Total Weeks of Surveillance	Percentage of Weeks The Drugs Were Detected				Percentage of Weeks With No Abuse	Percentage of Weeks Negative For Methadone
		Heroin	Barbiturates	Amphetamines	Cocaine		
40 mg (N=21)	64	64.1[a]	1.6	17.2	6.3	23.4[d]	22.4
30 mg (N=21)	71	39.4[b]	1.4	16.9	1.4	31.0[e]	35.2
20 mg (N=23)	67	34.3[c]	—	6.0	—	44.8[f]	22.4
Total	202	45.5	1.0	13.4	2.5	33.2	26.7

Note: Comparisons between "a" and "c" produce a statistically significant difference . . . $X^2=11.582$; $P= < .001$.
Comparisons between "a" and "b" produce a statistically significant difference . . . $X^2=8.169$; $P= < .01$.
Comparisons between "d" and "f" produce a statistically significant difference . . . $X^2=6.609$; $P= < .05$.

55

patients under treatment. Further details of their history are given in the Table.

Division of Program Into Three Phases.—PHASE 1.—The addict patients were stabilized with methadone hydrochloride in an unlocked hospital ward, given a complete medical workup, psychiatric evaluation, a review of family and housing problems, and job-placement study. After the first week of hospitalization, they were free to leave the ward for school, libraries, shopping, and various amusements—usually, but not always, with one of the staff. Patients lacking a high school diploma started in classes that prepare students for a high school equivalency certificate. For the present study the time in this initial phase was arbitrarily set at six weeks.

During this phase of hospitalization, the treatment unit was kept small (four to nine patients). This was felt necessary because most patients started the treatment with serious anxieties and doubts. The limitation of patient load allowed the staff to individualize the daily ward activities and deal with the special problems of each patient.

PHASE 2.—This began when subjects left the hospital and became outpatients, returning every day for methadone medication. They were asked to drink their medication in the presence of a clinic nurse, and to leave a daily urine specimen for analysis. When indicated, this rule has been relaxed; reliable patients who have been on the program for several months have been given enough medication for a weekend at home or a short trip. Continued contact with the hospital staff was provided as required. The most important services needed during this phase of treatment were help in obtaining jobs, housing, and education.

PHASE 3.—This phase is the goal of treatment, the stage in which an ex-addict has become a socially normal, self-supporting person. The two patients who are considered to have arrived at this phase are still receiving maintenance medication since the physicians in charge of their treatment feel that withdrawal at this time would be premature. Supervision of their medication is as careful as in phase 2; the only distinction between patients in phases 2 and 3 is in the degree of social advancement.

PHASE 1A.—This phase designates a special group of four patients who are being maintained on high doses under close and continuing observation to reveal any delayed toxic effects of methadone (Table). So far, none have been found. These patients live on a metabolic ward, and so are still classified in phase 1, but as measured by social adjustment they have progressed to phase 2 or 3, since all are either employed or going to school. The ward serves mainly as their residence, which they are free to leave as they wish subject only to the general routine of hospital activities.

Narcotic Medication.—Patients have differed markedly in tolerance to narcotics at the beginning of treatment, and in the rate with which they have adapted to increasing doses of medication. Individualization of treatment thus has been necessary. A rough estimate of initial tolerance was made from each new patient's history of drug usage, with allowance for exaggeration since addicts coming to a maintenance program usually fear that physicians will not prescribe enough medication, and with recognition of the fact that the number of "bags" used by an addict is not a reliable measure of narcotic tolerance. The diacetylmorphine content of a "bag" obtained on the street today is low and variable. This estimate provided a guide to initial dosage, but the only sure way to measure tolerance is to observe the reaction to test doses of narcotic drugs. The schedule, therefore, differed for each patient.

On admission patients usually have shown mild or moderately severe symptoms of abstinence, the last shot of diacetylmorphine having been taken some hours before. These patients were relieved promptly by one or two doses of morphine sulfate (10 mg) or dihydromorphione (Dilaudid) hydrochloride (4 mg), given intramuscularly, and then started on oral methadone hydrochloride therapy (10 to 20 mg, twice daily). Patients coming to treatment without symptoms were started on a regimen of methadone without other medication, but were

Maintenance Therapy of Ex-Addicts With With Methadone Hydrochloride, Summary of First 15 Months (February 1964 to May 1965)

Ethnic Group*	Age† Years'		Previous Treatments‡				Ar-rests	Education	Best Job§	Military Service‖ Years	Time on Program, Months	D¶	P#	HS**	Present Activity
	FD	A	F	S	M	P									
E	16	22	–	3	3	–	6	8th grade	Truck driver	–	15	150	1a	Cert	Preparing for college (Sept. 1965)
E	18	31	3	3	2	–	8	1 year high school	Odd jobs (few months each)	–	15	180	1a	Cert	Horticulture school
P	21	33	2	–	4	–	14	2 years high school	Office clerk	– –	10	100	1a	Cert	Employed (rehabilitation work)
E	20	30	1	2	3	1	1	Graduated high school	Store manager	A3	10	180	1a	–	Employed (usher cashier in theater)
E	17	22	–	–	6	–	4	2 years high school	Shipping clerk	–	11	100	3	–	Employed (parking lot foreman)
E	21	25	–	–	–	12	1	2 years college	Musician	–	10	100	3	–	Employed intermittently (musician)
E	18	25	–	–	2	–	6	Graduated high school	Radio operator in military service	N4	3	100	2	–	Employed (office work)
N	17	32	1	–	2	–	9	2 years high school	Clothes presser	–	1½	100	1	NS	Seeking employment
N	22	37	–	1	1	–	3	2 years high school	Truck driver	A4	1½	80	1	NS	Seeking employment
P	15	23	–	–	–	–	1	2 years high school	Head usher	A3	1½	90	2	Cert	Working as waiter
N	16	27	1	–	4	–	1	3 years high school	Stock clerk	A5	1½	130	1	NS	Army
E	18	22	3	–	3	2	4	1 year college	Mason	–	1	100	1	–	Seeking employment

58

Group*	FD†	A†	F‡	S‡	M‡	P‡		Education	Job§	Military∥		Dose¶	Phase#	HS**	Status
P	25	35	1	—	2	—	3	1 year high school	Paint sprayer	-	½	110	1	—	Employed
P	20	32	1	—	4	—	9	2 years high school	Supervisor of shipping department	—	1	100	1	NS	Employed
N	18	30	2	—	—	—	6	3 years high school	Shipping clerk	AF4	¼	70	1	NS	Seeking employment
E	18	24	—	—	10	—	0	8th grade	Installing window screens	—	3	115	2	NS	Employed
P	14	30	—	—	—	—	2	2 years high school	Office clerk	M3	3	70	2	NS	Welfare (seeking employment)
P	19	25	—	—	16	—	10	2 years high school	Office clerk	AF 2½	3	110	2	NS	(Employed (hospital record room)
E	17	19	—	1	1	1	0	Graduated high school	None	—	3	120	2	—	Vocational school (barber)
P	13	20	—	—	—	1	2	3 years high school	Stock boy	—	3	50	2	NS	Employed (hospital laundry)
E	19	26	—	—	2	—	8	2 years high school	Construction laborer	—	1½	100	2	NS	Seeking employment
N	14	30	—	—	—	—	2	8th grade	Shipping clerk	AF4	1½	10	2	Cert	Leather goods company interpreter

* For comparison with other treatment series, patients classified into three groups: Western European ancestry (E) Puerto Rican and Cuban (P), and Negro (N).

† Age first used diacetylmorphine (FD); age at admission (A).

‡ Number of admissions to Federal Hospital—Lexington, Ky (F); state hospitals—Manhattan State, Central Islip (S); municipal hospital—Manhattan General, Metropolitan, Riverside (M); private clinics and groups, including Synanon (P).

§ All but two patients were employed at time of admission. Job indicated is best position ever held.

∥ Time in Army (A), Navy (N), Marines (M), or Air Force (AF).

¶ Dose methadone hydrochloride given orally, mg/day.

Phases of treatment: 1a—four patients, residents on metabolic ward of Rockefeller Institute; 1—new patients being stabilized on methadone therapy, they sleep in hospital but may leave during day for school, shopping, or job; 2—patients newly discharged, living at home or rooming house, needing social support; 3—ambulatory patients who are self-supporting.

** High school equivalency status: If not a high school graduate each patient was encouraged to enroll in night school to prepare for high school equivalency certificate. Those who have completed this course, passed examination, and received certificate are indicated by "Cert"; those now in night school indicated by "NS."

59

watched carefully for appearance of symptoms after admission. After the first 24 hours most patients could be maintained comfortably on the oral medication alone. The dose of methadone hydrochloride was increased gradually over the next four weeks to stabilization level (50 to 150 mg/day). Two patients in whom tolerance at the expected rate failed to develop have been held at lower doses (Table). With some patients, treated early in the study, the buildup of dosage was too rapid; they became overly sedated for a few days, and two of them had transient episodes of urinary retention and abdominal distention. Other patients, given too little, have become abstinent, exhibiting malaise, nausea, sweating, lacrimation, and restlessness. With more accurate prescription, patients have not become euphoric, sedated, or sick from abstinence at any stage of treatment. They have simply felt normal, and have not asked for more medication.

After the patients reached maintenance level, the morning and evening doses were combined by progressive reduction of the evening medication with an equal addition to the methadone taken in the morning. After discharge from the hospital patients could thus be maintained by a single daily visit to the outpatient clinic. The patients who have had difficulty in spanning a 24-hour period with a single dose have been given medication to take at home; this has been a minor problem, limited to those who could visit the clinic only in the evening. In all cases it has been made clear to the patients (and accepted by them as a condition of treatment) that the amount of medication and the dosage schedule were the responsibility of the medical staff. Physicians did not discuss dosage with the patients, although of course they listened carefully to any report of symptoms that might suggest excess or lack of medication.

Laboratory Control.—The urine of every patient was collected daily in the hospital and at each clinic visit, to be analyzed for methadone, morphine (the chief metabolite of diacetylmorphine), and quinine (a regular constituent of the street "bag"). The thin layer chromatographic method of Cochin and Daly[1] was used, after preliminary extraction of the alkaloids from urine with cation exchange resin. The sensitivity of the procedure was such that it would give a definite positive if a patient had taken an average "bag" of diacetylmorphine during the preceding 24 hours.

RESULTS

The most dramatic effect of this treatment has been the disappearance of narcotic hunger. All of the patients previously had made efforts to remain drug-free after withdrawal, but were unable to resist the craving. Drug hunger became intolerable for most of them shortly after discharge from a withdrawal unit and return to their neighborhood. It became especially severe when they were exposed to emotional stress. With methadone maintenance, however, patients found that they could meet addict friends, and even watch them inject diacetylmorphine, without great difficulty. They have tolerated frustrating episodes without feeling a need for diacetylmorphine. They have stopped dreaming about drugs, and seldom talk about drugs when together. Patients have even become so indifferent to narcotics as to forget to take a scheduled dose of medication when busy at home.

The extent to which the patients have ceased to behave as addicts, and their reliability in reporting illegal drug use, were verified by the results of urinalysis. Negative results in almost all analyses showed that use of diacetylmorphine has been rare and sporadic, although the patients have had ample exposure to addict friends and pushers. Remarkably, the episodes of drug taking were reported by the patients spontaneously, and their reports have correlated with the laboratory evidence.

An interesting phenomenon, which has been seen in several patients, was the production of symptoms typical of drug deficiency by acute emotional stress. Anxiety in some susceptible patients caused malaise, nausea, yawning, and sweating, indistinguishable from the effects of abstinence, even though the patients were being maintained on large doses of medication. After experiencing relief with reassurance but without additional medication, susceptible patients have become less alarmed by these symptoms, and the episodes have occurred less frequently. In two other patients symptoms suggesting abstinence have appeared in the course of mild respiratory-tract infections. These symptoms, not associated with anxiety, were difficult to evaluate, but in any event disappeared in a few days without need for increase in medication. These observations suggest that the effectiveness of methadone can vary with changes in psychological and metabolic state.

The degree of tolerance established by methadone was titrated in six patients by giving diacetylmorphine, morphine, dilaudid, or methadone intravenously in a double-blind study. The drugs were given in randomized order and various doses six hours after the last administration of methadone. Stabilization with methadone, as here described, was found to make patients refractory to 40 to 80 mg diacetylmorphine (which would cost $10 to $25 if purchased on the street). Larger amounts were not systematically tested; probably blocking would extend to greater doses since two patients with high tolerance showed little reaction to intravenous injection of 200 mg of diacetylmorphine—a huge amount, possibly enough to kill a nontolerant individual.

Unscheduled, but perhaps necessary, experiments in drug usage were made by four patients. These subjects found that they did not "get high" when "shooting" diacetylmorphine with addict friends on the street. Both the patients and their friends were astounded at their lack of reaction to the drug. They discontinued these unrewarding experiments without need for disciplinary measures, and have discouraged other patients from repeating the experiment. So long as patients take methadone as scheduled, they apparently cannot feel the euphoria of an addict taking a street bag of diacetylmorphine.

Complications.—The chief medical problem has been constipation. The tonus of the sigmoid and the defecation reflex remain depressed even in patients with high tolerance to the narcotic effects of methadone, while the motility of the upper gastrointestinal tract appears to be unaffected. Five patients, given a barium sulfate meal and followed with daily x-ray examinations for a week, showed normal or only slightly delayed passage of barium through the small intestine, but in three of the five, the evacuation of barium from the colon was abnormally slow. Fecal impaction has occurred when patients have made no effort to defecate for several days. Patients therefore were instructed to take a hydrophilic colloid every day, and a supplementary laxative or enema if bowels have not moved for three days. With these precautions patients have had no further difficulty.

Apart from constipation, patients have shown no major ill effects ascribable to use of methadone. The tendency of addicts to leukocytosis (9,000 to 14,000 white blood cells/cu mm with 60% to 80% polymorphonuclear cells[2] continued, apparently unaffected by this medication. Bone marrow biopsies in four patients after eight months of treatment were normal. No effect of methadone on renal function was disclosed by repeated urinalyses. Liver-function tests, when originally normal, remained so. Results of basal metabolic rate, thyroid uptake of sodium iodide I 131, red blood cell uptake of labelled triiodothyronine, and plasma protein-bound iodine were normal in three patients who had been stabilized on methadone hydrochloride (100 to 150 mg/day) for four to six months. Some patients have reported excess sweating in hot weather, but no one has been unable to work for this reason.

Mental and neuromuscular functions appear unaffected. Patients have performed well in school and at various jobs. Studies of motor skill (accuracy in tracking moving targets) showed normal coordination. We have not yet been able to find a medical or psychological test capable of distinguishing patients on methadone therapy from normal controls. They can, of course, be distinguished by urinalysis.

There has been no problem so far in holding patients. Only two of the patients who started treatment have been discharged. These uncooperative and disruptive psychopaths were transferred to withdrawal units. Two others who were admitted specifically for tolerance tests at an early stage of the study were returned (as originally planned) to the withdrawal unit from which they came; both subsequently have asked to return to the program.

A fifth patient signed out after only four days on the ward, and also asked to return.

COMMENT

Previous efforts to treat addict patients with narcotic medication, have been handicapped by lack of sufficiently long-acting agents. The Council's report[1] noted that in 1919 to 1923 experience, "in all instances it was eventually found necessary to give drugs to addicts for self-administration." This is inherent in the pharmacology of parenterally administered morphine, which was used in these clinics and would probably apply to other agents with short periods of action such as diacetylmorphine, dihydromorphine, or meperidine. If addict patients are to be maintained with any of these drugs, they would need several injections per day; otherwise they would return to the street for additional drugs.

Projected into large-scale treatment, a medical use of short-acting narcotic drugs would require dispensaries staffed to give thousands of injections per day, with rooms or park benches in the neighborhood for addicts to wait between shots. Alternatively, physicians would have to yield control of drug administration to the addicts themselves. Neither alternative is acceptable. With methadone, however, the situation is much different since patients can be stabilized with a single daily dose, taken orally, under medical control. Maintenance of patients with methadone is no more difficult than maintaining diabetics with oral hypoglycemic agents, and in both cases the patient should be able to live a normal life.

We believe that methadone has contributed in an essential way to the favorable results, although it is quite clear that giving of medicine has been only part of the program. This drug appears to relieve narcotic hunger, and thus free the patient for other interests, as well as protect him against readdiction to diacetylmorphine by establishing a pharmacological block. A previous attempt by one of us (M.N.) to treat addict patients without narcotic medication ended in failure.[3] Other clinics, attempting to rehabilitate patients after withdrawal, have had equally poor results. These, however, are indirect arguments. When the treatment program is sufficiently well established, the necessary control studies with social support, but without medication, must be made.

This study was supported by the Health Research Council grant U-1501 of New York City, and by the National Association for Prevention of Addiction to Narcotics.

Major contributions to this investigation were made by the following: Mary Jeanne Kreck, MD, bone marrow biopsies and tests of narcotic tolerance; Joyce Lowinson, MD and George Lowen, MD, expansion of the program at Manhattan General Hospital; Nathan Poker, MD, measurements of intestinal motility; David Becker, MD, and Eugene Furth, MD, tests for thyroid function; and Norman Gordon, MD, Alan Warner, and Ann Henderson, measurements of motor skills of patients, and ratings with intelligence tests and mood scales.

Sodium iodide I 131—*Iodotone-1 131. Oriodide-131, Radiocaps-131, Thertodide-131, Traceretal-131.*

REFERENCES

1. Cochin and Daly: Rapid identification of analgesic drugs in urine with thin layer chromatography, 1962.

2. Isbell, *et.al.*: Liability of addiction of 6-dimethylamino-4-diphenyl-3-heptatone (methadone, "amidone" or "10820"), 1948.

3. Berle and Nyswander: Ambulatory withdrawal treatment of heroin addicts, 1964.

Chapter 4.

Rehabilitation of the Street Addict*

Vincent P. Dole
Marie E. Nyswander

The street addict is a special and troublesome kind of drug-dependent individual[1]—a person identified with the slums of a large city, alienated from normal society, a thief and a chronic jailbird. He (or she) supports an expensive habit without legal income and so, inevitably, is involved in crime. The life of a heroin user is not a pleasant one, however, even though heroin does provide some periods of euphoria. Increasing doses and more frequent injections of the drug are needed for relief of abstinence symptoms, while the euphoric state becomes more difficult to attain. Heroin fails to satisfy the user on a long term basis. Heroin addicts—like alcoholics and heavy smokers—try from time to time to escape the slavery of their habit. In their dissatisfaction with the habit lies motivation and the hope of any program of rehabilitation.

The social trap in which the street addict is caught sharply distinguishes him from the middle class user (who may ruin his family, but maintains respectability) or the addicted physician or nurse (who diverts narcotic supplies to personal use) or the patient with chronic disease given narcotic medicine by medical prescription. All of these individuals have in common a physical dependence on narcotic drugs, but the problems of rehabilitation are widely different.

Any program that ignores the social deficits of the

* This article was reprinted with permission from the *Archives of Environmental Health,* **14,** 477-480, 1967.

street addict will fall short of making him a productive citizen in free society. Acquisition of the drug habit is only the first step in the social deterioration of the street addict and, likewise, stopping the use of heroin is only the beginning of rehabilitation. When an adolescent becomes addicted to heroin, his maturation ceases. The normal experiences of school, family life, vocational training, and assumption of responsibility are blocked, and his energies become diverted to the means of getting money for heroin. If he was not delinquent before becoming addicted, he becomes so; his alienation from society widens with exposure to the addict world and jail. This is the path that must be retraced in therapy.

Suppose, for the purpose of discussion, it could be possible to cure heroin addiction instantly and completely by giving a medicine. Let us imagine that this utopian treatment would end all craving for narcotics and establish a state of perfect physical health. This, obviously, would be a valuable adjunct to treatment, but it would not repair the deficit caused by several years of addiction during the critical period of a young person's life. The patient, although cured pharmacologically, would still lack a job and lack the self-assurance and work record that would make him employable. To the world, perhaps even to his family, he would still be a junkie. Rehabilitation is a slow process; this, indeed, is true of learning in general, but the cured addict has the extra burden of having been a failure and having lost faith in himself. A pharmacological cure is no more than a beginning. To become a productive and responsible member of society, the ex-addict needs help from someone who understands the nature of his struggle.

Methadone is not quite the magic medicine outlined above. It does provide a blockade against heroin effects,[1] and it relieves the insidious drug hunger of detoxified addicts, but it does not suddenly banish all interest in heroin. Many patients must pass through a period of experimentation in which they return to the old neighborhood and try heroin again. For some, one test is enough; the lack of euphoria in a properly blockaded patient eliminates the appeal of this drug. For some others, the experiments will continue for a time, even though the block-ading action of methadone prevents euphoria. It would seem that the habit pattern of heroin taking is deeply es-tablished in some addicts and can be extinguished only by a number of negative experiences. With the metha-done blockade, however, the patient is protected against readdiction to heroin; not only does methadone block euphoria from heroin, it also eliminates the secondary ab-stinence symptoms that otherwise follow after heroin taking and lead the addict back to regular use.

With time, with discussion of his problems, and with monitoring of the urine by objective tests,[2] the patient can be carried through the transitional period of intermit-tent drug taking. Meanwhile, many important changes are taking place in his relationship to society and in his attitude toward himself. If, as is true of many street addicts, he came from a deprived background, where drugs were widely used, and had become addicted through curiosity, he may have no residual psychopatho-logical symptoms once the pressure of heroin addiction has been removed. Such a patient will pass through a series of stages during the first year of rehabilitation and (with methadone blockade) will have a good chance of be-coming a productive member of the community. This is not merely an expression of hope; the expectation is based on the experience of the Methadone Maintenance Research Project over a period of 2½ years involving, at the current census, a total of 124 patients who had been intractable street addicts. No patient in the program has become readdicted to heroin while blockaded with metha-done; two thirds of the patients under treatment for three months or longer are steadily employed or at school.

First, consider the sequence of events in an uncompli-cated process of rehabilitation (if addiction ever can be described as uncomplicated) and then the additional problems caused by an underlying psychopathology in-dependent of addiction—problems that remain when the use of heroin has been discontinued (e.g., psychopathic personality, anxiety neurosis, schizophrenia).

In the treatment of primary, or uncomplicated, addic-tion with methadone, four stages can be distinguished, each with characteristic problems and therapeutic responses. The first stage, called phase 1 in previous reports, [3,4] is a period of induction and uncertainty. The addict comes to treatment with mixed feelings and many doubts. He can be helped substantially by reassurance from older patients who have experienced similar anxieties on entry into the program and who have succeeded in starting a new life. An early and favorable sign in the response of the new patient is the development of pride in personal hygiene. His clothing is washed and pressed; he shaves each morning and helps maintain the ward. Perhaps he has no usable clothing and no money. For such patients the purchase of inexpensive but decent clothes and a raincoat is an essential step in rehabilitation, since he must present an acceptable appearance for employment interviews, and for his self-respect. Some time during the second or third week, if the methadone is given in proper doses (enough to prevent abstinence symptoms, but not so much as to produce narcotic effects), the patient comments on the disappearance of drug hunger and begins to talk with other patients about non-drug topics of current interest.

During phase 1 the patient is receptive to many educational approaches; groups go with counselors or older patients to museums and to sporting events; patients read a surprising variety of books; they participate in YMCA events; some go to night school or start vocational training. They are, nonetheless, still insecure. They need the reassurance of frequent contacts with professional and nonprofessional members of the staff; the street is only a few days or weeks behind them.

After six weeks' residence in the medical ward (an arbitrary time fixed for the pilot study), the patient has been stabilized on medication, his initial medical and psychological examinations have been completed, and he is ready for discharge to the outpatient clinic. He enters phase 2a. The most urgent problem at the time of discharge is housing, since many street addicts are homeless and destitute. For such individuals an interim period of support on public welfare is essential; the patient must be enabled to live in a rented room and begin to establish a new life. Some patients—the younger ones with unfinished schoolwork or others with defined vocational interests—may return to school; scholarships and money for vocational rehabilitation can be obtained from various agencies for qualified students. Other patients are encouraged to seek jobs. Since they are likely to be overwhelmed by nervousness and memories of previous failure, it is helpful if a member of the staff accompanies the applicant on his first visit to the employment office. This support may seem unnecessary—and perhaps it has been in some cases, since agencies have confused the patient with the staff member in the interview, but both the older patients and the counseling staff insist that this support is desirable. The physician can provide an essential reassurance for prospective employers by describing the program and giving guarantees of medical control.

Phase 2a, the stage following discharge from the hospital, may last six weeks to six months. It is followed by phase 2b, in which the patient has established a socially acceptable routine of life and may have a steady job. The episodes of experimental drug taking characteristic of the earlier phase have ended or become infrequent. The main problems of the patient in phase 2b relate to his difficulties in finding employment; to schoolwork; to the burdens of newly assumed responsibilities; and, for some patients without family or close friends, to loneliness. Counselors, not necessarily trained in social work but good listeners, are invaluable.

It is important to recognize that some patients, driven by feelings of guilt for their past life and by a desire to please the staff, will attempt to overperform. Some patients have taken multiple jobs and have worked to exhaustion to purchase new furniture and clothes for their families: others have combined an ambitious program of schoolwork with a new job. These overperforming patients must be helped to find a reasonable pace, since the deficit of years cannot be remedied in a moment. Like many of us, they need help in finding a balance between work and recreation.

Phase 3 may not ever be reached; but, if it is, the patient will have established a new routine of life, socially acceptable and consistent with his abilities. He will have developed a long range outlook for the future; he will have a bank account and friends. At this stage he no longer needs support from older patients or counselors. He looks to the physician as a medical advisor, not as a guardian. The chief danger in this stage is his complacency, since a successfully treated patient ceases to consider himself as an addict. He is likely to feel that continued taking of medication is a needless inconvenience. Admittedly, the question as to whether or not the blockading medication should be continued into phase 3, or even indefinitely, is still unanswered. It is clear, however, that the decision as to continuation should be made by the physician and not by a patient who feels that maintenance of the blockade is inconvenient.

The problem patients—the disturbed individuals with psychopathology independent of addiction—respond less well. These patients may not be recognizable in the initial interview or in phase 1, since addiction and the resultant social pressures cause anxiety and distortions in attitude that cannot be well separated from more fundamental disturbances. In the course of treatment, however, some patients fail to progress as expected. Psychopathic individuals cause disturbances in the ward and in the outpatient clinic, sometimes episodes of violence. Schizoid individuals remain isolated and may or may not be able to hold a job. Patients with anxiety neurosis may not find a sufficiently protected environment. They may report symptoms of abstinence and be convinced that the medication has been reduced when, in fact, the dose has remained constant and the recurrent symptoms are emotional. Other patients may continue to use alcohol to excess or to have continuing problems of barbiturate, tranquilizer, or amphetamine abuse.

The problem patients, fortunately, have been a minority in the group that we have treated. The relatively low incidence of disturbed patients in our series may result from a favorable selection. Our patients were chosen mainly from the deprived groups—Puerto Rican and colored persons coming from the slums. For many of these individuals, addiction was more a matter of exposure to drug use in adolescence than of psychopathology. Another group of patients, drawn from middle class areas in which addiction is a more extreme deviation, presumably would show a higher proportion of disturbed individuals.

Now consider a question that might be asked about any program for street addicts: What can be expected of the treatment? What are the measures of success or failure that will permit different therapies to be compared and appropriate treatment to be prescribed for different patients?

Most of us would agree that the greatest success is achieved when an addict becomes a productive member of society. For some patients—those with disabling psychopathology—this goal may be impossible, and, for them, life in a protected environment certainly is preferable to the anti-social existence of a street addict. But it does seem that for many patients a brief period of hospitalization may be sufficient to initiate the process of rehabilitation. Prolonged confinement of these patients in institutions would seem to be unnecessary and expensive and might defer the beginning of their rehabilitation.

CONCLUSION

Many street addicts can be rehabilitated by stopping heroin usage by methadone blockade and by giving common sense support. This approach, however, is not a cure for every addict; an undetermined proportion of addicts have additional psychopathological problems and need more specialized facilities for treatment.

This study was supported by grants for the Health Research Council, Department of Hospitals, and the Community Mental Health Board, New York.

Generic and Trade Names of Drugs

Methadone—*Dolophine.*

REFERENCES

1. Dole, *et.al.:* Narcotic blockade: a medical technique for stopping heroin use by addicts, 1966.

2. Dole, *et.al.*: Detection of narcotic drugs, tranquilizers, amphetamines and barbiturates in urine, 1966.

3. Dole and Nyswander: A medical treatment for diacetyl-morphine (heroin) addiction, 1965.

4. Dole and Nyswander: Rehabilitation of heroin addicts after blockade with methadone, 1966.

Chapter 5.

Successful Treatment of 750 Criminal Addicts

Vincent P. Dole,
Marie E. Nyswander
Alan Warner

In November 1963, on the initiative of the Health
Research Council of New York City, a study of heroin addiction was started at Rockefeller University Hospital.
The council recognized the need for new methods of
treatment. Thousands of heroin addicts were filling the
jails of New York City. It seemed reasonable to ask
whether some medication might control the drug hunger
of these criminal addicts, and enable them to live in the
community as decent citizens.

Clinical studies conducted in the metabolic ward
during 1964 and extended to Beth Israel Medical Center
in 1965 suggested that this result might be achieved by
using the familiar drug methadone hydrochloride in a
new way. By establishing tolerance to methadone, and
subsequently maintaining the tolerant state with a
constant daily oral dose, we found it possible to block the
action of heroin, and eliminate the hunger for narcotic
drugs.[1] Patients, thus blockaded, felt no narcotic effects,
but lost their compulsive desire for heroin. They stopped
being criminals, and in the majority of cases became productive members of society. A preliminary report of the
clinical findings was published in 1965.[2]

At the time of this report, the potential value of

*This article was reprinted with permission from the *Journal of
the American Medical Association,* **206**(12), 2708-2711, 1968.

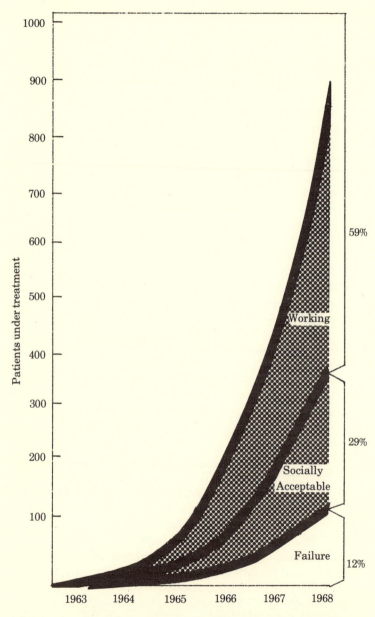

Fig. 1. Growth of the methadone maintenance treatment program. In addition to patients in treatment, approximately 1,000 addicts are awaiting admission to program.

treatment for large scale use remained indeterminate. The results, although encouraging, were limited to the treatment of a few patients for a few months. The present report summarizes the much more extensive experiénce of the past four years (Fig 1). The number of criminal addicts who have been rehabilitated with methadone treatment is large enough to empty a moderate sized jail, and there are at least 1,000 more addicts waiting for treatment. Detailed records of medical and social status have been kept for all patients, and analyses of urine for narcotic drugs, barbiturates, and amphetamines have been made at least weekly.[3]

All patients admitted to treatment from the beginning of the research (January 1964) to the time of this report (June 1968) are included in the statistics, except for a special group of patients who received combined treatment for addiction and tuberculosis, and a few patients who had been started on methadone therapy elsewhere and were accepted as transfers. For some analyses, such as measures of social stability and productivity, the tabulation has been limited to patients who have been in treatment for more than three months.

A notable feature of the treatment program has been the absence of compulsion or confinement. It has not been found necessary in the methadone program to apply prison techniques for control of behavior. Some addicts who had been notorious troublemakers in prison-type programs have become ordinary patients with methadone treatment. Not all have responded favorably, of course; some patients have been discharged for disruptive behavior, or because of nonnarcotic drug abuses. All of these failures including patients who had been in treatment for only one day—are included in the statistics (Table 1).

PROCEDURE

Addicts with a history of at least four years of mainline heroin use and repeated failures of withdrawal treatment were admitted to treatment in the order that they applied, subject to the following conditions: age 20 to 40 (upper limit raised to 50 in the third year of the

Table 1.
Discharges from January 1964 to May 1968*

	Time on Program, mo			
Cause	<1	1-6	6-12	>12
Behavior	5	23	13	13 (50%)
Drug abuse				
Heroin	0	0	0	0 (0%)
Nonheroin	2	2	0	5 (8%)
Medical				
Disability	4	8	7	8 (25%)
Death	2	1	5	1 (8%)
Voluntary	2	2	1	5 (9%)
	(14%)	(33%)	(24%)	(29%)

* There were 863 total admissions and 109 total discharges (13% of admissions).

study), no legal compulsion (i.e., methadone treatment not a condition of probation or parole), no major medical complication (e.g., severe alcoholism, epilepsy, schizophrenia), and resident of New York City. During the first 18 months only men were admitted to the program; subsequently a woman's unit has been in operation, with admission by the same procedure except that the intake office attempts to bring in married couples to the two units at approximately the same time.

The treatment program is divided into three phases, related to the progress of rehabilitation with methadone maintenance continuing throughout. During phase 1, a six week period of hospitalization on an open medical ward, the patients are brought to a blockading level of methadone. The new patient should be given this medication in relatively small, divided orally administered doses (e.g., 10 mg twice daily), and brought to maintenance level (80 to 120 mg/day) gradually, over a period of four to six weeks. Some experience in regulation of dose is necessary: if the medication is increased too rapidly, the patient will become over-sedated during the first few weeks, and may experience urinary retention and constipation, whereas if the dose is inadequate, a patient who had been using a large amount of heroin will have unnecessary withdrawal symptoms. There appears to be a wide margin of safety in administration of methadone to patients who have been heroin addicts, but of course the physician must avoid giving an excessive dose to a new patient. When in doubt, the safe rule is to give the medication in divided doses and observe the effects over the first 24 hours.

As the dose is gradually increased over a period of four to six weeks, the medication makes the patient refractory to narcotic drugs and eliminates (or greatly reduces) any narcotic drug hunger, presumably by maintaining a blockade of the sites of narcotic drug action. There should be no euphoria or other undesirable side effects (except mild constipation) if the medication is given in proper dosage. If the patient appears to be sedated during this induction phase the dose of methadone should be held constant or reduced until further tolerance is developed.

More recently, we have been testing a strictly ambulatory treatment, and have obtained favorable results, confirming the previous reports of Brill and Jaffe[4] and of Wieland.[5] New patients are started on small doses of methadone and are gradually brought up to stabilization level, as closely supervised outpatients. This is much less expensive than hospitalization and, with proper supervision, equally successful.

Phase 2 begins for the patients when they are discharged to the outpatient clinic, and continues for at least a year. The newly discharged patients return for medication to the outpatient clinic each weekday, and are given medication to take home for the weekends. Later, as justified by good conduct, the patients are permitted to come at less frequent intervals, taking out doses of medication for the intervening days. At least once per week (with rare exception) each patient is required to drink a full dose of the medication in the clinic, and thus demonstrate that he has maintained his tolerance by taking medication during the intervals. Each time that a patient comes to the clinic he is required to leave a urine specimen for analysis.

Phase 3 is reached when the subject has become a stable and socially productive member of the community, and can be treated as an ordinary medical patient. To be classified in this category, he must be acceptably employed (either in a job or at school, or if a woman, as a homemaker), and have no further problems with drugs or alcohol. The stability of rehabilitation must be proven by one year of normal life in the community. Medically the treatment of these patients remains the same as the treatment of patients in phase 2; they also take at least one dose of medication in the clinic each week, and leave a urine specimen.

Patients who have been discharged for misconduct, or who have asked to leave the program, have been withdrawn from medication by gradual reduction in dose over a period of about a month. This is done easily and without discomfort. We have not, however, considered it desirable to withdraw medication from patients who are to remain in the program, since those who have been discharged have experienced a return of narcotic drug hunger after removal of the blockade, and most of them have promptly reverted to the use of heroin. It is possible that a very gradual removal of methadone from patients with several years of stable living in phase 3 might succeed, but this procedure has not yet been adequately tested.

The supportive services provided by the methadone program and community agencies have been related to the needs of the patients. Some patients, when freed from the burden of heroin addiction, have ceased all antisocial activity; they obtained jobs without further assistance and began to support their families. These exceptional individuals needed nothing from the program except medical supervision. More frequently, the slum-born, minority group criminal addict needed help to become a productive member of society. Many of these invividuals came to us from jail with no vocational skills, no family, and no financial resources. They were further handicapped by racial discrimination and by their police records.

RESULTS

Drug-related crime has been sharply reduced by the blockade of narcotic drug hunger. Prior to treatment 91%

Table 2.

Convictions* of 912 Patients on Methadone Therapy, January 1964 to May 1968 (939 Patient-Years)

	Felony	Misde- meanor	Lesser Offenses
Narcotics	3	10	0
Dangerous drugs	0	4	0
Nondrug crimes	0	27	7
Rate per 100 patient-years	0.3	4.4	0.7

* Convictions for offenses committed while patients were receiving treatment. Pretreatment conviction rate (all offenses) was 52 per 100 patient-years.

of the patients had been in jail, and all of them had been more or less continuously involved in criminal activities. Many of them had simply alternated between jail and the slum neighborhoods of New York City. The crimes committed by these patients prior to treatment had resulted in at least 4,500 convictions (for felonies, misdemeanors, and offenses), a rate of 52 convictions per 100 man-years of addiction. The figure is obviously a minimum estimate of their pretreatment criminal activity since convictions measure only the number of times an addict has been caught. For every conviction, the usual addict has committed hundreds of criminal acts for which he was not apprehended.

Since entering the treatment program, 88% of the patients show arrest-free records. The remainder have had difficulties with the law. Some of these individuals, however, were arrested merely on suspicion, on charges such as loitering, or by inclusion in a group arrest. In such cases, if the charges were subsequently dismissed, the episode has not been considered a criminal offense in our statistics. The remainder, 5.6% of the patients, were guilty of criminal offenses and were convicted. In all, there have been 51 convictions in 880 man-years of treatment experience (a rate of 5.8 convictions per 100 man-years). Table 2 shows a more detailed analysis of these data.

We believe that the record of convictions of patients in treatment is essentially complete since a patient receiv-

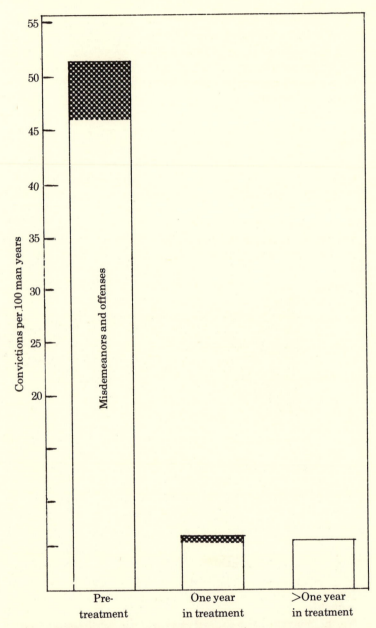

Fig. 2. Reduction in criminality of 912 former heroin addicts, as measured by 90% drop in rate of convictions.

ing methadone cannot absent himself for longer than a week without being missed. Moreover, legal representation is available for arrested patients. It provides both an accurate definition of the charge, and an incentive for the arrested person to report his difficulty. As to the estimate of arrests and convictions of patients before treatment, we have only a minimal and incomplete figure. The reduction in crime, therefore, is at least 90% (Fig 2).

All patients convicted of crimes and removed from treatment by imprisonment were discharged from the program. Some of them have been, or will be, readmitted on completion of their jail sentences. A few other patients were discharged voluntarily. Of a total of 863 admitted to treatment, ten (1.2%) were discharged from methadone treatment at their own request because they

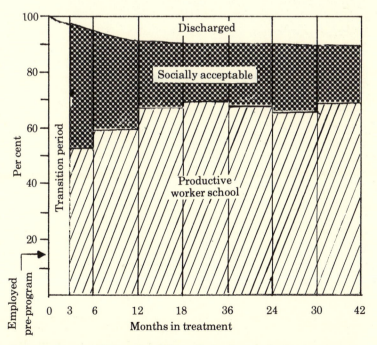

Fig. 3. Status of 723 male addicts admitted to methadone treatment. Rehabilitation was measured by productive employment and crime-free status over four-year period.

wished to leave New York; these patients are not considered either successes or failures since their outcome is not definitely known. The remainder (12%), all of whom we report as failures of the program, can be classified both by the length of time in treatment and the reason for discharge (Table1). In most cases the misconduct that led to discharge involved uncooperative or antisocial behavior, or nonnarcotic drug abuse (including alcoholism). For these individuals—fortunately the minority—stopping heroin use with blockade treatment was not enough to open the way for rehabilitation. Possibly more elaborate programs, combining blockade treatment with psychotherapy and sheltered environment, might have succeeded.

Since blockade with methadone makes heroin relatively ineffective, a patient cannot use heroin for the usual euphoria, nor will he experience abstinence symptoms after an experiment with the drug. He can, however, remain drug-oriented in his thinking, and be tempted to return to heroin. Many patients have made sporadic attempts to use heroin again, especially during the first six months of treatment. Their habits of association with addicts, and of heroin taking in certain environments, were not eliminated by the blockade. For such individuals, the negative experience of experimenting with heroin and feeling little or no euphoria may contribute to the extinction of conditioned reflexes that underlie drug-seeking behavior.[6] Needless to say, the staff does not encourage such dangerous experiments, but we recognize that for some individuals this type of self-experimentation might be a necessary step in reeducation and should not be regarded as a failure of treatment. Fortunately, experiments of this kind were the exception rather than the rule. The majority of patients have stopped heroin use completely after starting methadone treatment. This fact has been verified by repeated analyses of urine. For example, in a group of 174 patients, in which the analyses were done three times weekly for the first year of treatment, 55% did not show a single positive for self-administered narcotics. On the other hand, a minority of these patients, about 15%, continued to use heroin intermittently (e.g., on weekends) even though the euphoric effect was blocked. These tended to be isolated, schizoid individuals who were unable to find new friends or participate in ordinary activities.

The greatest surprise has been the high rate of social productivity, as defined by stable employment and responsible behavior (Fig 3). This, of course, cannot be attributed to the medication, which merely blocks drug hunger and narcotic drug effects. The fact that the majority of patients have become productive citizens testified to the devotion of the staff of the methadone program—physicians, nurses, older patients, counselors, and social workers. The success in making addicts into citizens also shows that an apparently hopeless criminal addict may have ambition and intelligence that can work for rather than against society when his pathological drug hunger is relieved by medical treatment.

This investigation was supported by grants from the Health Research Council (City of New York Department of Health) and the New York State Narcotic Addiction Control Commission.

Generic and Trade Names of Drugs

Methadone hydrochloride—*Adanon Hydrochloride, Althose Hydrochloride, Amidone Hydrochloride, Dolophine Hydrochloride.*

REFERENCES

1. Dole, *et.al.:* Narcotic blockade, 1966.
2. Dole and Nyswander: A medical treatment for diacetylmorphine (heroin) addiction, 1965.
3. Dole, *et.al.:* Detection of narcotic drugs, tranquilizers, amphetamines and barbiturates in urine, 1966.
4. Brill and Jaffe: The relevancy of some newer American treatment approaches for England, 1967.
5. Wieland: Methadone maintenance treatment of heroin-addiction: Beginning treatment on an outpatient basis, paper read before Annual Meeting of American Psychiatric Association, Boston, 1968.
6. Wikler: Conditioning factors in opiate addiction and relapse, 1965.

Chapter 6.

Methadone as a Primary Drug of Addiction*

Joseph D. Sapira
John C. Ball
Emily S. Cottrell

Methadone is a synthetic analygesic first produced at the I. G. Farbenindustrie in Germany during the Second World War, as a byproduct of research on meperidine. There was a morphine shortage in Germany at the time, but methadone was not used, apparently because the large doses studied resulted in a substantial incidence of side effects.

After the war the U. S. State Department's Technical Industrial Intelligence Committee investigated this research program and was more favorably impressed by methadone than the German authorities had been. The drug was subsequently studied in this country, and its potent analgesic properties confirmed. It was placed on the market under the trade names Dolophine, Adanon, Methadon-Lilly, Amidone, and Amidon.

Preliminary studies of its addiction liability were performed under the auspices of the National Research Council's Drug Addiction Committee, and it was demonstrated experimentally that methadone produced drug dependence of the morphine type.

In addition to its use as a narcotic analgesic, metha-

* This article was originally published under the title "Addiction to Methadone Among Patients at Lexington and Fort Worth" in the *Public Health Reports,* **83**(8), 691-694, 1968. It is reprinted here with permission.

87

done has been used to treat narcotic addicts during withdrawal. It is used because it substitutes for heroin and morphine, and the methadone withdrawal syndrome, although somewhat protracted, is less intense on a daily basis than that of heroin or morphine. Recently, the drug has been used to treat narcotic addicts in a maintenance program[1,2,3].

We studied persons who habitually self-administered methadone without medical supervision. We sought to determine if methadone abuse exists, what the clinical characteristics of methadone addicts are, and if methadone abusers are different from abusers of other narcotic analgesics.

MATERIALS AND METHODS

Discharge records for drug addicts leaving the Lexington, Ky., or Fort Worth, Tex. Public Health Service Hospitals during fiscal years 1962-66 were reviewed. We found that 227 discharges involving 214 patients with a first drug diagnosis of methadone addiction occurred during this 5-year period. Sample 1 was comprised of 72 methadone addicts discharged from the Lexington hospital during fiscal year 1962. This sample was chosen, on the basis of controlled data from that year for 3,229 nonmethadone addicts. This allowed evaluation of differences between methadone and nonmethadone narcotic addicts[4].

Sample 2 was selected from all men discharged from the Lexington hospital during the 32-month period ending August 1967 with a first drug diagnosis of methadone addiction. It consisted of 25 patients after others whose charts had incomplete or conflicting information were eliminated.

RESULTS

Of the 72 methadone addicts in sample 1, 18 percent were women, as were 17.8 percent of the 3,229 patients in the control group. The mean age of the 59 men in sample 1 was 46.6 years. The mean for men in the control group was 35.5 years, and 45.7 years in sample 2.

Fifty-seven men in sample 1 were white. This unusual-ly high incidence of white patients compared to the control population (X^2 = 49.9, P < 0.005) was observed for the entire period 1962-66. Only one patient in sample 2 was nonwhite.

Male methadone addicts per male population 21 years and older were calculated for each state in this study. In sample 1, 15 states—Nevada, Arkansas, Virginia, Mis-sissippi, Massachusetts, Alabama, New Mexico, Colo-rado, Tennessee, Michigan, Louisiana, South Carolina, Georgia, Oklahoma, and North Carolina—had a metha-done addiction rate among men at least twice that pre-dicted on the basis of their known male addict rate. For the period 1962-66, five states—Nevada, Virginia, Ok-lahoma, Mississippi, and South Carolina—had metha-done addict rates for men at least triple their predicted rates. These states are concentrated in a "methadone belt" centered in the southeast. The results are not the product of a low total rate of narcotic use among men in these states, since 11 of the 15 states with highest methadone rates in 1962 were among the 20 states ranked highest for male narcotic addicts per male population 21 years and older.

Of the 72 methadone addicts in sample 1, 70 were vol-unteer patients; of the 3,229 addicts in the control group, 2,723 were volunteers. There was a comparatively greater propensity for methadone addicts to volunteer for treatment (X^2 = 8.03, P < 0.05). Similarly, 96 percent of the 214 patients with first drug diagnosis of metha-done addiction in 1962-66 were volunteers, as were 96 per-cent of those in sample 2.

In sample 1, 81.4 percent of the methadone addicts who voluntarily entered the hospital left against medical advice without completing treatment. This high inci-dence of early signout among volunteer methadone addicts was also seen for the other years of the study period, averaging 84.8 percent for the 5-year study period and 80 percent for sample 2. Thus, less than one of five methadone addicts who volunteered for treatment com-pleted the program. This is even more striking since the mode for length of stay throughout this entire period was

7 ± 2 days for the methadone addicts. Patients being re-admitted made up 69.5 percent of sample 1 and 80 percent of sample 2.

A review of additional diagnoses entered on the charts of all methadone addicts discharged from 1962 to 1966 revealed no instances of painful disease for which methadone might be legitimately prescribed by a physician. In sample 2 all prior admissions were also reviewed, and although several patients began receiving drugs in a medical setting, there were no instances of painful disease for which continued analgesia would be required.

During the entire 5-year period, 42.2 percent of the methadone addicts discharged had a second drug diagnosis and 5.7 percent had a third drug diagnosis. These data confirm the clinical impression that use of methadone per se does not lead to the cessation of alternate drug-seeking behavior. Of the 96 second drug diagnoses, 52 were for depressants (sedatives, hypnotics, and alcohol), 22 for opiates (synthetic and naturally derived narcotic analgesics), and two for amphetamines. Of the 13 third drug diagnoses, 10 were for depressants and three for opiates.

Eight physicians and four nurses were among the 214 methadone addicts. This contrasts with the high representation of health professionals among meperidine (Demerol) addicts[5]. Assuming that health professionals have a choice of any legally available drug, there does not seem to be any functional consensus that methadone has clear advantages over other synthetic narcotic analgesics.

Of the 25 male methadone addicts in sample 2, the mean number of years of opiate addiction was 17, with age at onset 28 years (mean = 28.8, median 26.9 range 15-66 years). Methadone had been abused for an average of 5.9 years: use started as early as 1950, with the range in methadone use being from 1 to 15 years.

Nine of these addicts administered their drugs intravenously; nine, orally; and seven, subcutaneously. Seventeen obtained methadone from physicians, seven from pushers, and one from a drugstore.

Twenty had from one to 14 previous hospitalizations

History of 25 male methadone addicts at the Lexington Public Health Service Hospital

Case No.	Occupation	Age	Route of methadone administration	Source of methadone	Years of methadone use	Years of opiate use	History of heroin use	Arrest history	Number of admissions to Lexington hospital
1	Odd jobs	35	Intramuscular	Physician	8	11	Yes	Yes	8
2	Farmer	56	Intravenous	do	3	36	No	No	15
3	Cook	73	Oral	do	1	50	Yes	Yes	15
4	Illegal	31	...do	do	15	15	Yes	Yes	5
5	Driver	30	Intravenous	do	3	7	Yes	Yes	5
6	Illegal	29	...do	Pusher	1-3	12	Yes	Yes	3
7	Unemployed	44	Oral	Physician	1-5	24	No	Yes	3
8	Retired	75	...do	do	9	9	Yes	No	2
9	Truck driver	35	Intravenous	Pusher	6	14	Yes	Yes	4
10	Illegal	50	...do	Physician	3-6	17	No	Yes	3
11	...do	56	Oral	do	4	25	Yes	Yes	10
12	...do	36	Intravenous	Pusher	5	8	Yes	Yes	4
13	Salesman	46	...do	do	8	8	Yes	Yes	2
14	Illegal	27	Oral	do	1	10	Yes	Yes	2
15	Retired	70	Intravenous	Physician	2	53	Yes	Yes	6
16	Physician	51	...do	Drugstore	1	2	No	No	1
17	Unemployed	53	Intramuscular	Physician	14	24	No	Yes	10
18	...do	40	Intravenous	Push	2	2	No	Yes	1
19	Disabled	35	Intramuscular	Physician	3	3	No	No	2
20	Unemployed	46	...do	do	1	2	No	Yes	1
21	...do	36	Oral	do	7	7	Yes	No	1
22	Illegal	36	...do	do	6	13	Yes	No	2
23	Plumber	54	Intramuscular	do	1	4	No	Yes	2
24	Clerk	43	...do	Pusher	9	16	Yes	Yes	4
25	Unemployed	55	Oral	Physician	1-3	18	Yes	Yes	1

for drug addiction (see table). In addition to a history of unsuccessful treatment for opiate addiction, the methadone addicts of sample 2 had engaged in antisocial behavior. Twenty patients had an arrest history. The first arrest, at a mean age of 21 years, commonly preceded opiate addiction. Three had been Federal prisoners, and 12 had a history of venereal disease. Eighteen of the 25 had smoked marihuana, and 14 had abused heroin. At the time of last hospitalization, eight patients were divorced or separated. Finally, most terminated treatment at Lexington against medical advice; only six stayed more than 19 days.

Nine of the 25 methadone addicts were engaged in fairly steady employment, seven were principally in illegal endeavors, six were unemployed, and three were disabled or retired. The marginal character of their employment was not because of lack of education, as their median education was 10.3 years as compared to 10.9 years for the U.S. white population 25 years and older in 1960.

DISCUSSION

Although methadone is not the drug of choice among American narcotic addicts, 214 methadone addicts have been admitted to the Lexington and Fort Worth hospitals in recent years. Methadone addiction appears to be discomforting enough to prompt persons to seek treatment, as evidenced by the significantly higher voluntary admission rate of these addicts compared with the entire narcotic addict population. This was true even though most methadone addicts had been unsuccessfully treated on at least one other occasion.

There was no evidence to support the belief that methadone abuse per se facilitates subsequent rehabilitative efforts since during the period of study more than four of five methadone addicts who voluntarily requested treatment at the Lexington hospital left against medical advice. Not only did they not complete the course of therapy, but some of them were probably not completely detoxified since the mode for their length of hospital stay was 7 ± 2 days for each year in the study period.

SUMMARY

During fiscal years 1962-66, 214 patients at the Lexington, Ky., and Fort Worth, Tex., Public Health Service Hospitals had a first drug diagnosis of methadone addiction. Compared to all other narcotic addicts, methadone addicts tended to be older, white, and residing in states of the "methadone belt" (Virginia, Tennessee, Georgia, Alabama, Mississippi, Louisiana, Arkansas, Oklahoma, New Mexico, and Nevada).

No evidence was found to support the theory that nonmedical use of methadone decreases drug-seeking or antisocial behavior. Methadone addicts had about twice as many second and third drug diagnoses as the general narcotic addict population.

REFERENCES

1. Dole, *et.al.*: Narcotic blockade: A medical technique for stopping heroin use by addicts, 1966.

2. Dole and Nyswander: A medical treatment for diacetylmorphine (heroin) addiction, 1965.

3. Dole and Nyswander: Rehabilitation of the street addict, 1967.

4. Ball: Two patterns of narcotic drug addiction in the United States, 1965.

5. Rasor and Crecraft: Addiction to meperidine (Demerol) hydrochloride, 1955.

PART TWO
Maintenance Therapy: Recent Experiences and Issues

Chapter 7.

A Comparison of Two Stabilization Techniques*

William F. Wieland
Carl D. Chambers

THE ISSUE

The original utilization of the methadone maintenance modality included an initiation phase which
required the addict-patients to be hospitalized for six to
eight weeks. During this inpatient phase of treatment,
the patient was not only stabilized with the drug, but
was also prepared psychologically and socially for reintegration into the community. Unfortunately, the shortage
of specialized hospital space and personnel experienced
in treating narcotic addicts severely limit the use of a modality based upon such an inpatient phase. If the inpatient initiation phase could be demonstrated as *not* essential in the total effectiveness of this modality, several desirable consequences would follow. For example, a large
amount of money would be released to provide expanded
concurrent services to addict-patients, a greater number
of treating facilities and a wider variety of agencies
would be able to incorporate the modality, and most important, many more narcotic addicts could be treated.
The authors believe such demonstration can now be empirically presented.

THE EXPERIENCES

Both inpatient and outpatient stabilization techniques

* This article was reprinted with permission from the *International Journal of the Addictions,* 5(4), 645-659, 1970.

Table 1
Selected Characteristics for 32 Narcotic Addicts Stabilized with Methadone (August, 1966-February, 1968)

	Addict Patient Identifiers			Basic Demographic				Basic Disease Attributes					Methadone Maintenance		
	Age	Race	Sex	Born in Pa.	Years Educ.	Mar. Status	Prior Job	Age 1st Use	Heroin Addict	Years of Use	No. of Cures	No. of Arrests	Initiation Type	Initiation Date	Daily Dose	Months of Treatment
1.	38	W	M	Yes	13	M	Yes	18	Yes	20	5	1	In	8-66	200	36
2.	26	N	M	Yes	13	M	No	22	Yes	4	1	1	In	3-67	60	29
3.	27	W	M	Yes	12	S	No	21	Yes	6	3	2	In	3-67	200	29
4.	30	W	M	Yes	12	M	Yes	15	Yes	15	9	12	In	4-67	160	28
5.	25	W	M	Yes	16	M	No	17	Yes	8	3	3	In	5-67	130	28
6.	26	N	F	No	12	Sep.	No	22	Yes	4	1	3	In	7-67	40	26
7.	22	W	M	Yes	10	M	No	17	Yes	5	0	2	In	7-67	120	26
8.	37	W	F	Yes	11	D	No	17	Yes	20	3	5	In	9-67	80	24
9.	21	W	M	Yes	12	S	No	13	Yes	8	7	22	In	10-67	180	23
10.	39	N	M	No	11	M	No	20	Yes	19	3	12	In	10-67	120	23
11.	29	N	M	Yes	12	S	No	16	Yes	13	1	9	In	11-67	120	22
12.	35	W	M	Yes	12	D	Yes	16	Yes	19	5	9	In	11-67	170	22
13.	28	N	M	Yes	13	S	No	16	Yes	12	11	11	In	1-68	70	20
14.	32	W	F	Yes	12	M	No	20	Yes	12	0	2	Out	7-67	120	26
15.	23	W	M	Yes	10	M	No	18	Yes	5	0	8	Out	9-67	100	24
16.	41	W	M	Yes	11	M	Yes	20	Yes	21	2	1	Out	9-67	100	24
17.	23	W	M	Yes	7	D	No	20	Yes	3	1	16	Out	9-67	180	24
18.	23	W	M	Yes	12	S	Yes	20	Yes	3	1	0	Out	9-67	40	24

19.	21	W	M	Yes	10	M	No	16	Yes	5	2	6	Out	10-67	100	23
20.	35	W	M	Yes	11	M	Yes	18	Yes	17	4	12	Out	10-67	160	23
21.	39	W	M	Yes	10	M	Yes	19	Yes	20	1	37	Out	10-67	180	23
22.	28	W	M	Yes	12	D	No	17	Yes	11	3	6	Out	10-67	100	23
23.	52	W	M	Yes	12	M	Yes	25	Yes	27	6	31	Out	10-67	140	23
24.	37	W	M	Yes	12	M	Yes	19	Yes	18	1	10	Out	10-67	80	23
25.	32	W	F	No	12	M	Yes	23	Yes	9	2	3	Out	10-67	80	23
26.	23	W	M	Yes	16	Sep.	No	21	Yes	2	2	0	Out	10-67	90	23
27.	30	W	M	Yes	10	M	No	15	Yes	15	1	6	Out	10-67	120	23
28.	53	W	M	Yes	10	M	No	20	Yes	33	4	0	Out	10-67	140	23
29.	39	W	M	Yes	10	Sep.	No	21	Yes	18	6	6	Out	10-67	140	23
30.	34	W	M	Yes	9	S	Yes	15	Yes	19	2	10	Out	10-67	160	23
31.	37	W	M	Yes	11	M	No	22	Yes	15	5	19	Out	10-67	140	23
32.	41	W	M	Yes	12		No	22	Yes	19	5	11	Out	11-67	120	22

have been utilized in the Philadelphia Narcotic Addict Rehabilitation Program. The plan of the study was to compare these inpatient and outpatient initiation techniques. During the time when both initiation techniques were being utilized, August 1966 to February 1968, 32 narcotic addicts were stabilized with methadone and were still in active treatment during August 1969. Of these 32 addicts, 13 were initiated and stabilized as inpatients and 19 were initiated and stabilized as outpatients. This study is a statistical comparison between the 13 inpatient and the 19 outpatient initiates.

The criteria for admission were similar to those of Dole and Nyswander, namely, a history of at least four years of addiction, over twenty years of age, and voluntary acceptance of treatment. Most patients received the methadone three times per week with a range of one to five times per week. The clinic was closed on weekends.

ADDICT-PATIENT PROFILES

The 32 heroin addicts reported in this study (Tables 1 and 2) can be readily characterized as hard-core addicts. They had typically begun opiate abuse while still in their teens (median age of onset was 19), had, from the age of onset, been using heroin an average of 13 years, had undergone an average of 3.1 medical detoxifications, and had also experienced enforced non-medical detoxifications as the result of being incarcerated several times. No significant differences were produced relevant to these attributes when the addicts were separated into two groups by controlling for the technique of initiation.

In spite of their addictions, the majority were married and living with their spouses and over one-third of them were legally employed at the time they began treatment. Indicative of geographical stability, almost all of the addicts had been born in Pennsylvania. The level of attained education was as high as the base populations from which they came; over half had completed high school and 16% had pursued education beyond high school. Two things did, however, separate them from

Table 2

Comparisons Between Addict-Patients Initiated as
Inpatients and Outpatients

	Initiation Technique		
Attributes	**Inpatient** **N = 13**	**Out-patient** **N = 19**	**Total** **N = 32**
1. Ages			
Range	21-39	21-53	21-53
Mean	29.5	33.8	32.1
2. Race			
White	(8) 61.5%	(19) 100.0%	(27) 84.4%
Negro	(5) 38.5%	(—) —	(5) 15.6%
3. Sex			
Male	(11) 84.6%	(17) 89.5%	(28) 87.5%
Female	(2) 15.4%	(2) 10.5%	(4) 12.5%
4. Born In Pennsyl-vania			
Yes	(11) 84.6%	(18) 94.7%	(29) 90.6%
No	(2) 15.4%	(1) 5.3%	(3) 9.4%
5. Education (Years)			
Range	10-16	7-16	7-16
H. S. graduates	(10) 76.9%	(8) 42.1%	(18) 56.3%
6. Marital status			
Single	(4) 30.8%	(2) 10.5%	(6) 18.8%
Married	(6) 46.2%	(13) 68.4%	(19) 59.4%
Divorced/separated	(3) 23.1%	(4) 21.1%	(7) 21.9%
7. Working before treatment			
Yes	(3) 23.1%	(8) 42.1%	(11) 34.4%
No	(10) 76.9%	(11) 57.9%	(21) 65.6%
8. Age 1st opiate use			
Range	13-22	15-25	13-25
Mean	17.7	19.5	18.9
9. Years of use			
Range	4-20	2-33	2-33
Mean	11.4	14.3	13.1
10. No. prior treatments			
Range	0-11	0-6	0-11
Mean	4.0	2.5	3.1
Total with "cures"	(12) 92.3%	(17) 89.5%	(29) 90.6%
11. No. arrests			
Range	1-22	0-37	0-37
Mean	6.9	9.7	8.6
Total with arrests	(13) 100.0%	(16) 84.2%	(29) 90.6%

their base populations. The sex and race distributions were not representative for the Philadelphia base populations. Both males and whites were over-represented with most of the patient population (75%) being white males.

Of all of the attributes analyzed within the frame of reference of initiation technique, only race produced a significant difference. No Negroes were among the addicts initially taken into the program and stabilized as outpatients. This occurred as the result of the means whereby addicts arrived at the clinic. During the first few months that the technique was utilized, patients came to the clinic as medical referrals from physicians or as referrals from addicts already under treatment. White addicts predominated at this stage of the program because of the bias of the two referral sources.*

Clinical Improvement

All of the 32 addict-patients were evaluated by a psychiatrist, the program director, at the time of initiation and at various intervals throughout treatment. Marked and sustained clinical improvement, as judged by interview ratings of mood, attitude and emotional stability, was noted for 25 (78.1%) of these patients. There was no significant difference between those patients who began treatment as inpatients and those who began as outpatients. Ten (76.2%) of the inpatients and 15 (78.9%) of the outpatients had shown marked and sustained clinical improvement (Table 3).

Employment

The employment status of an addict-patient being maintained with methadone is one of the major indices routinely cited as indicating the effectiveness of the modality. Replicating this effectiveness, legitimate employment did significantly increase among these 32 patients (Table 4).

---

* This racial imbalance did not continue. Of the 148 addict-patients who have been maintained with methadone to date, 59(39.9%) have been Negroes. At the present time, 67.9% of all initiations into treatment are Negro addicts.

Table 3
Incidence of Clinical Improvement Among
Methodone Maintenance Patients After
a Minimum of 20 Months of Treatment

Stabilization Techniques[a]	Marked and Sustained Clinical Improvement	
	N	%
Inpatient initiation (N = 13)	10	76.2
Outpatient initiation (N = 19)	15	78.9
Total initiations (N = 32)	25	78.1

[a] Statistical difference: x^2 = .089; P = Not significant.

As expected, the dominant means of obtaining money prior to treatment were illegal. Among all of the patients, 56.3% reported most of their money was obtained illegally. Among those with no legal job, however, 85.7% were supporting themselves illegally. After treatment, 77.8% of those who had previously supported themselves illegally secured and maintained full-time legitimate employment (Table 5).

After a minimum of 20 months of maintenance with methadone, 78.1% (N = 25) of the addict-patients of both sexes held full-time legitimate jobs. The salaries ranged from $100 to $1500 per month with an average of $565. Employment status was *not* associated with initiation technique utilized during stabilization (Table 6).

The seven patients who remained unemployed after being maintained with methadone had stopped stealing and other illegal forms of obtaining money. Obtaining treatment had permitted four of them to live within the

Table 4
Employment Status of 32 Heroin Addicts Before and
After Maintenance with Methadone

Employment Status[a]	Before Treatment		After Treatment	
	N	%	N	%
Unemployed	21	65.6	7	21.9
Employed	11	34.4	25	78.1
Total	32	100.0	32	100.0

[a] Statistical difference: x^2 = 12.444; P = <.001.

Table 5
Primary Means of Support Before and After a Minimum of 20 Months of Methadone Maintenance

| | Primary Means of Support | | |
Subjects	Before Treatment	After Treatment	Current Earned Monthly Income
Inpatients			
1. 38-WM	Musician	Musician	$580
2. 26-NM	Illegal	Machine Operator	385
3. 27-WM	Illegal	Clerical	320
4. 30-WM	Mechanic	Mechanic	600
5. 25-WM	Welfare	Welfare	None
6. 26-NF	Illegal	Service	200
7. 22-WM	Illegal	Laborer	440
8. 37-WF	Illegal	Waitress	320
9. 21-WM	Illegal	Laborer	525
10. 39-NM	Illegal	Porter	330
11. 29-NM	Illegal	Welfare	None
12. 35-WM	Waiter	Waiter	500
13. 28-NM	Illegal	Clerical	465
Total	23.1% employed (N = 3)	84.6% employed (N = 11)	X earned income $425
Outpatients			
14. 32-WF	N.I.L.F.[a]	N.I.L.F.-Spouse[a]	None
15. 23-WM	Illegal	Laborer	340
16. 41-WM	Proprietor	Proprietor	1500
17. 23-WM	Illegal	Bartender	100
18. 23-WM	Stevedore	Stevedore	600
19. 21-WM	Illegal	Cook	400
20. 35-WM	Typesetter	Typesetter	480
21. 39-WM	Proprietor	Bartender	430
22. 28-WM	Illegal	Laborer	320
23. 52-WM	Truck Driver	Truck Driver	330
24. 37-WM	Skilled Manual	Foreman	1000
25. 32-WM	Sales	Sales	700
26. 23-WF	N.I.L.F.[a]	N.I.L.F.-Family[a]	None
27. 30-WM	Illegal	Welfare	None
28. 53-WM	Illegal	Truck Driver	576
29. 39-WM	Illegal	Welfare	None
30. 34-WM	Butcher	Butcher	600
31. 37-WM	Illegal	N.I.L.F.-Spouse[a]	None
32. 41-WM	Illegal	Sales	450
Total	42.1% employed (N = 8)	73.7% employed (N = 14)	X earned income $600

[a] Not in the labor force.

Table 6
A Comparison of Employment Status Distributions After
a Minimum of 20 Months of
Maintenance with Methadone[a]

Employ- ment Status	Inpatient Initiation		Outpatient Initiation		Total Addict- Patients	
	N	**%**	**N**	**%**	**N**	**%**
Legally employed	11	84.6	14	73.7	25	78.1
Public assistance	2	15.4	2	10.5	4	12.5
Not in labor force	0	—	3	15.8	3	9.4
Total	13	100.0	19	100.0	32	100.0

[a] Employed vs. Other Categories: $x^2 = .090$; P = Not significant.

limits of public assistance grants and the other three to
live within their spouse's or families' incomes.

Heroin Cheating

These 32 heroin addicts had been abusing the drug an
average of 13.2 years. After a minimum of 20 months of
maintenance with methadone, nine (28.1%) were detected
through urine surveillance as occasional "cheaters" with
heroin.* Although the prevalence of heroin cheating by
the patients may seem high, the amount of cheating was
not. For example, urines from the nine heroin "cheaters"
were analyzed an average of 15.3 times during the last 60
days of this evaluation period and heroin was detected
an average of only 2.0 times. Stated differently, of the
138 urinalyses for these nine patients, only 18 (14.5%)
revealed heroin abuse (Table 7).

No significant differences were noted between those
addict-patients initiated as inpatients and those initiated
as outpatients. Four of the inpatients (30.8%) and five
of the outpatients (26.3%) were found to occasionally
cheat with heroin. Likewise, no significant differences in

* A urine specimen is collected for analysis during each visit to
the clinic. An average of 2.9 urins per week for each patient are analyzed.

Table 7
Prevalence of Heroin "Cheating" among Addict-Patients
Maintained with Methadone for a
Minimum of 20 Months[a]

Stabilization Techniques	No Detected Heroin Abuse During Past Two Months		Some Heroin Abuse During Past Two Months	
	N	%	N	%
Inpatient	9	69.2	4	30.8
Outpatient	14	73.7	5	26.3
Total	23	71.9	9	28.1

[a] Statistical difference: $x^2 = 0.016$; P = Not significant.

the amount of cheating was revealed. The inpatients were tested an average of 13.5 times with heroin being detected an average of 2.5 times per patient. The outpatients were tested an average of 16.8 times with positive heroin an average of 1.6 times per patient.

The occasional cheating with heroin was not related to the daily methadone dose. Addict-patients were stabilized at doses which ranged from 40 to 200 mg/day. Cheating was observed in patients on the minimal dose as well as in patients on doses as high as 160 mg.

Cheating was only marginally associated with the employment status of the patient. Of all the male addict-patients who were working (N = 23) 73.9% were not cheating. Of the males who were not working (N = 5) 60.0% were not cheating. These differences are not, however, statistically significant. There were likewise no significant differences between the two types of initiates.

Although a number of patients have used other drugs and alcohol on occasion, none of this group became seriously involved. However, alcoholism or concurrent drug addiction have occurred in a small number of subsequent patients.

Arrests

As with most narcotic addicts, multiple arrests were common among these 32 patients prior to treatment. Of the 32, 90.6% (N = 29) reported they had been arrested. Those with arrest histories (N = 29) reported an average of 15.9 arrests of which 8.6 were arrests for drug behavior. Under treatment, however, the prevalence of arrests significantly decreased to only 18.8% (N = 6). Of the six who were arrested after treatment began, the mean number of arrests was only 1.0, and none had been arrested for a drug related offense (Table 8).

The significant decreases noted in arrests while being maintained with methadone were not associated with the initiation technique utilized to stabilize the patients (Table 9).

CONCLUSIONS

This study has empirically demonstrated the effectiveness of the out-patient technique for stabilizing and maintaining narcotic addicts with methadone. One group of 19 heroin addicts, who had been addicted an average of 14.3 years and had histories with an average of 9.7 arrests and 2.5 prior formal treatments, were initiated, stabilized, and maintained with methadone as outpatients. This group was statistically compared with 13 heroin addicts who were initiated and stabilized as inpatients. The 13 inpatients had comparable addiction, arrests, and prior treatment histories. *Analyses of four measures of personal and social rehabilitation failed to produce any significant differences between those addict-*

Table 8
Prevalence of Arrests Before and After a Minimum of 20 Months of Treatment with Methadone Maintenance[a]

Arrest History	Arrested Before			Arrested After		
	N	%	X Arrests	N	%	X Arrests
Yes	29	90.6	8.6	6	18.8	1.0
No	3	9.4	—	26	81.2	—
Total	32	100.0	—	32	100.0	—

[a] Statistical difference: $x^2 = 27.671$; $P = 0.001$.

patients who initiated treatment as inpatients and those who received all of their treatment as outpatients.

1. A majority of all the addict-patients, 78.1%, manifested marked and sustained clinical improvement, as evaluated by psychiatric interview, while being maintained with methadone. There was *no* significant difference between the inpatient and outpatient initiates in the incidence of clinical improvement.

2. A majority of all the addict-patients, 78.1%, have been employed in economically sufficient work roles while being maintained with methadone. This constituted a statistically significant increase when compared to such work roles prior to methadone maintenance. There was *no* significant difference between the inpatient and outpatient initiates in the incidence of economically sufficient work roles.

3. As measured by no positive urines during the most recent two month period, a majority of all the addict-patients, 71.9%, had ceased cheating with heroin. There was *no* significant difference between the inpatient and outpatient initiates in the incidence of heroin cheating.

4. A majority of all the addict-patients, 90.6%, had extensive arrest histories prior to the initiation of treatment. The 29 addict-patients with arrest records had been arrested an average of 15.9 times of which 8.6 were drug related. Only three of the 29 had *no* drug related arrests. While being maintained with methadone, this incidence of arrests decreased significantly to only 18.8% of all the addict-patients. No drug related arrests occurred while under treatment. There was *no* significant difference between the inpatient and outpatient initiates in either the incidence of arrests prior to treatment or the incidence of arrests while being maintained with methadone.

Table 9

Prevalence of Arrests Within Stabilization Technique Before and After a Minimum of 20 Months of Treatment with Methadone Maintenance [a]

Stabilization Techniques	Arrested Before Treatment			Arrested After Treatment		
	N	%	X Arrests	N	%	X Arrests
Inpatient	13	100.0%	6.9	4	30.8	1.0
Outpatient	16	84.2	9.7	2	10.5	1.0
Total	29	90.6	8.6	6	18.8	1.0

[a] Statistical differences: before—x^2 = 0.019; P = Not significant. After—x^2 = 0.960; P = Not significant.

In summary, significant increases occur in clinical improvement and legitimate work roles, significant decreases occur in arrests and in heroin abuse while being maintained with methadone. In none of the above was the personal or social rehabilitation significantly related to either of the initiation techniques. This evidence strongly suggests that successful rehabilitation through the mechanism of methadone maintenance does not depend upon the technique utilized for initiation and stabilization.

These findings have several implications. For instance, monies currently budgeted for expensive inpatient services, both physical plant and staff, could be utilized to expand programs to treat more addicts. Furthermore, an additional and often hidden type of narcotic addict can be serviced with the outpatient modality. For example, the addict who is maintaining a legitimate work role while addicted frequently cannot or will not jeopardize that work role for an extended inpatient initiation phase of treatment. Finally, it is apparent that any re-entry difficulties routinely associated with inpatient treatment are automatically eliminated.

As methadone maintenance cannot be viewed as the total solution to narcotic addiction, neither can outpatient initiation to the total solution to stabilization with methadone. Access must exist to inpatient facilities for the infrequent cases where physical or psychiatric pathologies coexist with the addiction that require more intensive care. In the Philadelphia Program, where all addicts are now stabilized as outpatients, it has been found that approximately 10% will require some temporary inpatient care during their stabilization phase. Hepatitis and severe psychiatric symptoms have been the primary reasons for hospitalization. In no case has hospitalization continued beyond that minimally required to control the coexisting pathology.

At the present writing, a total of 148 narcotic addicts have been stabilized as outpatients. To date, no apparent deviation from the success pattern demonstrated by the initial 19 addict-patients has been noted. Only 20 (13.5%) of the 148 patients have terminated treatment, which is similar to the figure reported by other programs. Of the 20 terminations, nine (45.0%) became unavailable for treatment through moving out of the city (N = 7), incarceration (N = 1), and death (N = 1). Four others, 20.0%, were suspended from the program for continuous rule-infractions, and six, 30.0%, were terminated at their own request but against medical advice. One patient was detoxified and discharged with his treatment completed. He was still abstinent a year after his discharge.

COMMENTS

This study was conducted to demonstrate that outpatient stabilization and maintenance with methadone was equally as effective. The treatment histories of 32 hard-core heroin addicts, 13 of whom were initiated as inpatients and 19 as outpatients, were compared. Regardless of the stabilization technique, methadone maintenance produced significant clinical improvements and increases in work performance while producing significant decreases in heroin abuse, criminal behavior and arrests. No significant differences in the two groups were noted, leading the authors to conclude that successful use of methadone maintenance was not dependent upon an inpatient phase of treatment.

Chapter 8.

Characteristics of Patient Retention/Attrition*

Carl D. Chambers
Dean V. Babst
Alan Warner

THE ISSUE

The retention power of the methadone maintenance modality is without equal in the addict rehabilitation field. It is almost as if this type of patient will continue in treatment regardless of what we do or do not do for them. Attrition does, however, occur and data is now available which isolates those attributes most associated with continuing in treatment.

THE EXPERIENCE

The Sample

The study population was 679 patients admitted to the Dole-Nyswander program from its initiation in 1964 to March, 1968. Our strategy was to compare those patients who remained in treatment for at least two years with those who did not. Within this study population, 541 or 80% continued in treatment a minimum of two years and 138 or 20% attrited prior to this minimum period. Even those who terminated earlier than the two-year follow-up period remained in treatment an average of 12.6 months (median was 12.7 months).

* Presented at the Third National Conference on Methadone Treatment, New York City, November, 1970.

The Reasons for Termination

An analysis of the primary reasons recorded for the 138 treatment terminations indicated 112 (81%) were involuntarily terminated; 22 (16%) voluntarily terminated themselves and 4 (3%) were administrative terminations. A more complete distribution of the reasons for termination is as follows:

The Comparisons

Utilizing a single factor or dependent-independent variable analysis where all attributes were collapsed to 2 by 2 contrasts produced some unexpected differences and failed to produce some differences one would anticipate.

Still utilizing a single factor or dependent-independent variable analysis but regrouping the data for another perspective reenforced the unanticipated results derived from our first analysis. For example;

> 1. Continuing in treatment was *not* related to the sex of the patient—80% of the male patients and 80% of the female patients remained in treatment for at least two years.

Table 1.
Primary Reason for Treatment Terminations

I. Involuntary Termination		81.2%(N=112)
1. Uncooperative Behavior	17.4% (N=24)	
2. Antisocial Behavior	7.2% (N=10)	
3. Unreachable Psychopathology	7.2% (N=10)	
4. Drug Abuse	8.7% (N=12)	
5. Alcohol	10.9% (N=15)	
7. Medical Disability	2.2% (N=3)	
8. Death	12.3% (N=17)	
II. Voluntary Termination		15.9% (N= 22)
1. Voluntary Discharge	14.5% (N=20)	
2. Loss to Contact	1.4% (N=2)	
III. Administrative Terminations and Unknowns		2.9% (N=4)
1. Administrative	.7% (N=1)	
2. No Information	2.2% (N=3)	
Total		100.0% (N=138)

5

2. Continuing in treatment was *not* related to the marital status of the patient—86% of the patients with intact marriages and 79% of the patients who were not married remained in treatment for at least two years.

3. Continuing in treatment was *not* related to the multiple abuse of drugs—83% of the patients who had not been multiple drug abusers and 77% of those who had been multiple drug abusers remained in treatment for at least two years.

4. Continuing in treatment was *not* related to the abuse of alcohol—82% of those who had no history of alcohol abuse and 75% of those who had abused alcohol remained in treatment for at least two years.

5. Continuing in treatment was *not* related to the ethnicity of the patients—82% of the white, 77% of the black and 81% of the Puerto Rican patients remained in treatment for at least two years.

6. Continuing in treatment was *not* related to the education of the patients—79% of the high school graduates and 80% of those who were not high school graduates remained in treatment for at least two years.

7. Continuing in treatment was *not* related to the age at onset of heroin use—79% of those who began before age 21 and 80% of those who began at or after age 21 remained in treatment for at least two years.

8. Continuing in treatment was *not* related to the number of prior treatments experienced by the patients—81% of those with 2 or less treatments and 79% of those with 3 or more prior treatments remained in treatment for at least two years.

9. Continuing in treatment was *marginally* related to the conviction history of the patients—78% of those who had never been convicted and 80% of those with convictions remained in treatment for at least two years. However, the number of convictions was significantly related to continuing in treatment—85% of those with two or less convictions and only 72% of those with three or more convictions remained in treatment for at least two years (Significant at .01).

10. Continuing in treatment *was* related to the length of abuse of narcotics—90% of those who had abused 5 or less years but only 77% of those who abused more than 5 years remained in treatment for at least two years (Significant at .01).

11. Continuing in treatment *was* related to the employment status of the patient at time of admission—88% of those who were legally employed at admission but only 77% of those who were not employed remained in treatment for at least two years (Significant at .01).

An expanded distribution of these attributes with a control for the sex of the patient permits a more focussed associational analysis. For example;

Table 2.

Characteristics of Methadone Maintenance Patients by Length of Time They Remain in Treatment

Attributes At Time of Admission Into Treatment (1964-1968)	Less Than Two Years (N=138)	Two Years or More (N=541)
I. Demographic Characterisitcs		
1. Age: Range	22-52 years	19-60 yrs
1. Age: Mean	33.2 years	32.6 yrs
2. Race: Whites	34%	39%
3. Sex: Males	86%	85%
4. Education: High School Graduates	30%	29%
5. Marital: Married at Admission	15%	22%
6. Occupation: Semiskilled or Above	76%	81%
7. Job Status: Employed at Admission	13%	25%(P= .01)
8. Work History: At Least 36 Months of Continuous Employment	49%	50%
II. Arrest History Characteristics		
1. Never Convicted	9%	8%
2. Three or More Convictions	75%	66%(P= .05)
III. Drug Abuse Characteristics		
1. Onset Age (Heroin) Age 18 or Less	39%	43%
2. Multiple/Concurrent Drug Abuse	54%	45%
3. History of Drinking Problem	29%	19%
4. Five or More Prior Treatments	49%	51%
5. Six or More Months on Waiting List	49%	47%

1. In general and regardless of sex, the fewer the number of convictions, the greater the chance of remaining in treatment. This item had the greatest outcome differentiating power of all of the attributes when a statistical technique common in parole prediction was employed—the Mean Cost Rating technique. In brief, the MCR technique measures the extent an item has the ability to differentiate between categories with high and low outcome rates.

2. In general and regardless of sex, those patients who had concurrently abused amphetamines with the opiates were less likely to remain in treatment.

3. At least among the males, those most recently accepted into treatment were the ones most likely to terminate. The opposite is true for the female patients.

4. At least among the males, being employed at the time of admission into treatment has a positive association with remaining in treatment. Employment at admission is neither a positive nor negative association to outcome among the female patients.

5. In general and regardless of sex, *having* a problem with alcohol has a negative association with remaining in treatment. *Having had* such a problem, however, is no more negatively associated with outcome than never having had a problem.

6. Of all the race-sex cohorts, Puerto Rican females most frequently remain in treatment and black females have the highest attrition rate.

7. Among males, the younger the age at admission, the greater the positive association with remaining in treatment. Among females, the most advantageous age is between 25 and 29, and the least is under age 25.

A complete expansion of the characteristics can be reviewed in Table 3.

Our previous research and clinical experiences have led us to assume we can predict which types of patients might do better than others. We generally assume those patients with the least chance of remaining in treatment share combinations of the following characteristics:

a. Early onset age
b. Long drug history
c. Concurrent drug or alcohol abuse
d. Multiple convictions

In general, the combining of these characteristics suggests the following:

1. Being a multiple drug abuser or an alcohol abuser is probably more negatively associated with remaining in treatment than the length of time the patient has been abusing drugs.

2. Being a multiple drug abuser or an alcohol abuser is probably more negatively associated with remaining in treatment than the age at which the patient began abusing drugs.

3. Having been arrested and convicted a number of times is probably more negatively associated with remaining in treatment than being a multiple drug or alcohol abuser, the time when the patient began abusing drugs and the length of time the patient had been abusing drugs.

Utilizing these data, a configural analysis was performed to verify the potency of the number of convictions as a predictor for remaining in treatment. The configural analysis is, of course, derived entirely from a statistical base.

Table 3.
Expanded Characteristics of Methadone
Maintenance Patients and Their Association
with Remaining in Treatment

Admission Characteristics	Males		Females		
	No. of Patients	%in Program 2 Years Later	No. of Patients	%in Program 2 Years Later	MCR for Males
Total	579*	79.6%	100	80.0%	—
Number of Previous Convictions					
2 or less	178	84.8	38	81.6	.181
3-6	260	81.5	32	87.5	
7 or more	140	69.3	30	70.0	
Job Status at Admission					
Working	139	88.5	10	80.0	.135
Not working	428	76.6	86	80.2	
Year Admitted					
1964-65	64	84.4	5	40.0	.096
1966	181	82.9	30	80.0	
1967-68	332	77.1	65	83.0	
Other Drugs— Addict or Heavy Use					
No problem	291	82.8	37	81.1	.094
Barbiturates	31	77.4	7	85.7	
Amphetamines	11	72.7	2	50.0	
Other	199	76.9	38	79.0	
Alcohol					
No problem	246	81.7	43	83.7	.093
Had problem	23	82.6	5	80.0	
Has problem	74	73.0	10	70.0	
Ethnicity					
White	214	82.2	46	80.3	.081
Black	237	76.8	43	76.7	
Puerto Rican	109	80.7	8	87.5	
Other/No data	19	79.0	3	100.0	
Age at Admission					
24 years or younger	58	86.2	10	70.0	.071
25-29 years	149	81.9	19	89.5	
30-34 years	161	78.9	22	77.3	
35 years or older	203	76.4	47	80.8	

Marital Status
Married	111	85.6	27	85.2	.069
All others	449	78.6	70	78.6	

Medical Complications
None	307	80.8	41	85.4	.029
Some	251	78.9	55	80.0	

Longest Job Ever Held
Less than 12 months	113	79.6	24	70.8	**
12-23 months	98	75.5	17	88.2	
24-35 months	77	84.4	13	84.6	
36 months or more	291	79.7	46	80.4	

Months Waited Before Admission
0-2 months	105	79.0	25	80.0	**
3-5 months	151	81.5	24	79.2	
6 months or more	233	78.5	43	83.7	

Age When Started Using Heroin Daily
16 years or younger	135	83.0	16	81.2	**
17-18 years	121	79.3	16	81.2	
19-20 years	113	74.3	18	83.3	
21-22 years	77	83.1	11	90.9	
23-24 years	53	83.0	9	55.6	
25 years or older	80	76.2	30	80.0	

Number of Previous Hospitalizations
2 or less	173	80.9	032	84.4	**
3-4	103	73.8	25	76.0	
5 or more	301	80.7	42	78.6	

Last Grade Completed
Some college	61	86.9	5	60.0	
Some high school	404	78.5	79	78.5	
Eighth grade or less	62	85.5	3	100.0	

* Not all items total 579 since unknown were not included.
** MCR not computed as not enough consistent relationship was observed by inspection to warrant its computation.

The first step in carrying out a configural analysis is to take the item most related to outcome. In this case, it is number of previous convictions. This best item is then cross-classified with each of the next most related items and with outcome to determine which factors provide the most differentiation within each subgroup. For example, those with 2 or less previous convictions is the first subgroup in the configuration.

The factor that best differentiated as to outcome

Table 4.

Multiple Factor Classification for Male Patients
Based upon Clinical Anticipation

Years of Abuse	Multiple Use	No. of Convictions	Age at Onset	No. of Patients	% in Program 2 Years Later
5 Years or Less	No Problem	—	—	24	95.8
5 Years or Less	Mult. Use	—	—	18	83.3
6-11 Years	No Problem		19 yrs or less	49	89.8
6-11 Years	No Problem		20 yrs or more	40	80.0
6-11 Years	Mult. Use		19 yrs or less	65	80.0
6-11 Years	Mult. Use		20 yrs or more	47	74.5
12-15 Years		6 or less	—	95	80.0
12-15 Years		7 or more	—	36	58.3
16 Years or More		6 or less	20 yrs or more	49	91.8
16 Years or More		6 or less	19 yrs or less	63	79.4
16 Years or More		7 or more	20 yrs or more	23	69.6
16 Years or More		7 or more	19 yrs or less	35	65.7

Table 5.
Configural Classification for Male Patients Based
Upon A Combination of Single and Multiple Factor Predictors

	Admission Characteristics	No. of Patients	% in Program 2 Years Later
2 or less previous convictions	No problem with other drugs or alcohol	76	88.2%
	Concurrent use of other drugs and/or alcohol abuse	102	82.4%
	Employed at admission	49	93.9%
3 to 6 previous convictions	Not employed at admission	160	78.1%
	Semiskilled or better	125	76.8%
7 or more previous convictions	Unskilled	45	55.6%

117

Table 6
The Relationship Between Detected Abuse and Length of Time on Methadone Maintenance

Detected Abuse	Less Than 18 Months 64 Addict-Patients	18 Months or More 55 Addict-Patients
Heroin	41.1%	28.5%
Other Narcotics	10.1%	8.7%
Barbiturates	10.0%	13.2%
Amphetamines	13.7%	15.3%
Negative Methadone	17.5%	17.3%
No Abuse Detected	36.3%	45.0%

Table 7
The Incidence of Cocaine Abuse During an Eight Week Surveillance Period

No Positives	67.2% (N=80)
Positive 1-4 Weeks	29.4% (N=35)
Positive 5-8 Weeks	2.5% (N=3)
No Tests	.8% (N=1)
Total	100.0% (N=119)

Total does not equal 100.0 due to rounding error.

Table 8
The Distribution of Cocaine Abuse Among the 119 Addict-Patients

Cohorts	Positive For Cocaine At Least One Week During the Eight Week Surveillance
Low Dose Patients (N=48)	27.1%
High Dose Patients (N=71)	38.0%
White Males (N=67)	17.9%
Black Males (N=42)	54.8%
White Females (N=5)	40.0%
Black Females (N=5)	40.0%
Total Patients (N=119)	31.9%

within this subgroup was concurrent use of other drugs and/or alcohol abuse. This type of operation was repeated within each subgroup, and as can be seen in Table 5, different factors were used within each subgroup.

This statistically derived classification does differentiate between types as to outcome and the differences are in the direction expected.

Based upon the configural analysis, the potency of the number of convictions as our best predictor of remaining in treatment was reenforced.

Utilizing all three techniques, the patient with 7 or more convictions and who had no employment skill to market was the least likely to remain in treatment (55.6%). One would assume ancillary services should be marshalled and focussed toward the buffering against these attributes. Conversely, the patient with the fewest convictions and no multiple drug or alcohol problem was the most likely to remain in treatment (95.8%).

Chapter 9.

The Incidence and Patterns of Drug Abuse during Maintenance Therapy*

Carl D. Chambers
W. J. Russell Taylor

THE ISSUE

The literature would lead one to believe drug abuse ceases once the stabilized patient "tests his medicine" and the effects are "blocked" or when the substitute narcotic eliminates "drug-craving." Recent empirical work does not entirely substantiate these assumptions.

THE EXPERIENCE

During 1969, the research, urine surveillance and clinical components of the Narcotic Addict Rehabilitation Program—a N.A.R.A. Title IV Project—at the Philadelphia General Hospital, collaborated in the completion of a number of interrelated studies designed to gain the fullest appreciation of the drug abuse phenomena among methadone maintenance patients. These studies were designed to secure answers to a series of questions which seemed to be critical issues in the ambulatory treatment of voluntary patients:

1. What is the extent of the abuse of heroin, other narcotics, barbiturates and amphetamines among stabilized patients?
2. What is the extent of cocaine abuse which is not detected during routine urine surveillance?

* A version of this paper was presented at the 33rd Annual Meeting of the *Committee on Problems of Drug Dependence,* National Research Council, National Academy of Sciences Division of Medical Sciences, Toronto, Canada, February 1971.

3. What is the reliability of drug abuse data obtained from patients?

4. What success do therapists have in the detection of drug abuse and in discriminating among the various types of abuse?

This report is a brief overview and summary of the results of these various inquiries.

THE EXTENT OF DRUG ABUSE AMONG STABILIZED PATIENTS

A study population of 119 stabilized patients was isolated which included all the patients who had been on the maintenance program for at least six months. There were no attributes which would suggest these 119 patients were significantly different from those patients typically serviced in methadone clinics: the median age was 33, 60.5% were white, 8.4% were females, the median year of addiction was 15, 89.1% had prior treatment histories and 85.7% had arrest histories.

Urine specimens collected during each clinic visit over a nine-month surveillance period (April-December 1969) became the core data for the analysis. Data derived from each specimen were grouped together by weeks within the surveillance period. The technique of analysis results in statements of the average number of weeks in which a study population abuses specific drugs.

Results

1. The extent of drug abuse among these 119 stabilized patients was greater than anticipated. Heroin was being abused 35.3% of the time, the other narcotics were being abused 9.5% of the time; barbiturates were being abused 11.5% of the time and amphetamines were being abused 14.4% of the time. "Clean urines," specimens in which no drug abuse was detected, occurred only 41.1% of the time. Of marked significance, urines in which *no* methadone was detected occurred 17.4% of the time.

2. At least within this study population, certain forms of drug abuse appeared related to the daily methadone dose. For example, those patients receiving 60-100 mgs,

Table 1
The Percentage of the Total Weeks of Surveillance
During Which the Various Abuses were Detected

Detected Abuse	119 Addict-Patients
Heroin	35.3%
Other Narcotics	9.5%
Barbiturates	11.5%
Amphetamines	14.4%
Negative Methadone	17.4%
No Abuse Detected	41.1%

abused heroin more often, more frequently presented specimens which were negative for methadone and less frequently had specimens for which no abuse was detected.

3. A significant relationship was found to exist between certain forms of abuse and race of the patients. Black patients were found to abuse heroin more frequently than white patients (47.1% versus 27.5%) and the white patients more frequently had specimens for which no abuse was detected (44.8% versus 34.6%). The races did not differ significantly on abuse of other narcotics, barbiturates, amphetamines or the submission of urines negative for methadone.

A further discrimination of the race variable was obtained by simultaneous control for sex. Heroin abuse was found to be occurring 48.0% of the time among black males but only 26.7% of the time among white males. The only other significant difference occurred with "clean urines." White males submitted "clean urines" 45.8% of

Table 2
The Relationship Between Detected Abuse and
Daily Methadone Doses

Detected Abuse	60-100 mgs. 48 Addict-Patients	110-220 mgs. 71 Addict-Patients
Heroin	45.7%	28.3%
Other Narcotics	10.2%	8.8%
Barbiturates	11.4%	11.5%
Amphetamines	11.5%	16.4%
Negative Methadone	21.0%	14.9%
No Abuse Detected	33.7%	45.5%

Table 3
The Relationship Between Detected Abuses and
the Race of the Patients

Detected Abuse	72 White Addict-Patients	47 Black Addict-Patients
Heroin	27.5%	47.1%
Other Narcotics	10.1%	8.4%
Barbiturates	12.5%	9.9%
Amphetamines	16.1%	11.6%
Negative Methadone	15.8%	18.8%
No Abuse Detected	44.8%	34.6%

the time while black males did so only 33.5% of the time. Although abuse patterns were determined for the female patients of both races, the cohorts were believed to be too small for meaningful comparisons.

4. A minor relationship was found to exist between the abuse of heroin and the age of the patients. Those patients who fell in and below the median age—33 years—abused heroin more frequently than did older patients (39.7% versus 31.1%). The two age groups did *not* differ in their abuse of the other narcotics, barbiturates, nor the incidence of urines negative for methadone. Age was *not* a factor in the incidence of "clean urines."

5. A significant relationship was found to exist between the abuse of heroin and the length of time on the methadone program. Those patients who fell below the median length of treatment, less than 18 months, abused

Table 4
The Relationship Between Detected Abuse and
the Race/sex of the Patients

Detected Abuse	67 White Males	42 Black Males	5 White Females	5 Black Females
Heroin	26.7%	48.0%	38.3%	39.4%
Other Narcotics	10.3%	8.4%	9.0%	8.4%
Barbiturates	12.7%	10.2%	10.6%	7.1%
Amphetamines	16.1%	11.2%	16.9%	14.9%
Negative Methadone	15.1%	19.4%	25.2%	13.9%
No Detected Abuse	45.8%	33.5%	30.7%	43.3%

Table 5
The Relationship Between Detected Abuse and the
Age of the Addict-Patients

Detected Abuse	Through Age 33 58 Addict-Patients	Age 34 and Above 61 Addict Patients
Heroin	39.7%	31.1%
Other Narcotics	10.6%	8.4%
Barbiturates	10.8%	12.1%
Amphetamines	16.5%	12.4%
Negative Methadone	17.9%	16.9%
No Abuse Detected	39.9%	42.2%

heroin more frequently than those who had been in treatment for a longer period of time (41.1% versus 28.5%). Those patients who had been under treatment for the longer periods also submitted urines more frequently in which no abuse was detected (45.0% versus 36.3%). Length of treatment was *not* a factor in the abuse of the other narcotics, barbiturates, amphetamines or the incidence of urines negative for methadone.

THE EXTENT OF COCAINE ABUSE

A modification of the urinalysis procedures permitted an expanded surveillance to include the detection of cocaine use. Surveillance for this abuse was not available, however, except for eight weeks during the nine-month study period. During those eight weeks, 38 of the 119 patients (31.9%) were found to have used cocaine at least once.

The majority of cocaine abusers used the drug less than 50% of the time. Patients on the higher methadone doses more frequently used cocaine than those on the lower doses (38.0% versus 27.1%). As with heroin abuse, black males significantly more often abused cocaine than any of the other race/sex cohorts.

RELIABILITY OF INTERVIEW DATA

Each patient was interviewed at the beginning of every month during the study period and asked to indicate the extent of any drug usage during the previous

Table 6
The Relationship Between Detected Abuse and
Length of Time on Methadone Maintenance

Detected Abuse	Less Than 18 Months 64 Addict-	18 Months or More 55 Addict-
Heroin	41.1%	28.5%
Other Narcotics	10.1%	8.7%
Barbiturates	10.0%	13.2%
Amphetamines	13.7%	15.3%
Negative Methadone	17.5%	17.3%
No Abuse Detected	36.3%	45.0%

month. Comparisons were then determined between the data obtained by interview and by urinalyses. Our experiences clearly demonstrate the futility of attempting to elicit information from these patients concerning their abuse of drugs. For example, during one of the monthly comparisons (May 1969), only 34.2% of those who were *detected* abusers had *admitted* any abuse. With regard to specific drugs, 51.6% of the heroin abusers, 25.0% of the barbiturate abusers and 20.0% of the amphetamine abusers had admitted the abuse.

THE ABILITY OF THERAPISTS TO DETECT DRUG ABUSE

During the same period the reliability of interview data was assessed, the counselor/therapist responsible for each of the patients was asked to indicate which of their clients were abusing heroin, barbiturates and am-

Table 7
The Incidence of Cocaine Abuse During an Eight Week Surveillance Period

No Positives	67.2% (N=80)
Positive 1-4 Weeks	29.4% (N=35)
Positive 5-8 Weeks	2.5% (N=3)
No Tests	.8% (N=1)
Total	100.0% (N=119)

Total does not equal 100.0 due to rounding error.

Table 8
The Distribution of Cocaine Abuse Among the
119 Addict-Patients

Cohorts	Positive For Cocaine At Least One Week During the Eight Week Surveillance
Low Dose Patients (N=48)	27.1%
High Dose Patients (N=71)	38.0%
White Males (N=67)	17.9%
Black Males (N=42)	54.8%
White Females (N=5)	40.0%
Black Females (N=5)	40.0%
Total Patients (N=119)	31.9%

phetamines. Comparing these judgements with the urinalyses indicated 70.6% of the judgements relating to heroin abuse were inaccurate as were 51.7% of those relating to barbiturate use and 19.3% of those relating to amphetamine abuse. Thus, the counselor/therapists could detect the amphetamine abusers with a high degree of accuracy. This was not true with heroin and barbiturate abusers. There was *no* significant difference between the professionals and the ex-addict counselor/therapists in their ability to detect abuse.

Comments and Discussion

It is apparent that within this study population, the types and frequencies of drug abuse were much greater than those which one would expect from reviewing the literature.

The data also suggest that while maintenance doses of methadone through the cross-tolerance mechanisms can be expected to prevent the euphoric effects of low-dose self-administered narcotics, it cannot be expected to "blockade" all attempts to "get over" the medicine. Quite unexplainable within current thinking, some patients stabilized on high doses—in excess of 180 mgs.— report euphoric effects of even low doses of intravenous heroin. Such anecdotal reports are easily verified or refuted in carefully designed and controlled laboratory experiments.

A discrepancy between the data and the literature relevant to the extinguishing of "drug craving" also appears to exist. The high incidences of a variety of drug abuses among these patients stabilized a minimum of one year indicate that drug craving, at least as translated into "drug seeking" and "drug taking," most certainly had neither been extinguished nor significantly diminished.

In spite of the above, 52.9% were maintaining an intact marriage, 44.5% were legally employed on at least a part-time basis, and while 85.7% had been arrested prior to treatment, only 1.7% had been arrested at any time during their methadone treatment period (a median of 18 months).

Methadone *does* effectively eliminate the patients' fears of the abstinence syndrome. While in a maintenance program, the patient need never be afraid of going into withdrawal or becoming "sick." Methadone *does not*, however, eliminate the patients' desires for and pursuit of a "high," their attachment to and involvement with the "needle" nor their enjoyment with and acceptance of the "street life." A relatively common practice among maintenance patients is to trade a portion of their take-home medication for drugs from which to receive a "high." He, therefore, has the best of both lives. Only highly skilled clinicians providing a full range of ancillary services will be able to buffer the rehabilitant against these non-medicine influences.

We seem to be at a stage of development where most methadone maintenance clinicians and program administrators are proposing the abolition of urine surveillance because of its supposed retarding effects in a therapeutic relationship and because of its high cost. On the basis of our studies, we must vigorously oppose such a proposal. We believe adequate laboratory surveillance of urine to detect the possible self-administration of such abuse-potential drugs as the amphetamines, the barbiturates, cocaine and heroin to be a necessary adjunct to the appropriate and effective management of any addict rehabilitation program. While the various patterns of drug abuse are illustrative of the problems inherent in the rehabilitation of narcotic addicts, to what extent and in what ways they may be detrimental to the total therapeutic process has yet to be documented. We do believe, however, that the type and frequency of the drug abuse can be a very potent message to the therapist which he must learn to interpret and to act in accordance with it. For example, cocaine abuse among those patients who were abusing only cocaine, almost disappeared when they were confronted with the information that a urine test had been developed to detect the abuse.

Chapter 10.

Self-Administered Methadone Supplementation

Carl D. Chambers
Janet J. Bergen

THE ISSUE

A substantial number of patients receiving maintenance therapy report regular supplementation of their
daily methadone dose. Until now, the dimensions of this
anti-therapeutic self-treatment and the characteristics of
those involved have been unknown.

THE EXPERIENCE

A substantial number of patients in methadone maintenance programs have been found to self-administer
supplementary doses of methadone on a daily basis. This
daily supplementation occurs even among those patients
believed to be stabilized. Quite obviously, when the
addict-patient begins to treat himself, the likelihood of
therapeutic success and rehabilitation are diminished.
The probability of adverse side effects e.g. the death of
the patient from therapeutic or accidental overdose is
also increased. Severe respiratory depression could occur
because of an unannounced therapeutic increase by the
physician's order or an excessive self-administered supplementary dose by the patient himself.

Unfortunately, the existence of methadone supplementation is not readily detectable, and an awareness of
such behavior does not normally become apparent to the
clinician. For example, moderate self-administered
increases would not produce any acute physiological

changes which would be readily observable. Those patients who are detected supplementing are usually those who inject the extra methadone rather than take it orally. These "injectors" will, on occasion, present themselves at the clinic in an intoxicated state, with abcesses at the injection site or with new sclerotic veins. The standard urine surveillance procedure in most programs—the cation exchange, fractional extraction and thin-layer chromatography procedure—would not reflect this supplementation. Thin-layer chromatography will detect only the presence of methadone in the urine-not the quantity. Detection of this form of abuse most frequently occurs upon verbally confronting the patient.

This study was designed to ascertain the incidence of *admitted* self-administered methadone supplementation among all the patients serviced in the Narcotic Addict Rehabilitational Program Maintenance Clinic located at the Philadelphia General Hospital.

During November-December of 1969, there were 173 registered and active methadone maintenance patients in the clinic. All 173 patients were interviewed by their counselor/therapist with reference to supplementation of their daily medication. Each patient's case record was reviewed and data were abstracted to provide a frame of reference for comparing those patients who admitted supplementation and those who denied this abuse.

Results

1. *Self-administered methadone supplementation within this study population was a behavior of the younger white male patients.* Of the 17 admitted supplementers, 16 (94.1%) were white males with a median age of 26. There were no white females or black males who admitted to supplementation, and only one black female, 34 years of age, admitted this abuse behavior. Stated somewhat differently, the incidence of self-reported supplementation within the study population was 9.8%; 18.8% among white male patients, 7.6% among black female patients and absent among white females and black males.

Table 1.
Identifiers of the Methadone Supplementers

Race/Sex/ Cohorts	Patients on Methadone		Self-Administered Supple-menters		Incidence of Supple-mentation
White Males	85	49.1%	16	94.1%	18.8%
White Females	11	6.4%	0	—	0
Black Males	64	37.0%	0	—	0
Black Females	13	7.5%	1	5.9%	7.6%
Total	173	100.0%	17	100.0%	9.8%

2. *The supplementers were not recent initiates to the methadone program.* With the possible exception of one patient—a 21-year-old male who had been in treatment only 2 months—these supplementers would be considered "stabilized." The time in treatment ranged from a low of 2 months to 27 months with a median of 16 months.

3. *The supplementers were not "therapeutically-ignored" patients.* All of these patients were being seen in the clinic a minimum of 3 times per week, and 58.8% (N = 10) were reporting to the clinic 5 times per week. Eight or 47% were recipients of concurrent chemotherapy, (e.g., sedatives, tranquilizers, anti-depressants) which required the attention of the physician and nurses in addition to the counselors.

4. *The supplementers were not patients being maintained on low doses of methadone.* In fact, all of the supplementers must be considered relatively high-dose patients. Only one patient was receiving less than 100 mg. per day. The doses ranged from 80 to 200 mg. per day, the median being 140 mg.

5. *The supplementers were not self-administering low doses of methadone.* The daily supplementation ranged from 10 to 400 mg., with a median of 100 mg. per day. In general, those patients who were low-dose supplementers—10 to 30 mg. per day—were securing 10 mg. methadone tablets and ingesting them orally; and those who were self-administering high doses were securing injectable methadone and using it intravenously.

6. *The supplementers were abusing other drugs while*

Table 2
Clinical Identifiers of the Methadone Supplementers

Age Race Sex	Months In Treatment	Weekly Clinic Visits	Concurrent Chemo-therapy	Prescribed Daily Dose (Mgs)	Supplement Dose (Mgs)	Supplement Route
1. 21-wm	27	5	No	180	200	IV
2. 21-wm	26	3	No	120	20	oral
3. 21-wm	21	5	Yes	140	100	oral
4. 21-wm	10	5	Yes	80	20	oral
5. 22-wm	2	5	No Data	120	150	oral
6. 22-wm	18	5	Yes	140	100	IV
7. 22-wm	19	5	No	120	30	oral
8. 23-wm	6	3	No	100	400	IV
9. 26-wm	13	3	Yes	180	100	oral
10. 27-wm	16	5	No	200	200	IV
11. 31-wm	4	5	No	100	20	oral
12. 34-bf	21	3	No	100	30	oral
13. 35-wm	25	5	Yes	160	200	IV
14. 39-wm	26	3	No	180	50	IV
15. 42-wm	10	3	Yes	160	100	oral
16. 44-wm	15	5	Yes	160	30	oral
17. 45-wm	12	3	Yes	180	10	oral
Mean = 29.1	15.9	4.1	Yes = 47.1%	142.4	103.5	Oral = 64.6%
Median = 26	16	5		140	100	

Table 3
Other Drug Abuse Among the Methadone Supplementers

Age Race Sex	Concurrent Drugs Abused			
	Barbitu-rates	Ampheta-mines	Heroin	Cocaine
1. 21-wm	—	Yes	—	—
2. 21-wm	—	Yes	Yes	—
3. 21-wm	Yes	Yes	Yes	—
4. 21-wm	—	Yes	Yes	—
5. 22 wm	—	—	Yes	Yes
6. 22-wm	—	Yes	Yes	—
7. 22-wm	—	Yes	Yes	—
8. 23-wm	Yes	Yes	Yes	—
9. 26-wm	—	—	Yes	—
10. 27-wm	—	Yes	Yes	—
11. 31-wm	Yes	—	Yes	—
12. 34-bf	—	—	Yes	—
13. 35-wm	Yes	Yes	Yes	Yes
14. 39-wm	—	Yes	—	—
15. 42-wm	Yes	Yes	Yes	—
16. 44-wm	—	—	Yes	—
17. 45-wm	Yes	Yes	—	—
Totals	Yes = 35.3%	Yes = 70.6%	Yes = 82.4%	Yes = 11.8%

supplementing methadone. Urinalyses indicated that all these supplementers were taking other drugs, e.g., opiates, amphetamines, sedatives and cocaine. Heroin was most frequently abused, with at least 82.4% (N = 14) of the patients being detected with it in their urines. The amphetamines were the next most frequently abused—70.6% (N = 12)—followed by the barbiturates—35.3% (N = 6)—and cocaine—11.8% (N = 2). In addition, urinalyses revealed these supplementers were multiple drug abusers. For example, 82.4% (N = 14) were taking at least two different types of drugs, most frequently heroin and amphetamines; 29.4% (N = 5) were using at least three different types; and at least one of the subjects, a 35-year-old white male who had begun his drug-taking career at age 16, was abusing all the drugs detected with the urinalysis procedure.

7. *The supplementers had not adopted or reestablished conventional work roles.* Of the 17, 13 (76.5%) were still unemployed after an average of 16 months of maintenance therapy. Twelve of the patients were receiving public assistance. Three of the welfare recipients admitted to supplementing this assistance by illegal activities

Table 4
Social Identifiers of Methadone Supplementers

Age Race Sex	Primary Sources of Support
1. 21-wm	Welfare
2. 21-wm	Employment ($400)
3. 21-wm	Welfare
4. 21-wm	Employment ($400)
5. 22-wm	Welfare
6. 22-wm	Welfare/Illegal Activity
7. 22-wm	Welfare/Illegal Activity
8. 23-wm	Welfare/Illegal Activity
9. 26-wm	Welfare
10. 27-wm	Illegal Activity
11. 31-wm	Employment ($200)
12. 34-bf	Welfare
13. 35-wm	Employment ($600)
14. 39-wm	Welfare/Employment
15. 42-wm	Welfare
16. 44-wm	Welfare
17. 45-wm	Welfare

and one other worked regularly, but did not report this work to his welfare caseworker. One of the 17 subjects reported that *all* of his support was derived from illegal activities.

Supplementers Versus Non-Supplementers

The study included special reference to any differences that might be discernible between the 17 addict-patients who supplemented their methadone doses and the 156 addict-patients who denied supplementation.

The major statistically significant differences which appear were as follows:

1. Whites more frequently supplemented than blacks;
2. Patients under age 25 more frequently supplemented;
3. Patients who continue illegal activities, who do not seek conventional employment and who become dependent upon Public Welfare assistance more frequently supplemented;
4. Patients who had been using narcotics less than 10 years more frequently supplemented;
5. Patients who had undergone 2 or more prior treatment attempts more frequently supplemented;
6. Patients "stabilized" at daily doses in excess of 110 mg. more frequently supplemented;

7. Patients who received concurrent psychotropic medications more frequently supplemented; and

8. Patients required to come to the clinic three or more times per week more frequently supplemented.

Comments and Implications

There are a number of factors which suggest that at least those who self-report regular methadone supplementation are the "sickest" of the patients. For example, almost half of them were receiving psychotropic medications, three-fourths were still abusing heroin after an average of 16 months maintenance therapy, three-fourths were detected amphetamine abusers, three-fourths were unable or unwilling to secure employment, preferring to receive welfare and/or continue illegal activities, etc. Methadone clinicians acknowledge that some 10% of their patients require 90% of their time and effort. It would appear that the methadone supplementers fall in this group of more personally- and socially-disorganized patients.

Methadone supplementation was not found to be predictive of other forms of drug abuse. Most methadone supplementers also abuse other drugs, primarily heroin and amphetamines, but most addict-patients who abuse drugs do not supplement their methadone.

The apparent relationship between high supplementation and high prescribed dosage contradicts a common rationale generally supplied by the supplementers for their abusive behavior—that they are simply not getting enough methadone to "hold them." Insufficient dosage, then, does not appear to be a factor in the etiology of methadone supplementation. It is interesting to speculate that this relationship may in part be due to these patients having had the pretreatment experience of abusing methadone solely for its euphoric effects; and/or, in part, to their having been exposed to a poorly-managed stabilization regimen, where rapid increases produced a euphoric reaction. While we are not in a position to address ourselves to the latter, we do have data that 76.5% (N = 13) of these supplementers had abused methadone prior to entering the maintenance program.

Table 5
Comparison of Characteristics of 17 Methadone
Supplementers With 156 Nonsupplementers

Characteristics	Supplementers		Nonsupplementers		Chi-Square Test For Difference
	N	%	N	%	
Total	17	100.0	156	100.0	
Ethnicity					X² = 11.97; P = <.001
Black	1	5.9	73	46.8	
White	16	94.1	83	53.2	
Concurrent Abuse					No Difference
Heroin	14	82.0	128	73.0	
Other Opiates	6	35.0	46	26.0	
Barbiturates	6	35.0	47	27.0	
Amphetamines	12	71.0	90	52.0	
Age					
Under 18	—	—	—	—	
18-20	—	—	2	1.3	
21-25	8	47.1	30	19.2	
26-30	2	11.8	23	14.7	
31-35	3	17.6	21	13.5	
36 and over	4	23.5	80	51.3	
Unknown	—	—	—	—	
Age (collapsed)					X² = 6.07; P = <.01
under 25 years	8	47.1	32	20.5	
over 25 years	9	52.9	124	79.5	

138

	N	%	N	%	
Sex					No Difference
Male	16	94.1	133	85.3	
Female	1	5.9	23	14.7	
Employment					X² = 4.30; P = <.05
Employed	4	23.5	78	50.0	
Unemployed	13	76.5	78	50.0	
Current Illegal Behavior					X² = 12.80; P = <.001
Yes	4	23.5	7	4.5	
No	13	76.5	149	95.5	
Welfare Assistance					X² = 9.90; P = <.001
Yes	12	70.6	50	32.1	
No	5	29.4	106	67.9	
Years of Drug Use					
None	—	—	2	1.3	
One	—	—	2	1.3	
2-3	—	—	24	15.4	
4-5	4	23.5	16	10.3	
6-8	5	29.4	8	5.1	
9-10	2	11.8	9	5.8	
11-15	—	—	33	21.2	
16-20	3	17.7	34	21.8	
21-25	2	11.8	21	13.5	
26-30	1	5.9	7	4.5	
Years of Drug Use (collapsed)					X² = 4.13; P = <.05
10 years and under	11	64.6	61	39.0	
Over 10 years	6	35.4	95	61.0	

Prior Treatments				
None	4	23.5	57	36.5
One	2	11.8	53	34.0
Two	5	29.4	31	19.9
Three	3	17.6	5	3.2
Four	—	—	—	—
Five	1	5.9	—	—
Six	—	—	—	—
Seven	1	5.9	—	—
More than 7	—	—	10	6.4
Unknown	1	5.9	—	—
Prior Treatments (collapsed)				$X^2 = 8.60$; $P = <.001$
0-One	6	35.3	110	70.5
Two or more	11	64.7	46	29.5
Concurrent Drug Therapy				$X^2 = 7.38$; $P = <.01$
Yes	8	47.1	29	18.6
No	9	52.9	127	81.4
Daily Methadone Dose (mg.)				
0-50	—	—	16	10.3
51-70	—	—	18	11.5
71-90	1	5.9	28	17.9
91-110	3	17.6	39	25.0
111-130	3	17.6	38	24.4
131-150	2	11.8	17	10.9
151-170	3	17.6	—	—
171-200	5	29.4	—	—
201-250	—	—	—	—
251-300	—	—	—	—
Unknown	—	—	—	—

Daily Methadone Dose (collapsed)				
110 mg. and under	4	23.5	101	64.7	X²= 9.25;
over 110 mg.	13	76.5	55	35.3	P = <.001

Weekly Clinic Visits				
None	—	—	1	.7
One	—	—	7	4.5
Two	—	—	32	20.5
Three	7	41.2	20	12.8
Four	10	58.8	—	—
Five	—	—	96	61.5

Weekly Clinic Visits (collapsed)				
0-two	—	—	40	25.6	X²=4.32;
Three or more	17	100.0	116	74.4	P = <.05

There is some evidence to support a hypothesis that the incidence of methadone supplementation is much greater than the 10 per cent which we have reported. For example, other studies reported in Chapters 9 and 11 incicate that only about one half of those who abuse drugs during treatment will admit to the abuse when questioned. For example:

> a. 40% admitted heroin abuse, but 78% were detected during urine surveillance
> b. 8% admitted barbiturate abuse, but 30% were detected during urine surveillance
> c. 5% admitted to amphetamine abuse, but 25% were detected during urine surveillance

The true incidence of methadone supplementation could, of course, be ascertained with techniques already available, e.g., gas chromatography analysis. While the procedures are admittedly expensive, we must recommend their periodic use to detect this form of treatment manipulation.

Several implications are indicated in this type of documentation of the dimensions of supplementation with methadone. Methadone maintenance at even very high methadone doses does not appear to repress "drug-seeking" in some persons. With these patients, the clinician never really has control of the treatment procedure since he does not control the manipulation of the medicine dose. If the supplementation is not known to the clinician, any detoxification procedure becomes potentially impossible. What specific relation these continued "drug-seeking" and "drug-taking" behaviors have with "drug-craving", which is supposedly eliminated during maintenance therapy, is as yet undocumented.

These data also indicate the ready availability of "diverted" methadone and the ease with which addicts are able to secure large supplies of injectable methadone from unsuspecting or unconcerned physicians. These 17 patients were able to secure almost 2,000 mg. of methadone every day from other methadone patients and by "making doctors." The issue of methadone diversion is addressed in Chapter 14.

Chapter 11.

High Versus Low Dose Maintenance Therapy: An Empirical Test

Chetwynd E. Bowling
Arthur D. Moffett
W. J. Russell Taylor

THE ISSUE

Considerable controversy exists within the field regarding dose levels of methadone required to produce "stabilization," "blockade" and to eliminate "drug craving." All clinicians seek these desired effects, but the data are thus far inconclusive and contradictory.

THE EXPERIENCE

The approach the therapist takes in planning the treatment of heroin-dependent patients is largely influenced by his subscription to either the psychogenic or pharmacodynamic theory of narcotic addiction. The psychogenic theory has been in vogue for a considerable length of time and reflects the view that opiate-dependent patients possess a basic "addictive personality" manifested by sociopathic behavior and the inability to control their drug-using impulse. The traits consistently associated with addicts as totally irresponsible thieves and liars provide some credibility for this "sociopathologic" theory. The failure to produce evidence which identifies a characteristic psychopathology or "addictive personality" that pre-exists narcotic usage renders the psychogenic theory untenable as a total explanation of the addiction. Reliance on the psychogenic theory of addiction with its concomitant conventional modes of abstinence therapy, including long prison terms and the use of some measure of psychotherapy by the more forward-looking detention centers have usually failed to convert "criminal addicts" into acceptable members of society. The pharmacodynamic theory of addiction postulates that it is the trial of addictive drugs, appreciation of the pleasurable effects obtained, the positive reinforcement obtained by repeated usage and the metabolic changes induced in the body, particularly the central nervous system, which bring about the opiate-dependent state. But not every one who tries addictive drugs continues to become dependent on them. Perhaps a fundamental defect does exist in the addict's personality, which leads him to repeated drug use to the point of becoming a full-fledged addict. Since narcotic addicts are a heterogeneous group, it is not difficult to speculate that both psychogenic and pharmacodynamic factors are possibly involved in fostering drug-dependence. A systematic examination of the psychodynamics of residents of areas with high addiction rates is required to help us develop preventive measures for this pressing problem.

Narcotic Substitution Therapy

Narcotic substitution therapy grew out of the concept of the pharmacodynamic or metabolic theory of drug addiction, and was first tried with heroin to treat "morphinomania" at the turn of the century. Its current use to facilitate the rehabilitation of heroin-dependent people has generated controversy within the medical profession which, has spilled over to an increasingly alert public. The methadone maintenance approach has been widely publicized by Dole and Nyswander and others. They propose that a "narcotic blockade" is created if "sufficient" methadone is prescribed. Addicts would not only lose their "craving" for heroin, but oral methadone would "block" the euphoric effects of this illicit drug even if it were subsequently to be self-administered parenterally. Unfortunately, there is no adequate empirical base for determining what doses are required to produce this "blockade," eliminate "craving," produce this more "rehabilitatable" addict' or, indeed, even to verify these postulations empirically.

Perkins and Bloch (1970) reported daily doses as high as 141 mg. and more (approximately 2 mg/kg or more) in patients who remained active in their program as compared with patients receiving 80 mg/day or less (approximately 1 mg/kg or less)—who had a significantly greater discharge rate because of continued illicit drug use, criminal activity and behavioral problems. Methadone maintenance programs have been started in every major city since the inception of the first Dole-Nyswander experiments with New York addicts half a decade ago.

Dosage Comparisons

The authors designed a study to secure dose-related data in the anticipation these issues could be brought into better focus.

The subjects for study were selected solely on the basis of daily methadone dosage. All were patients in the West Philadelphia Community Mental Health Consortium Narcotic Addict Rehabilitation Program located at the Philadelphia General Hospital. All methadone maintenance patients in the program receiving approximately 2 mg/kg daily oral dose or more (140 mg and above) were designated for the "high-dose" group and compared with all patients receiving about 1 mg/kg/day (70-80 mg), who were defined as the "low-dose" group. Demographic data, along with social parameters, were analyzed for change between the time the patients were inducted and the time the study was undertaken during methadone maintenance therapy. Drug abuse while on maintenance therapy was to be determined both by interview and by regular urine surveillance.

Fifty-seven patients were found to be receiving approximately 2 mg/kg daily oral dose of methadone or more (140 mg and above), while 74 patients were being maintained on about 1 mg/kg/day (70–80 mg).

Heroin was the drug of abuse in 92.7% of the "high-

Methadone Dosage and Going to Work

	"High-Dose" Group	"Low-Dose" Group
Gainfully Employed	41.8%	42.8%
Receiving Welfare	58.2%	53.2%
Dependent/Other	—	4.0%
Total	100.0%	100.0%

dose" group for a mean period of 12.6 years compared with 93.2% among the "low-dose" patients for a mean period of 10.2 years. The mean age for the "high-dose" group was 32.0 years compared with 30.9 years for the "low-dose" group; 32.8% of the "high-dose" group were single (never married) compared with 32.4% of the "low-dose" group; and 83.9% of the "high-dose" group were born in Pennsylvania compared with 82.4% of the "low-dose" group. The average number of years of schooling for the "high-dose" group was 10.3 and 10.8 years for the "low-dose" group.

Results

1. *Methadone dose does not appear to be significantly related to* "re-habilitability" *as measured by "going to work" after stabilization.* At the time of study, 41.8% were employed in the "high-dose" group compared with 42.8% for the "low-dose" group.

2. *The data do not indicate any significant differences in being arrested between "high-dose" and "low-dose" patients.* The arrests for both groups were very low. In the "high-dose" group, 52.6% reported arrests prior to maintenance therapy, but only 1.8% reported being arrested while on the program. Similarly, 48.6% of the "low-dose" group reported arrests prior to methadone treatment and 3.8% after treatment began. All arrest data were self-reported data and reflect only the formal arrests (e.g. bookings) and not total police contacts.

3. *Methadone dose does not appear to be significantly related to continued heroin use after stabilization.* Over half of all the study group were detected as heroin users at least once during a two-week test period. Heroin use

was detected in 55.2% of the "high-dose" group and 67.1% of the "low-dose" group. These differences are not statistically significant. Heroin abusers in the "high-dose" group more frequently denied their behavior when confronted by a counsellor/therapist.

4. *Methadone dose does not appear to be significantly related to non-heroin drug abuse after stabilization.* Over half of all the study group were detected amphetamine abusers—58.6% of the "high-dose" group and 51.3% of the "low-dose" group—and 23.2% of the "high-dose" group and 10.5% of the "low-dose" group were detected abusing barbiturates. None of the barbiturate abuse could be accounted for as a concurrent medication.

Mean time on methadone maintenance for the "high-dose" group was 22.6 months (range—5 to 40 months) compared with 12.9 months (range—1 to 47 months) for the "low-dose" patients. Some differences were discovered to exist. "High-dose" patients tended to be male (98.2% compared with 83.8%) and white (66.7% compared with 31.1%) and more had a diagnosed psychiatric disease (14.0% compared with 6.6%). The implications and significance of these differences are not known.

In summary, this study of non-selected addict-patients receiving methadone maintenance therapy produced *no* statistically significant differences between those receiving high doses and those receiving low doses in three areas typically associated with becoming "rehabili-

Drug Abuse During "High"-and "Low-Dose"
Methadone Maintenance

DOSAGE	"High-Dose" (N=57)				"Low-Dose" (N=74)			
	Ad-mitted		De-tected		Ad-mitted		De-tected	
ABUSE DRUG	N	%	N	%	N	%	N	%
Heroin	14	24.6	32	55.2	42	53.8	51	67.1
Amphetamines	10	17.5	34	58.6	11	14.1	39	51.3
Barbiturates	8	13.8	13	23.2	6	7.7	8	10.5
Extra Methadone	9	15.8	—	—	05	6.5	—	—

tated"—going to work, getting arrested and stopping drug use. *Of marked significance, daily methadone, regardless of the dose, taken for extended periods of time, did not stop drug-seeking and drug-taking behaviors.* In this study group of 131 stabilized methadone patients, 63.4% were still abusing heroin, 55.7% were abusing amphetamines, 16.0% were abusing barbiturates and 10.7% reported they were supplementing their daily methadone doses. We believe such extensive "cheating" casts some doubt on the commonly-held assumption that "sufficient" daily methadone will reduce "drug craving" to a level where the maintained patient will cease the use of illicit narcotics. While we are aware that "drug craving," "drug seeking" and "drug taking" are all different, one must assume that there is some relationship among all of them. Our data do suggest the immediate need for careful study of the content and context of this continued drug abuse among stabilized patients.

REFERENCE

1. Perkins and Bloch: Study of some failures in methadone treatment, 1970.

Chapter 12.

High Versus Low-Dose Maintenance Therapy: A Review of Program Experiences

Leon Brill

The "classical" methadone maintenance model is the one initiated by Dole-Nyswander at the Morris Bernstein Institute in 1965, using high or "variable dose" methadone at an average level of 80–120 mg. daily. This is the prototype which has multiplied so rapidly first in New York City and gradually in other parts of the United States and abroad. According to Dole-Nyswander, the goal of high-dose methadone stabilization is to relieve "narcotic hunger" and effect a "narcotic blockade." This concept is being questioned increasingly by workers in the methadone field, who prefer to speak rather of "cross-tolerance," "cross-dependence" or "substitution."

Another model was subsequently felt to be indicated, however, for addicts who did not appear to require prolonged periods of stabilization at such high dosage levels and were more attuned to goals of abstinence within a relatively short period of time. This evolution first occurred through the new technique of initiation and stabilization on an ambulatory basis. The goal here is not to establish a "blockade" or cross-dependence, but to stabilize patients on minimal doses for a population which requires some degree of chemical support analogous to tranquilizers.

During the development of the methadone program, applicants were interviewed who appeared not to need either the high doses of methadone or prolonged maintenance treatment. These patients were typically either well-integrated and highly motivated to give up heroin addiction, or else only recently addicted and fearful of regressing further. Still others wished at least to attempt detoxification before commiting themselves to long-term maintenance. Most of these patients had already tried conventional treatment approaches and found them lacking or were unable to obtain alternative treatment because of the lack of facilities.

HIGH-DOSE METHADONE

The following description of the Dole-Nyswander model and treatment rationale is offered as a basis for comparison with low-dose maintenance:

Dole-Nyswander originally set out to answer one question: Is there some medication that will permit chronic, compulsive long-term heroin users to become socially productive members of society? Ideally, such a medication would need to have the following characteristics: It should be orally effective, non-toxic and safe to give over prolonged periods; it should relieve chronic preoccupation with the use of heroin; and it should be possible to arrive at a stabilization dose that did not require frequent readjustments. If it had any abuse potential at all so that illicit diversion to non-patients could create a problem for the community, then its duration of action should be long enough to give all doses under direct observation. More important, it must be acceptable to patients.

It became clear from Dole-Nyswander's work that methadone, when used appropriately, possessed all these characteristics. Furthermore when patients were given extremely large doses of methadone, one additional effect was obtained—a remarkable degree of tolerance to methadone itself and all other opiate-like drugs was induced. As a rule, the tolerance to methadone was so marked that stabilized patients felt little or no subjective change when they took their daily dose. The experience of Dole-Nyswander was confirmed by the program administered by the author with a colleague. What was important was the tolerance induced to other intravenous narcotics. In this respect, the effect of methadone was somewhat analagous to that of cyclazocine in the cyclazocine program administered by the author. The repeated ineffective use of heroin in an effort to overcome the methadone blockade appeared to result in a gradual extinction of the instrumentally-reinforced, heroin-seeking behavior. With the passage of time, patients appeared to become more tolerant to the effects of methadone so that their improved productivity could not be attributed to the drug effects alone. The data also showed that the longer patients remained in the program, the better was their social adjustment. Patients were also weaned away from the needle, which appeared to be associated with their addict life-style and the "hustling syndrome." The use of high-dose stabilization was based on the idea of cross-dependence or cross-tolerance, which means that one opiate drug can be substituted for another without ill effects. It was this property, together with the fact that it was longer lasting than heroin (which is effective for about 4 hours and would therefore require perhaps 6 ministrations a day) and has a much lower excretion rate which led Dole-Nyswander to choose methadone as their stabilizing drug.

Dole and Nyswander's work emanated originally from their belief that opiate abuse generated a prolonged "narcotic hunger" or craving, which became the physical basis for a confirmed opiate addiction. The first efforts must therefore be directed to relieving this narcotic hunger. Morphine was first tried, but proved unsatisfactory because morphine-maintained patients remained sedated and apathetic. It appeared to be a continuation of the heroin behavior, with more of the positive effects sought for.

Methadone was used next, first by intramuscular injection, then orally. The first proved unsuitable since patients still appeared narcotized. Oral administration was far more dramatic and effective. Though craving was relieved and a heroin blockade set up, stabilized patients could still function effectively in the community. There was neither euphoria nor incapacitating sedation except perhaps in the earliest stages. The blockade could also protect patients against overdose from opiate drugs. Most patients could function well when stabilized on 80–120 mg., though some required less—perhaps 40 mg. and others as much as 200 mg. and more daily. Comprehensive physical tests failed to elicit physical toxicity from the effects of sustained use. It should be emphasized that the question of dosage is still very much an area for research, with many unanswered questions as to optimal dosage for different kinds of patients.

Procedure

Initially, the criteria for admission to a high-dose methadone program included: four to five years of confirmed narcotics use and a history of repeated failures in treatment, age 20–40 years old (upper limit raised to 50 in the third year of study), no legal compulsion, no major medical and psychiatric complications (e.g. severe alcoholism, epilepsy, schizophrenia) and residence in New York. In the first 18 months, also, only men were admitted to the program. These criteria were recently modified to 18 as a minimum age, and at least two years of confirmed use. Many of the prior medical and psychiatric exclusions were dropped by some programs. The treatment procedures established by Dole and Nyswander are detailed elsewhere in this volume.

The focus of the Dole-Nyswander program has been away from preoccupation with "assumed" underlying problems. Counseling services offered are therefore geared to the so-called "concrete" or "tangible" services to help patients resolve their daily problems of living as with jobs, schooling, training, welfare assistance and family problems. They have introduced a number of changes in their procedure in the last two years, among them ambulatory stabilization on methadone for the great majority of patients; and development of a "Rapid Induction" Center whose goal it is to stabilize addicts "right off the street" in time.

LOW-DOSE METHADONE PROGRAM

The following section describes the variety of procedures and rationales employed by different programs utilizing low-dose methadone approaches. Implicit in this discussion is the need for "differential diagnosis" to ferret out the varied uses for high-dose and low-dose maintenance.

Philadelphia Program

The philosophy of the Philadelphia Narcotics Addict Rehabilitation Program is that "everyone has a right to be drug-free, but not everyone is capable of, or willing to become abstinent."[1]

This philosophy was translated into clinic policy whereby all new patients were admitted to the detoxification program, with the exception of the few long-term addicts whose histories and present attitudes indicated that the prognosis for success was extremely poor. These latter patients were admitted directly to a methadone maintenance program.[1]

In part, the ambulatory detoxification program, if prolonged, merges into the low-dose methadone stabilization program. Low-dose methadone maintenance appeared to be a treatment of choice for those addicts who did not require or desire cross-tolerance or blockade as a deterrent to further heroin abuse. They seemed more clearly geared to the goal of abstinence and getting off all drugs as rapidly as possible. Still, they had not been able to make it in abstinence-oriented programs and required some degree of chemical support for their rehabilitation. Drug craving for these individuals could be suppressed at low-dose levels of up to 40 mg. daily. They apparently used methadone rather differently, also, as a kind of tranquilizer or anti-depressant while attempting to reconstruct their lives. It was estimated that approximately 20% of the Philadelphia patients were able to benefit from such low-dose regimes.[1]

From a treatment standpoint, the advantages of outpatient low-dosage stabilization and treatment are numerous. The addict remains in the community, need not sever whatever constructive ties exist in the form of job, family, and community ties, and can move more rapidly towards productive social functioning with the help of methadone support and any individual or group counseling services indicated. From a cost analysis standpoint, such a modality is far less expensive to operate than one using inpatient facilities and scarce hospital beds.

In a subsequent study of the Philadelphia program, Wieland summarized some of the problems associated with outpatient detoxification and redefined detoxification and low-dose maintenance as follows:

> 1. The dispensing of methadone doses of 50 mg. or less daily is now termed "low-dose maintenance." The term "detoxification" is used only when a patient is actually undergoing a gradual dose reduction, usually at the rate of 10 mg. per week.
> 2. Patients are more rapidly transferred to "high-dose maintenance" when their need becomes apparent.
> 3. All methadone is dispensed in liquid form mixed with Tang—as it always has been for high-dose patients.

Findings. The report describes the status of 52 low-dose maintenance patients as of September 1, 1970. All had been in treatment a minimum of three months. For comparison purposes, a matched sample of 52 high-dose patients was selected,—i.e. patients stabilized on 100 mg. daily or more. Results were based on a 60-day evaluation period during July–August 1970. It was concluded that low-dose methadone maintenance in selected cases produces fairly similar results to high-dose maintenance. Both groups showed a high incidence of amphetamine use and relatively high barbiturate abuse. Clinically, it was feared that much of this was moderate use for relief of sluggishness, obesity, insomnia. "One might conclude that dosage per se was less important than other factors such as typology of patients, ancillary services and attitude of program re:punitive discharge from treatment. . . . Despite the high incidence of drug abuse, criminal activity and arrest rates are markedly reduced. Both patients and families report overall improvement under treatment despite the lack of total rehabilitation."[2]

Chicago Multi-modality Program

Jaffe experimented with both low-dose and high-dose methadone maintenance as part of a multi-modality approach to treatment in Chicago. This program is described in the chapter on "Innovative Methadone Programs in the United States."

Vera Institute Program

The Vera proposal describing a varied approach to both treatment and research is detailed in the chapter on "Innovative Methadone Maintenance Programs."

West Side Medical Center

A private clinic maintained by an individual doctor, Dr. Rafig Jan, maintained two clinics in New York City for ambulatory maintenance at low-doses of patients. At the time of writing, the patient population comprised approximately 1,200. Dr. Jan didn't believe in high-level, variable dose maintenance, but rather in low-dose maintenance. He was not interested in establishing a heroin blockage and preferred to help patients avoid the "high," with less danger of sickness and overdose. Low-dose maintenance is more closely geared to the "working man" in the street, he felt, since it is easier to get off methadone and "there is a chance to talk to the doctor for emotional support." Elavil was offered in combination with the methadone to provide firmer support. Jan believed the low-dose approach is particularly suited for lower-class patients and minority groups, and stated he was undertaking research to substantiate his position.[3]

Narcotics Addiction Foundation of British Columbia, Vancouver

The NAF attempts to offer a rounded treatment program, which also includes varied uses for methadone detoxification, low-dose and high-dose maintenance as well as abstinence-oriented approaches. (Report of NAF,

1969) This study is described in the chapter entitled "International Programs in Methadone Maintenance."[4]

Elsewhere in Canada

Holmes reported on 62 patients "mostly male," who had been on methadone maintenance employing quite small dose levels of 10-40 mg. per day; 6 were out-patients, 10 had been steadily occupied and attending the clinic more than 12 months. Only half the female patients continued treatment and none more than 12 months. Holmes admitted to problems related to the small dosages given.[5]

Santa Clara Program of Dr. Abram Goldstein—Dose Studies

A major objective of the Santa Clara Program of Goldstein was to secure information about methadone dosages. A blind design was therefore essential. Dosage was never revealed to patients or discussed with them.

Results Irrespective of Dosage. By 33 weeks of operation, 206 patients had been admitted to the program. Twenty-nine patients (14%) left the program involuntarily; most had been incarcerated for crimes committed prior to entering the program, a few left the area to escape outstanding warrants or because their role as police informers had become known. Five patients (2%) left voluntarily, usually to move to another area; and two patients were officially transferred to methadone programs elsewhere. None were dropped from the program by staff action. At this particular time, therefore, there were 170 active patients, or 83% of the number admitted.[6]

Of the 48 active patients with tenure of 6 months or longer in the program, 88% had stopped using heroin. This statement means that they had achieved a record of consistently negative ("clean") urines over a period covering at least the previous four weeks. Heroin use dropped very abruptly within the first two weeks of the program, to less than 10% of its initial value. Then a slower decline continued for a period of approximately three months. The majority of patients at that time had ceased using heroin entirely, and the majority of the remainder used only small amounts sporadically. A few continued a low-level of daily use, although very much less than before they entered the program. All the results cited were influenced by the predominance of better-motivated, older, and more stable patients among the early admissions to the program.[6]

Uniform Dosage. In 93 patients, uniform procedures were employed. The purpose was to ascertain the feasibility of a uniform dosage schedule, for this would greatly simplify the conduct of large-scale methadone programs.[6]

The study of "side effects" yielded some surprises. Indeed, some of the most prominent ones were clearly withdrawal effects rather than side effects, for their frequency and severity were inversely related to methadone dosage, and they occurred principally in the evening, eight hours or more after the daily dose. Symptoms that fell into this category comprised the constellation recognized by addicts as "feeling sick," including insomnia, nausea and vomiting, muscle pains and anorexia.

There were also dose-related side effects. Dermatitis, constipation, impotence, difficulty achieving orgasm, and feeling "loaded" on methadone were the prominent ones. They all tended to improve after the first month, but constipation and the sexual disfunctions persisted in a small fraction of patients. Drowsiness was troublesome during the first month; surprisingly, there was no difference between 50 mg. and 100 mg. although the 30 mg. dose was significantly better. In any case, severe drowsiness disappeared by the second month. Suppression of craving for heroin and reduction in heroin use were achieved faster at the higher doses, but by the third month the doses were virtually indistinguishable in these respects.[6]

Excessive sweating was a very common complaint, but difficult to classify. It was present to some degree in three-quarters of the patients before methadone, and in moderate or severe form in 10-15%. By the third month it had become worse in 42% of the patients and better in about 30%, remaining unchanged in the remainder. There was no dose relationship.

Proposed Research Directions.

a. Dosage studies require randomized concurrent assignments to the dosage groups. Patients must not know their dosages, and baseline data must be obtained before starting methadone. Many "side effects" were found to be at higher frequency and greater severity before methadone than later.

b. Symptoms come and go even on constant dosage. One should be restrained in attempting to deal with complaints by manipulating dosage until the effects of different doses have been more clearly defined.

c. Virtually all patients can be built up to a uniform stabilization dose without regard for individual differences. The most successful method is to begin ambulatory induction at 30 mg. once daily and increase by 10 mg. every second day, stabilizing at 100 mg. after fifteen days.

d. Comparison of 30, 50, and 100 mg. daily doses revealed surprisingly few differences. The 100 mg. dose caused certain side effects more frequently and at greater severity than did lower doses. On the other hand, symptoms of the withdrawal type were less frequent, and suppression of heroin craving and heroin use was faster than at lower doses. Heroin use, however, declined very sharply in all dose groups, with little difference between the doses after the first few weeks. There was no dose effect upon attendance or dropout rate.

e. Contrary to what is often said, he found no change in the use of alcohol, amphetamines, or marijuana, and a sharp decline in the use of barbiturates, as compared with the pre-methadone data.

f. In many patients, the duration of action of methadone appeared to be too short, causing withdrawal symptoms in the evening. Goldstein was able largely to alleviate this problem by splitting the dose. If a longer-acting narcotic than methadone became available, it should be tried on a daily basis to see if a smoother action with less fluctuation could be obtained.[6]

Special Program for Adolescents Using Low-Dose Methadone

Nyswander and Millman offer the following description of a "slow detoxification" program for adolescent heroin addicts in New York City, which could appropriately be termed low-dose maintenance:—

The authors at Rockefeller University began a study of 25 adolescent heroin addicts two years ago, combining rehabilitative services with slow detoxification using low-doses of methadone.[7]

Patients admitted were under 18 years of age, and had a history of one to two years of continuous mainline heroin addiction. They had failed in other recognized treatment programs and had had previous arrests. All patients were selected from the metropolitan area: explicit parental consent was required in each case. Patients were treated as out-patients at the Rockefeller University Hospital. At the onset of treatment, the dose of methadone was low (10-20 mg/day in most cases), and was subsequently brought up to a maximum of 20-50 mg/day. Medical complications of the medication were negligible. A number of patients experienced constipation, relieved in all cases with a laxative. Several complained of drowsiness early in their course.[7]

Initially, all patients were required to come to the clinic each weekday to take their medication and leave a urine specimen. They were given medication on Friday to take home for Saturday and Sunday. The program undertook to provide a situationally-oriented form of counseling, vocational and educational guidance, and recreational leadership.

Of the original twenty-five adolescents, 23 are currently in the program. In the present group, the average age is 17, with a range between 13 and 22. Of these 23 patients, 11 have remained heroin-free, 7 have used heroin occasionally (1-3 times per month), and 5 are using the drug several times weekly. It is planned to withdraw methadone from all patients who appear to have a reasonable chance of doing well without medication. Two patients in this group have already been detoxified. They continue to come to the clinic for consultation and to leave urine specimens.

There has been little problem with abuse of other drugs. Two patients used amphetamines intermittently, one patient used barbiturates on weekends, and another has used cocaine on several occasions. Two patients reported single experiments with LSD.

As in the regular Methadone Maintenance programs, an ex-addict, himself on a maintenance program, may play a crucial role in counseling other patients. This may be particularly true in an adolescent program where the patients are able to identify with him. Frequently, it is this staff member who makes the initial contact with a prospective patient. A good number of the patients had cases pending in court when they were admitted to the program, and it was decided to take an active interest in these.

The combination of extensive rehabilitative services with slow detoxification using low doses of methadone thus appears to hold promise in the treatment of adolescent heroin addiction. The authors have demonstrated the ability to wean patients off heroin, and believe it is significant that no patients have become readdicted. More data is required before a statement may be made relative to the feasibility of detoxifying the majority of adolescents on the program.[7]

Comments

This chapter has compared the techniques of high-dose and low-dose methadone stabilization. Though the "traditional" Dole-Nyswander high-dose methadone stabilization program had postulated the existence of "narcotic hunger" for which a "narcotics blockade" needed to be established, it was soon learned the low-dose methadone maintenance could be a treatment of choice for those addicts who did not require or desire cross-tolerance or blockade as a deterrent to further heroin use, and were more clearly geared to the goal of total abstinence. They had not, however, been able to make it in abstinence-oriented programs and required some degree of chemical support for their rehabilitation. Drug craving could be suppressed at levels as low as 30-40 mg. daily—which was useful as a kind of tranquilizer or antidepressant.

This low-dose regimen could serve other useful purposes as with younger heroin addicts, or in holding patients waiting to get into a treatment program, or else could merge into a longer-term ambulatory detoxification over a period of weeks or months. Goldstein, in his Santa Clara, program undertook a comparison of three groups stabilized on 30 mg., 50 mg. and 100 mg. respectively. He concluded that there was a more rapid suppression of heroin use with 100 mg. than with lower doses, but the results in all three groups tended to converge after the first months on the parameters of retention, arrest and increase in productivity. Higher doses produced more undesirable side effects than did lower doses. Jaffe's studies point to the same conclusions. While no further generalizations can be made at this time, it would appear that varied uses for methadone are both possible and desirable and research in these areas must be continued. There are clearly groups of patients for whom lower doses are indicated based on both needs and aspirations; and others who as clearly require higher levels, in some cases ranging well above the average of 80-120 mg. for their rehabilitation. Methadone treatment can be a far more flexible treatment tool than was originally envisioned, and its varied uses in combination with other treatment approaches warrants further exploration.

REFERENCES

1. Brill and Chambers: A multimodality approach to methadone treatment, 1971.
2. Wieland and Moffett: Results of a low-dosage methadone treatment, 1970.
3. Jan: Personal Communication, 1970.
4. Narcotic Addiction Foundation: Narcotic Addiction Foundation of British Columbia 14th Annual Report, Treatment Supplement, Vancouver, British Columbia, 1969.

5. Holmes: Paper presented before Committee on Problems of Drug Dependence, 28th Meeting, National Research Council, National Academy of Sciences, 1966.

6. Goldstein: Blind controlled dosage comparisons with methadone in 200 patients, Proceedings Third National Methadone Conference, 1970.

7. Millman and Nyswander: Slow detoxification of adolescent heroin addicts in New York City, Proceedings Third National Methadone Conference, 1970.

Chapter 13.

Physiological and Psychological Side Effects Reported During Maintenance Therapy

Carl D. Chambers
Leon Brill
John Langrod

THE ISSUE

". . . in all probability it (methadone) produces, like morphine, long-lasting physiological and psychological abnormalities. Therefore, because of the toxicity . . . it should be used cautiously . . . . Systematic studies should be undertaken to assess potential and known undesirable effects of methadone maintenance as well as the desirable actions." (Martin, 1970)

THE EXPERIENCES

The physiological and psychological effects as well as the implications of sustained administration of any narcotic, including methadone, are indeed poorly understood. Carefully-designed chronicity studies are noticeably absent in the literature. A review of those studies which have attempted to address this issue reveals a state of the art characterized by methodological inconsistencies and design inadequacies. One would assume such basic design controls as sex, length of addiction, methadone dose, duration of treatment, etc. would be included in each assessment. Unfortunately, this is *not* always the case.

The sometimes contradictory findings of some of the better-designed studies are indicated below:

1. Cushman, *et. al.* (1970) undertook an investigation of the implications of a methadone maintenance regimen for the hypothalmic-pituitary-adrenal axis. In a comparative study between heroin addicts and methadone-maintained addict-patients, they confirm the clinical impression of normal adrenal cortical function in maintenance-therapy recipients.

2. Wallach, *et. al.* (1969) compared the effects of self-controlled opiate addiction and medically-supervised methadone maintenance therapy in women. Female "street addicts" typically report that they suffer from amenorrhea, anovulation and infertility. In a study of 90 women of reproductive age who were receiving maintenance therapy, 82 began to menstruate regularly within 1-2 months following initiation. There were 13 pregnancies and the pregnancies seemed little affected by the methadone administration. The investigators concluded that ovulation, conception and pregnancy occur without serious problem to mother or child.

3. Maslansky, *et. al.* (1970), reporting on the careful study of *four* pregnancies in maintained females indicated:

a. Placental transfer of methadone did occur, but this transfer resulted in only minimal withdrawal activity, which required no medical intervention.

b. No teratogenic effect of this placental transfer was observed.

c. Methadone usage did result in low-birth-weight infants.

4. Bloom and Butcher (1970) reported that female patients of childbearing age appear to be more fertile once they are stabilized on methadone. These investigators also reported significant increases in weight gain in both males and females, increased frequency of urination in females, a dose-related numbness of the hands and feet as well as swelling of the feet and ankles, and a blurring of vision among high-dose and younger patients.

5. To date, Goldstein (1970) has provided us with the most systematic dose comparison assessment of side effects during the initial phases of maintenance therapy. Twenty patients receiving 30 mg. per day were compared with 80 patients receiving 50 mg., and with 106 patients receiving 100 mg. for the initial three months of maintenance therapy. The following were his most salient findings:

a. Dermatitis, constipation, impotence, difficulty in achieving orgasm, and feeling "loaded" on the methadone were the most frequently reported side effects. All effects tended to decrease after the first month, with constipation and sexual dysfunctions being most persistent. These side effects did *not* appear to be dose-related.

b. Drowsiness was a common complaint for those patients receiving 50 or 100 mg. daily. *Severe* drowsiness disappeared by the second month.

c. Excessive sweating was a very common complaint which was *not* dose-related. Quite unpredictably, sweating increased in some patients and decreased in others with no relation to methadone dose.

d. Numbness, tingling and stiffness of the fingers, sometimes accompanied by pains radiating down the arms was reported by almost one third of the 206 methadone patients and did *not* appear to be dose-related.

6. Wieland and Yunger (1970) studied 70 addict-patients on daily maintenance doses ranging from below 50 mg. to above 100 mg., and reported they could find *no* significant differences in the incidence or type of side effects which could be considered dose-related.

7. Jaffe (1970) studied 126 addict-patients and reported that the incidence of constipation and sweating were dose-related.

A LARGE-SCALE ASSESSMENT OF THE REPORTED AND /OR OBSERVED SIDE-EFFECTS DURING THE STABILIZATION PHASE

The authors have been able to analyze the recorded self-reported and/or clinically-observed physical and psychological side effects for a population of certified narcotic addicts stabilized on methadone in the same facility under the direction of the same clinical staff. The study population consisted of 637 addicts consecutively admitted during 1970-1971 to the methadone maintenance program of the New York State Narcotic Addiction Control Commission. All had been certified as narcotic addicts within the prescriptions of the civil commitment laws, and all had been detoxified and were drug-free upon the initiation of the stabilization regimen.

Females would appear to be underrepresented in this study population of 637 addicts—only 19 (3.0%) were females.

Not all addict-patients reported or were observed to have experienced physical or psychological side effects during the stabilization phase of maintenance therapy—137 addict-patients (21.5%) had no recorded side effects. Although the female sample is small for statistically significant comparisons, females appear to have recorded side effects more frequently during stabilization—84.2% of all females as against 78.3% of the males.

Table 1.
Reported and/or Observed Side Effects During the
Stabilization Phase of Maintenance Therapy

Side Effects	484 Males		16 Females		500 Total	
	N	%	N	%	N	%
1. Gastro-Intestinal						
a. Nausea	88	18.2	2	12.5	90	18.0
b. Vomiting	65	13.2	—	—	65	13.0
c. Constipation	209	43.2	2	12.5	211	42.2
d. Anorexia	90	18.6	1	6.3	91	18.2
e. Weight Change	48	9.9	—	—	48	9.6
2. Neuro Psychiatric						
a. Depression	5	1.0	—	—	5	1.0
b. Sedation	2	.4	1	6.3	3	.6
3. Musclo Skeletal						
a. Cramps	9	1.9	2	12.5	11	2.2
b. Contractions	3	.6	—	—	3	.6
4. Cardio Vascular						
a. Perspiration	92	19.0	—	—	92	18.4
b. Edema	58	12.0	2	12.5	60	12.0
5. Respiratory						
a. Asthma	4	.8	1	6.3	5	1.0
6. Genito Urinary						
a. Oliguria	—	—	—	—	—	—
b. Difficulty Starting Stream	73	15.1	1	6.3	74	14.8
7. Sexual						
a. Loss of Libido	38	7.9	—	—	38	7.6
b. Impotence	—	—	—	—	—	—
c. Premature Ejaculation	—	—	—	—	—	—
d. Excessive delayed orgasm	1	.2	—	—	1	.2
8. Integument						
a. Rash	64	13.2	2	12.5	66	13.2
b. Pruritis	53	11.0	3	18.8	56	11.2
9. Other						
a. Insomnia	1	.2	2	12.5	3	.6
b. Neurotic Behavior	1	.2	1	6.3	2	.4
c. Headaches	2	.4	2	12.5	4	.8
d. Aches & Pains	1	.2	1	6.3	2	.4
e. Anxiety	2	.4	—	—	2	.4
f. Heartburn	1	.2	—	—	1	.2
g. Peeling of hands	—	—	1	6.3	1	.2

A distribution of the side effects recorded during stabilization is contained in Table 1. Empirically confirming our respective impressions, the most frequently recorded side effects are constipation (42.2%), excessive sweating (18.4%), anorexia (18.2%) and nausea (18.0%).

AN ASSESSMENT OF THE INCIDENCE OF REPORTING SELECTED SIDE EFFECTS AFTER TWO YEARS OF MAINTENANCE THERAPY

During 1969, one of the authors interviewed 52 male addict-patients who had been in the New York City Harlem Hospital Methadone Maintenance Treatment Program for at least two years. The interview was designed to elicit an evolution of five specific physical side effects experienced *after* the completion of stabilization. The five side effects specified for the respondents were: excessive sweating, constipation, sleepiness/drowsiness, impotence/delayed ejaculation and "aches in bones and joints." These specific side effects were chosen because they were the ones most frequently discussed among methadone patients and clinicians.

The Study Group

The 52 addict-patients in the study group were included on the basis of a single selection criterion—having been maintained on methadone for at least two years. Various characteristics of these addict-patients are contained in Table 2.

Results

Each of the 52 subjects was requested to indicate whether he had ever experienced each of the side effects and to what degree he was currently experiencing them. The distributions of their responses are contained in Table 3.

It is, of course, impossible to attribute conclusively *all* such non-specific side effects to the medication being received. It seems reasonable to predict, however, that

Table 2.
Characteristics of 52 Male Long-Term Methadone
Maintenance Patients Studied for Side Effects

1. Ethnicity
   Black 77%
   White 12%
   Puerto Rican 11%

2. Age
   30 and under 12%
   31-35 .... 39%
   36 and over 49%

3. Duration of Heroin Use
   1-15 years 43%
   Over 15 years 57%

4. Duration of Maintenance Therapy
   Range .... 24-42 months
   Mean .... 31 months

5. Daily Methadone Dose
   Less than 100 mg. 32%
   100 mg. 40%
   More than 100 mg. 28%
   Range .... 80-130 mg.
   Median Dose .... 100 mg.

most maintenance patients will experience excessive sweating and constipation; and for significant numbers, these side effects will persist throughout the therapy process. Newly-inducted patients should be made aware of the chronicity of these side effects so that physical and psychological adjustments can be made early in treatment.

The data *do not* indicate the incidence of the other three side effects—sleepiness/drowsiness, sexual problems and nonspecific aches in the bones and joints—to be in excess of those within the same age groups within the general population. For example, we would not believe it unreasonable to expect a third of all males over age 35 to have some concern about impotence; or for a third to complain of being excessively tired and sleepy; or for 6% of them to complain of vague ill-defined aches and pains. The data *do* indicate the possibility of methadone involvement, and this possibility should be pursued empirically.

Table 3.

**The Evolution of Reported Side Effects Among
52 Males Who Had Received Maintenance Therapy
For At Least 2 Years**

1. Excessive Sweating	
A lot now	43%
A little now	18%
In the past but not now	22%
At any time since stabilization	83%
2. Constipation	
A lot now	10%
A little now	31%
In the past but not now	16%
At any time since stabilization	57%
3. Sleepiness/Drowsiness	
A lot now	2%
A little now	25%
In the past but not now	10%
At any time since stabilization	37%
4. Impotence/Delayed Ejaculation	
A lot now	12%
A little now	20%
In the past but not now	16%
At any time since stabilization	48%
5. Aches in Bones and Joints	
A lot now	3%
A little now	3%
In the past but not now	10%
At any time since stabilization	16%

Comments and Implications

There are a number of researchable side effect questions which have been largely ignored in spite of the widespread acceptance of maintenance therapy. These questions include, but are not limited to the following:

1. *What is the psychological impact on the addict-patient during long-term maintenance therapy?* There is *some* evidence that long-term maintenance patients are measurably more depressed than normal subjects. There is also *some* evidence that anxiety measurably increases after 2 to 3 years of maintenance therapy. We are, however, unwilling to accept any existing evidence, experimental or anecdotal, as conclusive. Such measures of psychological impact demand our immediate attention.

2. *What are the physiological impairments experienced during long-term maintenance therapy?* There is *some* evidence both anecdotal and experimental, which suggests that no measurable physical handicaps result from long-term maintenance therapy. For example, motor coordination does not appear to be affected in most patients. In contrast, there is *some* anecdotal evidence that even long-term patients will become sedated quite unpredictably on their normal daily doses. There have been no well-designed large sample assessments of physical impairment. Such assessments, controlling for dose- and time-ranges should be of the highest research priority.

3. *What are the cognitive impairments experienced during long-term maintenance therapy?* The authors are aware of *no* significant attempts to measure experimentally any cognitive impairment resulting from the chronic administration of high doses of methadone. We believe experimental measures for such factors as attention span, abstract problem-solving, memory recall, etc. should be pursued immediately.

Until these questions are addressed experimentally, the long-term side effects of maintenance therapy will remain largely unknown. That such a situation should prevail after so long a clinical experience is unwarranted and demands immediate resolution.

REFERENCES

1. Martin: Commentary on the Second National Conference on Methadone Treatment, 1970.

2. Cushman, *et. al.*: Hypothalamic-pituitary-adrenal axis in methadone-treated addicts, 1970.

3. Wallach, *et. al.*: Pregnancy and menstrual function in narcotics addicts treated with methadone, 1969.

4. Maslansky, *et al.*: Pregnancies in methadone maintained mothers; a Preliminary Report, 1970.

5. Bloom and Butcher: Methadone side effects and related symptoms in 200 methadone maintenance patients, 1970.

6. Goldstein: Blind controlled dosage comparison with methadone in two hundred patients, 1970.

7. Wieland and Yunger: Sexual effects and side effects of heroin and methadone, 1970.

8. Jaffe: Methadone maintenance: Variation in outcome criteria as a function of dose, 1970.

Chapter 14.

Methadone Diversion: A Study of Illicit Availability

Peter V. Walter
Barbara K. Sheridan
Carl D. Chambers

THE ISSUE

There has been a natural reluctance among enforcement people to accept the notion that methadone patients should be permitted to take supplies of the drug away from the clinic. Their perception of the "addict" includes a belief that portions of this "medicine" will be diverted into the illicit subculture for abuse by non-patients. Methadone clinicians believe the patients should be "trusted" not to divert their methadone, besides which the patients need their medication to remain stabilized.

Clinicians involved with the methadone maintenance modality have consistently expressed a belief in the need for "take-home medication." Essentially this relates to the feeling that as an addict-patient begins responding to the medication and to any ancillary services, e.g., as he "gets better," he should not be required to come to the clinic as frequently. While this does have some therapeutic value and does free clinic space and staff for the less responsive addict-patient, it nonetheless sets the stage for diverting medication into the illicit subculture market. We believe the diversion of these medicines to be the major source for those persons who become addicted to methadone as their primary drug of abuse, for those who wish to "boost" the potency of their primary narcotic, or want to "treat themselves" or simply want some "insurance" against a "panic" or the loss of a regular drug supply. (The reader is directed to Chapters 6 and 19 for issues and experiences with primary methadone addicts.) Since there is no known illegal manufacture of methadone, one measure of the extent of medicine diversion is to assess the availability of these medicines to the general population of street addicts. This report is based upon one such assessment.

The Study Population

A study population of active heroin addicts was selected at random during August 1971 from those available in a known high-drug-use area of New York City—the Bedford-Stuyvesant section of Brooklyn. The *only* sampling criterion imposed was that each addict-respondent must have been an active addict, e.g., not in treatment, jail, etc., for at least six months prior to the time of the interview. Of the first 100 addicts selected, 95 met this single criterion, and these 95 became the study population. Each subject was interviewed by an ex-addict who had been employed specifically because of his familiarity with the addict population in this section of Brooklyn. A standardized interview schedule was utilized, and each interview was conducted in the presence of one of the authors.

An analysis of the demographic characteristics of the 95 addict-respondents revealed nothing which would suggest they were significantly different from the universe of "heroin street addicts" in New York City.

The Results

A series of questions was directed specifically to the availability of illicit methadone, the actual purchase of illicit methadone, the identification of the source of the illicit methadone and the uses of the illicitly purchased methadone. The following are our findings:

   1. Of the 95 active heroin addicts, 87 (91.6%) reported they had been offered the opportunity to purchase illicit methadone within the past six months (March-August 1971).

Descriptive Characteristics

1. Age Distribution
   - a. Range .... 17-47 years
   - b. Median ....   24 years

2. Sex Distribution
   - a. Males 70.5%
   - b. Females 29.5%

3. Ethnic Group Distribution
   - a. Black 46.3%
   - b. Puerto Rican 22.1%
   - c. White 31.6%

4. Heroin as Primary Drug
   - a. Yes 100.0%
   - b. No.....................................   0.0%

5. Duration of Narcotic Use
   - a. Range .... 9 Mos.-23 years
   - b. Median ....   4 years

6. Prior Formal Treatments
   - a. No formal treatment 47.4%
   - b. Some prior treatment 52.6%

7. Amount of Current Daily Narcotic Use
   - a. Range of "bags" .... ½-35 bags
   - b. Median number of "bags" ....   4 bags
   - c. Range of "costs" .... $0-$150.
   - d. Median "cost" .... $12.

2. Of the 95 active heroin addicts, 53 or 55.8% reported they had purchased illicit methadone within the past six months (March-August 1971). Of these 53 buyers, 50 or 94.3% reported purchasing the methadone for their personal use. The vast majority of the 53 buyers of methadone—79.2%—reported methadone was always available in their neighborhoods.

3. Of these 53 recent purchasers of illicit methadone, all reported the drugs were in "wafer" form—the 40 mg. non-soluable tablet manufactured and distribut-ed by Eli Lilly. Only one addict-respondent reported ever purchasing any liquid form methadone during the past six months.

4. The cost of the recently purchased illicit methadone was very stable. The prices ranged from $3.00 to $5.00 per 40 mg. wafer, the average price being $4.00.

5. Not unexpectedly, the reported source of most of the illicit methadone was from ambulatory patients enrolled in programs dispensing "take-home medication." Of the 53 active narcotic addicts who had illegally purchased methadone during the past six months, 39 or 73.6% reportedly purchased the drugs from active methadone patients. The

remainder of these recent purchasers were unable or unwilling to specify the source of the illicit methadone.

6. There were, of course, a number of reasons specified for the purchase of the methadone. The most frequently specified primary uses were:

41.4% ..... to "insure" against withdrawal distress
17.2% ...... to "clean up"
39.7% ...... to "boost" other drugs
1.7% ...... to "resell"

All of the 95 active heroin addicts were also questioned relative to any "selling" of methadone. Of these active addicts, 12 or 12.6% reported they had sold methadone, with 8 or 8.4% reporting at least some of these sales as occurring within the last six months. When questioned as to the source of the illicit methadone, the 12 "sellers" indicated their primary sources had been personal friends who were patients in methadone programs (50.0%), their own medications while in methadone programs (41.7%) or "making private doctors" (8.3%).

In summary, these data indicate a ready availability of illicitly-diverted methadone. Most of the methadone available, at least in this study area, is in the form of 40 mg. wafers manufactured by Eli Lilly and being tested by clinics in this study area. Most of the methadone purchased was for quasi-medical or self-treatment use by the purchaser. A stable price indicated the supply of the "medicine" was sufficient to meet the high demand for it.

Comments and Implications

These data have isolated a number of questions and issues which require immediate investigation.

1. Some assessment of patient involvement in the various programs demands the highest priority. At the present time, diversion is occurring from ambulatory detoxification programs, ambulatory maintenance programs, pretreatment or "holding" programs, etc. We have *no* empirical base from which to assign differential rates, or suggest controls. While these current data confirm that medicine diversion is extensive and constant, e.g., 41.1% of all active heroin addicts reported buying methadone from patients, they do not assess how many

patients or which programs are involved. We believe that the accumulation of such assessment data is currently our most important research need.

2. An assessment of the differential rates of diversion from programs utilizing the various *types* of methadone is of critical importance. This is a necessary adjunct to the testing of the administrative and therapeutic effectiveness of the new "wafers." It is our preliminary evaluation that the diversion of methadone is higher in those programs which dispense medication in pill and in wafer form than in those which utilize liquid in the form of a juice vehicle.[1] We hypothesize that this differential rate is primarily due to the ease with which the individual addict-patient can "split" various parts of his medication, e.g., one-half, one-fourth, etc. Active heroin addicts express a preference for the liquid, however, which they believe, correctly or incorrectly, contains more methadone for less money, e.g., an "average bottle" is 120 mg. for $10.00.

3. The motivation and rationale for both purchasing and selling illicitly needs to be comprehensively assessed. We know, anecdotally, that diversion permits both the seller and buyer to manipulate their "habits." Methadone "patients" can sell a portion of their "medicine" and purchase narcotics to "get over" the remainder of the "medicine" or purchase amphetamines or sedatives to "get around" the "medicine." At the same time, active heroin addicts can "boost" their relatively weak heroin with the methadone, "cut their habit" through a self-treatment regimen or "stash away" so they won't ever need to worry about "getting sick." We do not know the extent or distributions of these motivations and rationales within the various addict and patient populations. We are reminded of one study accomplished in a methadone maintenance program in Philadelphia where almost 20% of all patients were selling portions of their "take-home" medication to buy cocaine, which they incorrectly assumed would not be detectable in their urines.[2] When confronted with urine data revealing this abuse, half of the abuse ceased.

4. How one learns about methadone is becoming one

of the more salient issues demanding inquiry. "Getting a taste" for methadone during a legitimate detoxification regimen is probably much more widespread than our scarce data would indicate (see Chapter 19). The importance of determining how one becomes a primary methadone addict, how one maintains this addiction and how one responds to detoxification and other treatments is brought quickly into focus when one remembers there is no illegal manufacture of methadone. There is only illegal diversion of legal supplies.

5. A number of active heroin addicts report they "become tired" of the street life and begin to seek programs to "clean up." They place themselves on the waiting lists for a number of programs and begin to buy and use illicit methadone while they wait. Some, of course, "cut their habits" to a manageable level and go back to heroin, ignoring the call when a treatment slot becomes available. Others sustain themselves and enter treatment when the opportunity occurs. Still others enter into a number of programs and sell medicines from some or all of them. We do not know how to screen for, or adequately predict the behavior of any of our treatment clients. We still do not know when, in an active addict's career, he is most susceptible to buying illicit methadone, entering into treatment or abusing programs after entering treatment.

REFERENCES

1. Chambers: Current treatment activities and legislation: Philadelphia, 1971.

2. Chambers, *et. al.*: The incidence of cocaine abuse among methadone maintenance patients, 1972.

Chapter 15.

Methadone Poisoning: Diagnosis and Treatment*

Vincent P. Dole
Francis F. Foldes
Harold Trigg
J. Waymond Robinson
Saul Blatman

THE ISSUE

The risk of methadone poisoning among children and irresponsible adults always exists when a clinic permits medication to be taken home. The immediate diagnosis and treatment of this poisoning are vital. As more maintenance programs develop and more patients "take home" varying portions of their medication, the greater the chances the "average doctor" will encounter this type of poisoning.

THE EXPERIENCE

The average quantity of methadone prescribed for patients on a methadone maintenance program is 80 to 120 mg. per day (higher doses are prescribed in some cases) taken by mouth in 2 to 4 ounces of Tang or fruit juice, or in solutions prepared by dissolving noninjectable tablets in water.† When taken by the maintenance patients, whose special tolerance for narcotics decreases the pharmacologic effects of this medication, this dose produces no sedation, no impairment of respiration, or

* Reprinted with permission from the *New York State Journal of Medicine,* 541-543, March 1, 1971.

other adverse effects. However, the same dose will cause severe respiratory depression if taken by nontolerant subjects who are not on the methadone program, and is likely to be fatal in children. The ingestion of methadone under such circumstances constitutes an acute emergency, requiring immediate diagnosis and treatment. Fortunately, specific and effective antidotes are available for treatment of the respiratory depression caused by an excessive dose of methadone or other opiate drugs.

Diagnosis

The history of narcotic intake is of paramount importance since the symptoms of coma and apnea are nonspecific, and time is too short to defer treatment while waiting for confirmation by laboratory tests.

Methadone is dispensed in prescription-labeled bottles, with the name of the patient, the hospital, and the prescribing physician on each bottle. If a child has ingested a dose, an empty container (and in it traces of the orange juice-like fluid) may be found nearby. The patient responsible for the medication should, of course, be questioned, if available. A child, age two to six years, who takes a full dose of methadone will become progressively comatose over a period of one-half to three hours, and, if untreated, will die of respiratory failure within this time. No data are available on the time course of respiratory depression in older children or nontolerant adults, but the symptoms certainly would be similar.

Treatment

Artificial respiration. Artificial respiration is indicated immediately if breathing has stopped, or if its rate or depth has become too low to maintain effective ventilation. If equipment is available, an airway tube should be inserted and a respirator mask applied (such as an Ambu respirator with bag and nipple for oxygen supply). An endotracheal tube with inflatable cuff is desirable for comatose patients to protect against aspiration of vomitus, but no time should be lost in looking for the special equipment required and a trained anesthetist to insert the tube. Artificial respiration by the best means immediately available should be started without delay in any case of severely depressed respiration.

Antidotes. Naloxone hydrochloride (Narcan), dose 0.01 mg. per kilogram, given intravenously, is the antidote of choice. If naloxone is not available, nalorphine hydrochloride (Nalline), dose 0.1 mg. per kilogram, or levallorphan tartrate (Lorfan), dose 0.02 mg. per kilogram, are also effective antidotes for narcotic overdose.* These latter two agents, however, may augment the degree of respiratory depression if the diagnosis of narcotic poisoning is in error. They can be harmful if the depression of breathing is due to poisoning with barbiturate or to other disease processes. Naloxone is free from this danger, and therefore is safe to use when the diagnosis is in doubt.

If respiration has improved in response to the first injection of antidote, but is not yet adequate, the injection should be repeated in five minutes and again in ten minutes. If, however, the first injection has had no significant effect, the diagnosis of narcotic overdose may be in error. In case of such doubt, it is safe to repeat the injections of naloxone, but further administration of nalorphine or levallorphan should be deferred for at least thirty minutes while adequate ventilation is maintained by artificial respiration and the patient's clinical status is carefully evaluated.

Observation. Establish a routine of close observation to ensure that the subject will be examined carefully every fifteen minutes, or more often, during the first twenty-four hours. If the patient is a young child, the crib should be put beside the nurse's desk in a good light so that respiration can be observed continuously. Narcotic antagonists should not be used to attempt to arouse comatose but adequately breathing patients, but an antidote must be available near the bed to treat depression of respiration that might recur during the next forty-eight hours.

* To convert dose in milligrams per kilogram to dose in milligrams per pound, divide the dose in milligrams per kilogram by 2.2.

This is of great importance since the antidotal action of narcotic antagonists is only two to three hours, while the depressant action of methadone may last from twenty-four to forty-eight hours. A patient, especially a child, may be successfully resuscitated with a narcotic antagonist, and later relapse into fatal coma if dissipation of the effect of the narcotic antagonist remains unrecognized.

Further injections. After successful initial resuscitation, further injections of narcotic antagonists may be given intramuscularly. The intramuscular dose should be about 50 per cent greater than the intravenous dose. The onset of action of narcotic antagonists is slower (five to ten minutes) after intramuscular than after intravenous injection (one to two minutes). The difference in speed of onset of action is unimportant if the patient is being watched closely and if the narcotic antagonist is given before respiration has become seriously depressed again.

Intravenous drip. In treating comatose infants and small children, it is advisable to maintain a slow intravenous drip of glucose-saline solution, consisting of 5 per cent glucose, 2 parts, mixed with saline, 1 part, for the first twenty-four hours. This ensures adequate hydration and provides an avenue for intravenous medication, if needed for treatment of circulatory collapse.

Lavage. Theoretically, emptying the stomach by lavage would be indicated if the procedure could be done immediately after ingestion. However, if the victim is not seen until an hour or more, lavage would not only interfere with the much more important artificial ventilation but is also potentially dangerous since it may cause tracheobronchial aspiration in comatose patients. For these reasons, gastric lavage should only be performed after ventilatory resuscitation and tracheal intubation with a well-fitting cuffed tube.

Contraindications. Dialysis is contraindicated; the

amount of methadone in blood is negligible, even after a fatal ingestion. Central nervous system stimulants are also contraindicated; they are ineffective against the depressant actions of methadone and synergistic to the deleterious stimulant effects of this drug.

Prevention

Obviously, children and irresponsible adults should not be given the opportunity to poison themselves. The importance of secure custody of methadone must be emphasized by physicians prescribing this medication. In general, the medication has been responsibly handled by patients being treated by methadone maintenance programs. There have, however, been 3 serious poisonings of children, two of them fatal, from approximately 2 million doses dispensed in New York City during the past six years. Each case was due to carelessness on the part of the patient for whom the medicine had been prescribed; all of them could have been avoided, and the 2 fatal cases could have been saved if they had had prompt treatment with antidotes.

Consultation will be available in New York City at all times to any physician or hospital receiving a case of suspected methadone poisoning. It is important that the emergency room of every hospital be prepared to deal with this type of poisoning since the patient can die in transit if refused admission and sent to some other facility.

Telephone numbers to call for consultation in New York City:

1. Poison Control Center, New York City Health Dept. Tel. 340-4495
2. M. J. Bernstein Institute: Tel. 677-2300; ext. 233
3. Beth Israel Medical Center: Tel. 673-3000; ext. 2251; 2501
4. Montefiore Hospital: Tel. 920-4321
5. Harlem Hospital: Tel. 621-3125 or 621-3126
6. Rockefeller University Hospital: Tel. 360-1485

A kit for hospital emergency room or physician's office should include:

1. Antidote (one of following): naloxone (antidode of choice), levallorphan tartrate, and nalorphine hydrochloride.

2. Syringes 5 cc. with assortment of needles for intravenous and intramuscular injection. Tourniquet and sponges.

3. Airway tubes, assortment of sizes (numbers 1 to 5).

4. Ambu respirator with nipple for oxygen supply.

5. Flashlight.

6. Written instructions for diagnosis and treatment of poisoning with methadone.

PART THREE

Detoxification Therapy: Recent Experiences and Issues

Chapter 16.

A Description of Inpatient and Ambulatory Techniques

Carl D. Chambers

THE ISSUE

Considerable controversy exists regarding the need for the inpatient detoxification of narcotic addicts. Those who support the inpatient procedure point to the advantages of a drug-free environment and close medical supervision of the withdrawal process. Proponents of the ambulatory procedure acknowledge these advantages, but point to the increased number of addicts who can be serviced at lower costs.

THE EXPERIENCES

Methadone, for the chemotherapeutic management of narcotic detoxification, was first reported by Isbell and Vogel in 1949 (see Chapter 2). Their clinical experiments documented the effectiveness of methadone in the reduction and elimination of narcotic withdrawal symptoms, which prompted the adoption of this substitution treatment procedure at the two U.S. Public Health Service Hospitals at Lexington, Kentucky and Fort Worth, Texas. During the initial years of use, the regimen called for the methadone to be administered twice a day subcutaneously in a substitution dose of 1 mg. of methadone for 5 mg. of morphine. A detoxified state was accomplished in 7 to 10 days. Since that time, methadone substitution has been the primary chemotherapeutic procedure for the detoxification of narcotic addicts.

Although methadone has been the primary chemotherapy vehicle for detoxifying narcotic addicts, various techniques for its use have evolved. These techniques may be grouped into two general categories—techniques for detoxification on an inpatient basis and ambulatory techniques. Regardless of which techniques are utilized, at least three factors operate to affect the rapidity with which detoxification can occur: the "size of the habit," as indicated by the severity of the withdrawal symptoms, the existence of a concurrent addiction, e.g., sedative, tranquilizer, etc., and the general physical condition of the addict-patient.

A Description of Inpatient Techniques

Advocates of a required inpatient detoxification point to a high incidence of sociopathic personality disorders among opiate addicts or to the adverse social influences surrounding most addicts as necessitating close supervision and isolation during detoxification.

The first major assumption the clinician must have when confronted with the task of assessing the degree of dependence on narcotics is the generally unreliable nature of an addict's personal account of the amount of drugs he has taken. In most cases, the addict-patient really does not know the amount of drugs he has taken, or knowingly chooses to exaggerate the quantity in the hope of receiving more medication. If he is abusing illicit drugs, the quality varies to such an extent as to render the concept of quantity relatively meaningless.

When withdrawal symptoms appear:

> . . . Elixir of methadone is ordered to ameloriate opiate withdrawal. . . . In view of the rather small opiate habits that are currently seen at this hospital (Lexington), with the likelihood that this will be a continuing observation, a 10 mg. dose is appropriate in the vast majority of cases. Where activity of any opiate addiction is in doubt, 5 mg. doses would be appropriate; and where habits seem unusually large or medical problems demand minimal discomfiture, 15 mg. doses are appropriate. If significant opiate withdrawal is seen upon admission (mydriasis with progressive decreased reaction to light, gooseflesh, 'pilomotor

erection,' muscular twitches, hot and cold flashes, aching bones and muscles, anorexia), the dose selected as outlined above is ordered SOS x 3 to 4. (An SOS dose is a dose given by the nursing attendant when the significant opiate withdrawal is seen. After further observation, it may be repeated as many times as ordered if the significant withdrawal recurs).[1]

. . . . Following this, the patient is withdrawn at the rate of 5 to 10 mg. per day, depending on his condition and progress.[1]

. . . *Special Aspects of Opiate Withdrawal:* In occasional cases with severe medical or surgical problems (i.e. heart disease, tuberculosis, cancer, recurrent intestinal obstruction, etc.) the patient is given methadone to the point of tolerance to avoid abstinence; is maintained for several days (during which medical evaluation is accomplished) and then withdrawn at the rate of 5 mg. or less per day. In such cases, the methadone is frequently given q.i.d. rather than b.i.d.[1]

. . . In other cases, acute febrile or inflammatory illnesses will increase the tolerance to opiates transiently and increase the severity of withdrawal symptomatology, requiring more methadone.[1]

. . . In cases of addiction to both opiates and barbiturates with significant barbiturate tolerance requiring some time for withdrawal, the methadone may be withdrawn more slowly without prolonging the total withdrawal period. In addition, such cases are sometimes stabilized on a methadone schedule (small) when they have shown only scant or grade one opiate withdrawal (in order to facilitate their management).[1]

Concurrent addictions require concurrent, but different detoxification regimens. For example, the incidence of a concurrent barbiturate-sedative addiction among narcotic addicts has been documented as high as 35 percent.[2] This addiction will, of course, require a chemotherapeutic withdrawal with a sedative-hypnotic and a considerably longer period of treatment than the narcotic withdrawal.

. . . Withdrawal of persons with strong physical dependence may be life-threatening, and can only be accomplished satisfactorily, and with reasonable safety, in a drug-free environment where hospital and nursing facilities are available.[3]

* * *

. . . The gravity of the barbiturate abstinence syndrome is indicated by the occurrence of death following the withdrawal of secobarbital from a patient who had been using 50 gm. of the drug daily.[4]

The contraindication of abrupt withdrawal of barbiturates and the specific symptoms to expect from physically-dependent persons are widely documented in the literature. Even a rapid reduction of the dose to which the person has become tolerant is considered dangerous. The general procedure for the medically-controlled withdrawal process dates back to the pioneering work done by Isbell and his associates in 1950.[5,6]

The initial procedure is, of course, to establish with some degree of certainty the amount of drugs the person has been ingesting. The ascertainment of this is accomplished through a "test dose" procedure. A "test dose" is the administering of a specific amount of barbiturates and examining the patient for effects within specific time limits. The "test dose" procedure developed at the Lexington facility is as follows:

> ... A test dose is a specific amount of pentobarbital given, after which the patient is examined (50 to 90 minutes later) for effect (toxicity, decreased withdrawal, etc.). It is usually ordered for 8 a.m. so that the evaluation may be made during morning withdrawal rounds, and the usual amount is 200 mgs. This dosage would be appropriate when the initial estimate of pentobarbital tolerance is felt to be in the 400 to 1100 mg. range. Tolerance to less than 400 mg. of pentobarbital per day has not produced a significant abstinence syndrome and therefore is not searched for precisely. For this reason, a 100 mg. test dose is rarely used. (It is only used when the clinical estimate is vague and the patient is elderly or debilitated to the extent that a 200 mg. test dose producing intoxication might endanger his health or lead to injury. In these cases, if a 100 mg. test dose produces no intoxication, it is always followed in a few hours by a 200 mg. test dose.) Where the initial estimate of tolerance is 1200 to 1600 mg. or more, a 300 mg. test dose is better. Test doses greater than 300 mg. are rarely of any help.
> ... (See Section on evaluating test doses). When the history of intake is much greater than the estimated tolerance (or the physician believes the history is exaggerated); or when the history of intake is denied and the physician is suspicious, a test dose (or the larger test dose if it is a choice between 200 mg. and 300 mg.) can be ordered only if the patient sleeps poorly (less than five to six hours with the usual sedation). In general, it is better to err on the side of intoxicating the patient when dealing with barbiturate withdrawal although keeping intoxication to a minimum greatly facilitates nursing management.[1]

After the "test dose" procedure of gradually increasing doses of barbiturates has ascertained the "stabilization dose," a gradual reduction in daily intake from that dose is indicated. There is general agreement that the dosage of barbiturates should not be reduced more than 0.1 gram per day and, occasionally, reduction should be stopped for periods of three or four days. The appearance of anxiety, weakness, and insomnia indicates that reduction should be stopped and the patient maintained on the dosage level at which the symptoms appeared for several days. It usually requires 14 to 21 days to withdraw barbiturates safely.

Stated somewhat differently, the dose should be withdrawn at the rate of one therapeutic dose per day. If during withdrawal the patient becomes apprehensive, tremulous or insomnolent, dosage reduction should be discontinued for 1 or 2 days, or until the signs disappear.

> . . . the dosage should not be reduced more than 100 mg. (1-½ grains) daily. If abstinence signs or symptoms recur, the dosage should be temporarily increased. Close observation is required because of concomitant mental confusion, lethargy, muscular incompetence, apprehension and possible convulsions.[3]

A Description of an Ambulatory Technique

The methadone substitution philosophy for ambulatory detoxification is essentially the same as for inpatient detoxification—to stabilize the addict on a relatively low dose of methadone and then gradually reduce the dose until such time as the addict-patient requires no substitute medication to prevent the onset of withdrawal symptoms.

The major clinical benefit of ambulatory detoxification for the addict-patient is that, even during the treatment process, he can begin to learn new or reestablish old non-addict social patterns. This time can also be used for ego-building experiences such as meaningful family and peer relationships and reestablishing himself in an educational or occupational role. This benefit *can* also be the major clinical disadvantage. The ambulatory detoxification modality, more than any other, requires that each patient assume the largest share of responsibility for his individual treatment. The clinician has very little active control over the outpatient. He can only prescribe the appropriate "medicines" and counsel his clients as part of the "deaddiction process." The patient helps shape the treatment process by not abusing the illicit drugs which are so readily available. In essence, then ambulatory detoxification becomes a social-interactional and motivational process while inpatient detoxification has been primarily a medical process.

The following is a description of the ambulatory technique utilized in the Narcotic Addict Rehabilitation Program at the Philadelphia General Hospital.

Patients came to the clinic voluntarily after having been on a waiting list for three to six months. They were usually self-referred, having heard of the program from their peers. The only criteria for admission were addiction to a narcotic drug and residence in a defined geographical area. Psychotic patients and mixed addictions were not excluded from treatment. Psychiatric or medical admissions, including concurrent sedative addictions, to a hospital are arranged when indicated by the clinical conditions. This was the diagnoses, however, in less than 10 percent of the cases.

Most patients began detoxification treatment on 40 mg. per day, either 20 mg. b.i.d. or 10 mg. q.i.d. Those with small habits (1–3 bags per day) would only require 20 to 30 mg. per day, and those with large habits (over 7 bags per day) could require as much as 50 to 80 mg. per day. Patients were seen every day during the initial phase of treatment so the original dose could be adjusted if necessary.

The 10 mg. tablets of methadone were used in this program for several reasons: (a) low doses of methadone, if taken in a single dose, appeared to be effective for only 6-12 hours, and tablets provided a convenient way to prescribe divided dosage; (b) patients could space their dose as they perceived withdrawal distress, which varied from patient to patient or from day to day; and (c) patients knew exactly how much methadone they were getting, which reduced suspiciousness and mistrust. Liquid methadone could also be used, but the division and spacing of doses would be more difficult for the patients.

At each clinic visit, the patient was expected to see a counsellor, who was either a social worker or trained ex-addict, for a 20- to 30-minute session. The main therapeutic emphasis was on supportive counselling regarding present and future behavior, including such areas as drug abuse, employment, interpersonal relations, and general attitudes. Since the work role constitutes a major index of male normality, it was strongly encouraged and assisted, when indicated, by job counselling or vocational training. After the counselling session, the patient received a one-day's supply of methadone and left a urine specimen to be analyzed for methadone, morphine, quinine, barbiturates, amphetamines, and cocaine.

In a program where there is no selection process, each addict-patient must be evaluated by a psychiatrist before beginning treatment. The psychiatrist can assist the counsellor in devising an individualized treatment plan and managing the more serious psychiatric complications, such as schizophrenia and severe depression. He should also be available for frequent consultation by the counsellor.

Ideally, when the patient has ceased "cheating" with heroin or other drugs, and has shown some movement towards emotional and social rehabilitation, the dose of methadone can be decreased by 10 mg. per day. If he is working, the frequency of clinic visits can also be reduced to 2 or 3 times per week. With further progress, the dose can again be reduced by 10 mg. per day, and the frequency of clinic visits reduced to a minimum of once a week. In the event of emotional or behavioral relapse, either the dosage or the number of visits or both can again be increased until "restabilization" occurs. The process of reducing the dose can begin again when the clinical condition warrants it.

Any outpatient treatment for which detoxification is the goal must be highly individualized. Ambulatory detoxification with some addict-patients may be accomplished in two or three weeks, but it will more typically require 4 to 8 weeks or longer. In some cases, the process could require a number of months. In these cases, however, methadone would not merely be used to detoxify the patient, which could, of course, be accomplished more rapidly in an inpatient setting, but would in effect be used as a stabilizing drug, thus offering an extended period of time for rehabilitation to occur without any of the withdrawal problems associated with normal maintenance level doses. Used in this manner, it would permit ambulatory treatment without the usual institutional restraints in much the same way as the various psychotropic drugs have permitted the outpatient treatment of psychiatric patients.

Certain aspects of the outpatient treatment outlined above may be viewed as a reward-punishment system. These include variations in the frequency of clinic visits, adjustments in dosage, the possibility of temporary suspension from treatment, and the verbal responses of the counsellor. Recalcitrant patients may be required to accomplish some task in a given time period (e.g., obtain a job, cease cheating, etc.) or face suspension for a period of time (usually 30 days). This reward-punishment system provides a concrete frame of reference by which both the patient and his counsellor can judge the overall progress.

In a two-year experimental period at this clinic, *some 25% of the addicts who entered into the ambulatory regimen were discharged as detoxified.*

It is apparent that a large number of addicts "use" an ambulatory detoxification program in various ways. For example, there are those who will come only once or twice. These "crisis" cases quite probably only want methadone to hold them until they can secure heroin. This problem can be readily eliminated by requiring a waiting period before dispensing medicine. A second large group who "use" the program consists of those who want only to reduce their habit or to have an "easy" habit combining methadone and heroin. Some systemic benefit is derived from the first since the addicts do not need to steal as much to support their habit. The latter must be discovered and either terminated or transferred to a maintenance program where they no longer derive any euphoric effects from heroin. Urinalysis is the most effective tool for isolating those persons who only want an easy habit. The illicit diversion of medication seems to be a major concern among those who oppose the use of ambulatory detoxification. Illicit diversion of medication will not occur if only small amounts of medication are dispensed at frequent intervals, preferably on a daily basis.

In summary, if the *only* issue is whether detoxification is possible in an ambulatory setting, then one must confirm that this is indeed possible. These data have shown that one can expect some 25% of those who initiate a detoxification regimen to complete the detoxification successfully.

These results, however, clearly point to a major clinical disadvantage in the outpatient detoxification modality. As indicated, this modality, more than any other, requires that each patient assume the largest share of responsibility for this treatment. He must come to the clinic daily to receive his medication, no easy task in a large metropolitan city; must follow the prescribed ingesting regimen without supervision, and remain in treatment even though he isn't "being sick" until the detoxification process is completed.

At the operational level, a major consideration with outpatient treatment modalities is that they are much less expensive to operate than inpatient units. When organized properly, outpatient clinics, with proportionately smaller numbers of professional and clerical staff than required in an inpatient unit, would have the capability of dispensing medication, providing counselling as well as medical, vocational and educational services to a larger number of patients on a daily basis.

REFERENCES

1. Arnold: The techniques of withdrawal of opiates and barbiturates-sedatives, 1961.

2. Chambers: Barbiturate-sedative abuse: a study of prevalence among narcotic addicts, 1969.

3. A.M.A.: Dependence on barbiturates and other sedative drugs, 1965.

4. Fraser, *et. al.*: Death due to withdrawal of barbiturates, 1953.

5. Isbell: Addiction to barbiturates and the barbiturate abstinence syndrome, 1950.

6. Isbell, *et. al.*: Chronic barbiturate intoxication, 1950.

Chapter 17.

Characteristics of Attrition During Ambulatory Detoxification

Carl D. Chambers

THE ISSUE

Premature termination of treatment (attrition) is a problem in any program. Attrition from ambulatory programs is, of course, higher than from any other type of program. It is now possible to better understand and predict the addict-patients who, in spite of their avowed desire to detoxify, do terminate a detoxification process prior to its completion.

THE EXPERIENCE

This study was designed to ascertain what attributes of the addict or his background were associated with terminating treatment prior to attaining abstinence. This design presumes that if the attributes are known, clinicians can better predict which of their addict-patients will require a greater concentration of time and skill.

The plan of the study was to ascertain, wherever possible, any significant differences between those who terminated the detoxification process before its completion and those who remained in treatment. To accomplish these determinations a chi-square analysis was planned. A second technique, multi-variant analysis of low frequency events, was utilized with the same dependent variables in an attempt to isolate any predictors of attrition.

All addicts admitted to the ambulatory detoxification

195

clinic at the Philadelphia General Hospital between August 1 and November 1, 1968 were defined as the study sample. During this three month period, 86 addicts were admitted into treatment. A cutoff date of March 31, 1969 was chosen. This date provided an 8-month maximum and a 5-month minimum "at risk of attrition" period. Completing or active patients were defined as those who were still in treatment as of the cufoff date. Attriting or inactive patients were those who had terminated the detoxification process "against medical advice." This A.M.A. status was ascribed to any patient who quit coming to the clinic to receive his methadone medication and failed to respond to written or telephone suggestions that he continue in treatment.

Data isolating the variables utilized for these analyses were collected by a social worker at the initial treatment visit or during subsequent routine clinic visits.

PATIENT CHARACTERISTICS

As a group, the 86 addicts could be characterized as typically being Negro, male, under 30 years of age,

Table 1.
Characteristics of the Addict-Patients

		Distribution Among 86 Addict-Patients	
Attributes	N	% of Total
1. Negro	67	77.9
2. Male	73	84.9
3. < Age 30	51	59.3
4. > 8 Years Education	64	74.4
5. Employed	47	54.7
6. Married	49	57.0
7. > Age 20 First Addicted	75	87.2
8. No History of Prior Treatment	69	80.2
9. No History of Criminal Conviction	48	55.8
10. No History of Welfare	64	74.4
11. No History of Alcohol Abuse	75	87.2
12. No History of Concurrent Drugs	52	60.5

school dropouts, married and legally employed at the time they requested treatment. Most of these addicts had not become addicted until after the age of 20. Except for their addiction problems, these patients did not have many of the social casualty characteristics typically associated with being hard-core heroin addicts in the United States. For example, a majority did not report any prior formal detoxifications, they did not have histories of being on welfare, they had not been abusers of alcohol, they had not been convicted of any crimes, and they were not concurrently abusing other drugs with their heroin.

ATTRITION CHARACTERISTICS

Of the 86 addict-patients, 59 or 68.6% terminated the detoxification process against medical advice. During the study period, 10.2% of the dropouts terminated within the first month of treatment. The largest percentage of attrition occurred during the last two months of the study period with 55.9% of all the terminations occurring within this period. Length of treatment ranged from less than one week to more than 30 weeks with a median of 24-26 weeks.

Table 2.
Distribution of A.M.A. Terminations
by Month of Attrition

Month of Attrition	Distribution of Attritions	
	N	%
1. August*	6	10.2
2. September*	3	5.1
3. October*	9	15.2
4. November	6	10.2
5. December	—	—
6. January	2	3.4
7. February	18	30.5
8. March	15	25.4
Total	59	100.0

* Patients Were Admitted Only During These Months

Table 3.
Comparisons of Basic Demographic Variables by Attrition

Basic Demographic Variables		N	% of Total 86	Percent Attrition	Significant Differences
1. Race:	Whites	19	22.1	52.6	None
	Negroes	67	77.9	73.1	
2. Sex:	Males	73	84.9	68.5	None
	Females	13	15.1	69.2	
3. Age:	< 30	51	59.3	72.5	None
	> 30	35	40.7	62.9	
4. Education:	< 8	22	25.6	95.5	Yes-Inspection
	> 8	64	74.4	59.4	X² Test Inappropriate
5. Employed at Intake:	Yes	47	54.7	66.0	None
	No	39	45.3	71.8	
6. Married at Intake:	Yes	49	57.0	77.6	X² = 4.232;
	No	37	43.0	56.8	P = < .05

Table 4.
Comparisons of Social Casualty Variables by Attrition

Social Casualty Variables		N	% of Total 86	Percent Attrition	Significant Differences
1. Age First Addicted:	< 20	11	12.8	72.7	None
	> 20	75	87.2	68.0	
2. Criminal Conviction:	Yes	38	44.2	63.2	None
	No	48	55.8	72.9	
3. Ever on Welfare:	Yes	22	25.6	68.2	None
	No	64	74.4	68.8	
4. Prior Treatment:	Yes	17	19.8	76.5	None
	No	69	80.2	66.7	
5. Ever Abuse Alcohol:	Yes	11	12.8	63.6	None
	No	75	87.2	69.3	
6. Concurrent Drug Abuse:	Yes	34	39.5	35.3	$X^2 = 28.968$;
	No	52	60.5	90.4	$P = < .001$

Results

Three comparisons produced significant differences between those who attrited and those who completed the detoxification regimen.

1. Addict-patients with less formal education more frequently terminated prior to detoxification. Almost all (95.5%) of those with less than eighth-grade educations left A.M.A. compared with 59.4% of those with more than eighth-grade educations.

2. Attrition among married addict-patients was 77.6% but only 56.8% among patients who were not married.

3. Addict-patients who had been "heroin only" users prematurely terminated treatment more frequently than the abusers of multiple drugs.

MULTIVARIANT ANALYSIS OF LOW FREQUENCY EVENTS

Separating the patients into groups with either a low or high risk of A.M.A. termination through the multivariant technique, the following comparisons were produced. Those addict-patients with a *low risk* of A.M.A. termination were more likely to be the older patients averaging about 35 years and were more likely to be the patients who became addicted to heroin later in life having an addiction onset age of about 27. In comparison, the average age for *high risk* addict-patients was about 26 and they became addicted at about 21 years of age. The *low risk* group was more frequently married at the time they began treatment but had completed fewer years of formal education. Having a history of a criminal conviction and concurrently abusing drugs with heroin were more frequently associated with the *low risk* patients. With the exception of the abusing of other drugs concurrently with heroin, none of the differences are statistically significant.

To verify the significance of concurrent drug abuse with attrition, a further analysis combining the previously determined interactional effects of age, a history of a criminal conviction and the concurrent abuse of drugs with heroin was performed. The influence of this latter factor, concurrent abuse, was clearly demonstrated.

Attrition was found to be the highest where the addict was abusing only one drug, heroin, regardless of age or having a criminal conviction. Conversely, the lowest attrition was found among those addict-patients concurrently abusing drugs with their heroin and this was also the case regardless of age or having a criminal conviction.

At least by these methods of analysis and among those factors analyzed, concurrent or multiple durg abuse prior to the beginning of detoxification appears to be the most potent predictor for remianing in treatment until detoxification is realized.

SUMMARY

This study was designed to assess the background characteristics of those addict-patients who either remained in or dropped out of an outpatient methadone detoxification treatment program for hard-core heroin addicts. Of 86 heroin addicts admitted for detoxification during the study period, 59 (68.6%) terminated treatment against medical advice and prior to becoming detoxified.

The highest rate of attrition was found to occur between the sixth and eighth months of treatment.

Statistical comparisons between those who terminated A.M.A. and those remaining in treatment produced significant differences in only two demographic areas. First, the greater the amount of formal education, the greater the potential for remaining in treatment. Secondly, those addicts who were married at the time of initiating treatment were more likely to terminate treatment prior to detoxification. This first finding is, of course, compatible with similar studies relevant to the utilization of medical and psychiatric services. The second finding is meaningful only if one acknowledges the pressures on the family man to return to normal productive roles as soon as it is possible. In this case, it would be as soon as his addiction and/or detoxification became manageable.

Statistical comparisons were also made of a set of attributes associated with various states of social casualty. Only one of these comparisons produced a significant difference between those terminating A. M. A. and those remaining in treatment. The concurrent abuse of other drugs with heroin at time of initiating the detoxification process was more frequently associated with remaining in treatment than was the abuse of heroin alone.

A multivariant analysis was accomplished to isolate the predictors of attrition. The association between the number of drugs abused and attrition was reinforced through this level of analysis. To be abusing only heroin was the most potent predictor of attrition among these outpatients attempting to detoxify with the use of methadone. Although this finding cannot, of course, be conclusively interpreted, the author surmises that addicts who concurrently abuse multiple drugs will correctly perceive of their detoxifications as being more difficult and requiring more time. Heroin-only addicts, on the other hand, would experience fewer physical and psychological changes and would perceive of their detoxifications as being less difficult and requiring less time. It is, therefore, probable that the heroin-only abuser can more readily ascertain when his addiction and/or detoxification becomes personally manageable and is more likely to judge for himself when treatment should terminate. Further studies, including repetition and comprehensive follow-up studies, are required, however, before complete interpretation is possible.

Chapter 18.

Drug Abuse During Ambulatory Detoxification

Carl D. Chambers,
W. J. Russell Taylor
Peter V. Walter

THE ISSUE

A major clinical disadvantage in ambulatory detoxification is the lack of control over what drugs the addict-patient may continue to abuse. The addict-patient is fully responsible for the progression and success of the treatment regimen. The dimensions and patterns of drug abuse during ambulatory detoxification are now known.

THE EXPERIENCE

During December 1969, there were 65 heroin addicts undergoing ambulatory detoxification at the clinic operated by the West Philadelphia Community Mental Health Consortium at the Philadelphia General Hospital. These 65 addict-patients became the study population for this inquiry into drug "cheating."

Urine specimens collected during each clinic visit over a one-month surveillance period became the core data for the analysis. Each specimen was analyzed for the presence of heroin, barbiturates, amphetamines and cocaine. The data derived from each specimen were "pooled" by weeks within the surveillance period. This technique of analysis and grouping reduces the over-detecting of an incidence of abuse which could remain in the body during more than one specimen collection period. The data are presented in the form of statements of the average number of weeks or percentages of time in which the study population abused specific drugs.

The 65 addict-patients were separated into three groups on the basis of their daily methadone doses. This grouping categorizes the addict-patients by stage of detoxification, e.g., patients on 40 mg., 30 mg. and 20 mg. are at different stages of detoxification.

Results

The abuse of all drugs during the ambulatory detoxification of this study population was extensive. Not unexpectedly, the incidence of abuse decreased as the detoxification progressed.

1. Addict-patients at the initiation stage of detoxification, e.g., 40 mg. of substitute methadone daily, were abusing heroin 64.1% of the time.

2. Addict-patients at the middle stage of detoxification, e.g., 30 mg. of substitute methadone daily, were abusing heroin 39.4% of the time.

3. Addict-patients at the later stages of detoxification, e.g., 20 mg. of substitute methadone daily, were abusing heroin 34.3% of the time.

Similar decreases were noted in the abuse of amphetamines. Those addict-patients receiving 40 mg. of methadone were abusing amphetamines 17.2% of the time and those receiving 30 mg. were abusing amphetamines 16.9% of the time. By the time detoxification had progressed to the final stages—20 mg. of substitute methadone per day—the addict-patients were abusing amphetamines only 6.0% of the time.

For all intents and purposes, there was no abuse of barbiturates by any of these addict-patients.

If one reverses the frame of reference from the amount of time the urines were "dirty" to the amount of time "clean," it is possible to view these addict-patients as becoming non-abusers. At 40 mg., the subjects were "clean," only 23.4% of the time. At 30 mg., they were "clean" 31.0% of the time, and at 20 mg., they

Table 1
Incidence of Drug Abuse Among 65 Detoxification Patients

Daily Methadone Dose	Total Weeks of Surveillance	Percentage of Weeks The Drugs Were Detected				Percentage of Weeks With No Abuse	Percentage of Weeks Negative For Methadone
		Heroin	Barbiturates	Amphetamines	Cocaine		
40 mg (N=21)	64	61.1[a]	1.6	17.2	6.3	23.4[d]	22.4
30 mg (N=21)	71	39.4[b]	1.4	16.9	1.4	31.0[e]	35.2
20 mg (N=23)	67	34.3[c]	—	6.0	—	44.8[f]	22.4
Total	202	45.5	1.0	13.4	2.5	33.2	26.7

Note: Comparisons between "a" and "c" produce a statistically significant difference . . . X^2=11.582; P= < .001.
Comparisons between "a" and "b" produce a statistically significant difference . . . X^2 = 8.169; P= < .01.
Comparisons between "d" and "f" produce a statistically significant difference . . . X^2 =86.609; P= < .05.

were "clean" 44.8% of the time. One should not, however, lose sight of the correlate fact—even at the final stages of "detoxification," the addict-patients were "cheating" with some drug 55.2% of the time.

Quite unexpectedly, the data revealed that these addict-patients were not taking their methadone a fourth of the time. There was no apparent relationship between the stage of detoxification and having urines which were negative for methadone.

A complete distribution of the patterns of abuse for each of the 65 addict-patients is presented below:

The study population consisted of 50 males and 15 females. Both sex cohorts were equally divided among the three stages of detoxification. An analysis of the data controlling for the sex of the addict-patients at each detoxification stage revealed the following:

1. At the initiation stage of detoxification, e.g., 40 mg. of substitute methadone daily, there is no difference in the incidence of heroin, amphetamine or barbiturate abuse. For all intents and purposes there is no barbiturate abuse in either sex cohort. Females are more frequently detected abusing cocaine, however.

2. At the middle stage of detoxification, e.g., 30 mg. of substitute methadone daily, males more frequently than females are continuing to abuse heroin, although it has significantly decreased for both, and the abuse of amphetamines has remained the same for both sexes.

3. At the later stage of detoxification, e.g., 20 mg. of substitute methadone daily, both sex cohorts are still abusing heroin a third of the time, but amphetamine abuse has virtually disappeared in both.

Table 2
21 Detoxification Patients
Receiving 40 MG. of Substitute Methadone Daily

No abuse during 30-day surveillance	0	
Negative for Methadone only	2	9.5
Heroin only	4	19.0
Heroin/Amphetamine	2	9.5
Heroin/negative Methadone	5	23.8
Heroin/Amphetamine/Cocaine	3	14.3
Heroin/Amphetamine/negative Methadone	3	14.3
Heroin/Cocaine/negative Methadone	1	4.8
Heroin/Barbiturates/Amphetamine/negative Methadone	1	4.8
Total	21	100.0

Table 3
21 Detoxification Patients
Receiving 30 MG. of Substitute Methadone Daily

No abuse during 30-day surveillance	0	
Negative for Methadone only	4	19.0
Heroin only	5	23.8
Heroin/Amphetamines	3	14.3
Heroin/negative Methadone	2	9.5
Amphetamine/negative Methadone	1	4.8
Heroin/Amphetamine/negative Methadone	4	19.0
Heroin/Barbiturate/negative Methadone	1	4.8
Heroin/Amphetamine/Cocaine/negative Methadone	1	4.8
Total	21	100.0

4. At the later stage of detoxification, e.g., 20 mg. of substitute methadone daily, males were submitting urines which were totally "clean" 43.4% of the time while females were submitting "clean" specimens only 28.6% of the time. Male urines contained *no* methadone 26.0% of the time, and female urines were negative for methadone half the time.

The study population consisted of 20 whites and 45 blacks. These race cohorts were distributed among the three stages of detoxification as indicated in Table 7.

An analysis of the data controlling for the race of the addict-patients at each detoxification stage revealed the following:

1. At the initiation stage of detoxification, e.g., 40 mg. of substitute methadone daily, there was a statistically significant race difference in the abuse of heroin—Blacks abused heroin more frequently $(X^2 = 4.592; P = < .05)$. Blacks also abused the amphetamines and cocaine more often than Whites.

Table 4
23 Detoxification Patients
Receiving 20 MG. of Substitute Methadone Daily

No abuse during 30-day surveillance	4	17.4
Negative for Methadone only	5	21.7
Heroin only	5	21.7
Barbiturates only	1	4.3
Amphetamines only	1	4.3
Heroin plus negative for Methadone	4	17.4
Amphetamine plus negative for Methadone	1	4.3
Heroin/Amphetamine/negative Methadone	2	8.7
Total	23	100.0

Table 5
Incidence of Drug Abuse Among 50 Male Detoxification Patients

Daily Methadone Dose	Total Weeks of Surveillance	Percentage of Weeks The Drugs Were Detected					Percentage of Weeks With No Abuse	Percentage of Weeks Negative For Methadone
		Heroin	Barbiturates	Amphetamines	Cocaine			
40 mg (N=16)	50	64.0	2.0	16.0	2.0		22.0	20.8
30 mg (N=16)	53	43.4	1.9	17.0	—		24.5	37.7
20 mg (N=18)	53	35.8	—	7.5	—		43.4	26.0
50 Males	156	47.4	1.3	13.5	.6		30.1	28.2

Table 6
Incidence of Drug Abuse Among 15 Female Detoxification Patients

Daily Methadone Dose	Total Weeks of Surveillance	Percentage of Weeks The Drugs Were Detected					Percentage of Weeks With No Abuse	Percentage of Weeks Negative For Methadone
		Heroin	Barbiturates	Amphetamines	Cocaine			
40 mg (N=5)	14	64.3	—	21.4	21.4	7.1	28.8
30 mg (N=5)	18	27.8	—	16.7	5.5	27.8	50.0
20 mg (N=5)	14	28.6	—	—	—	28.6	50.0
15 Females	46	39.1	—	13.0	8.7	21.7	43.5

Table 7
The Distribution of Whites and Blacks
by Detoxification Stage

Detoxification Stage	Whites		Blacks		Total	
40 mg. per day	7	35.0%	14	31.1%	21	32.3%
30 mg. per day	4	20.0%	17	37.8%	21	32.3%
20 mg. per day	9	45.0%	14	31.1%	23	35.4%
Total	20	100.0%	45	100.0%	65	100.0%

2. At the middle stage of detoxification, e.g., 30 mg. of substitute methadone daily, race differences in the amount of heroin abuse had disappeared. Blacks and whites were both abusing heroin about 40% of the time at this dose level. Whites, however, had begun abusing amphetamines some 40% of the time while black abuse had decreased from 25% to 10% of the time.

3. At the later stage of detoxification, e.g., 20 mg. of substitute methadone daily, blacks were still abusing heroin almost half the time, but all other drug abuse had essentially ceased. Whites were abusing heroin less—28.6% of the time—but they continued to abuse amphetamines 14.3% of the time.

4. At the later stage of detoxification, e.g., 20 mg. of substitute methadone daily, whites were presenting totally "clean" urines only 23.8% of the time and blacks were doing so 31.5% of the time. Whites were presenting urines which contained *no* methadone 38.1% of the time and the blacks were doing so 21.7% of the time.

Comments and Implications

One would expect some "cheating" in an ambulatory detoxification program. These data indicate drug abuse is extensive and that it continues throughout the "detoxification regimen." From these data, one should not expect more than one-half of the patients in such programs to cease abusing drugs even during the time one attempts to detoxify them.

We believe the most disturbing finding to be that these patients submit urines which contain *no* methadone

Table 8
Incidence of Drug Abuse Among 20 White Detoxification Patients

Daily Methadone Dose	Total Weeks of Surveillance	Percentage of Weeks The Drugs Were Detected				Percentage of Weeks With No Abuse	Percentage of Weeks Negative For Methadone
		Heroin	Barbiturates	Amphetamines	Cocaine		
40 mg	20	45.0	—	—	—	25.0	40.0
30 mg	15	40.0	—	40.0	—	33.3	33.3
20 mg	21	28.6	—	14.3	—	23.8	38.1
Total	56	37.5	—	16.1	—	26.8	37.5

Table 9
Incidence of Drug Abuse Among 45 Black Detoxification Patients

Daily Metha- done Dose	Total Weeks of Sur- veillance	Percentage of Weeks The Drugs Were Detected					Per- centage of Weeks With No Abuse	Per- centage of Weeks Negative For Methadone
		Her- oin	Bar- biturates	Amphet- amines	Co- caine		
40 mg	44	72.7	2.3	25.0	9.1	15.9	20.5
30 mg	56	39.3	1.8	10.7	1.8	30.4	35.7
20 mg	46	37.0	—	2.2	—	47.8	21.7
Total	146	48.6	1.4	12.3	3.4	31.5	26.7

almost one-fourth of the time they are supposedly being "detoxified" with prescribed *daily* doses of methadone. One can only assume they are selling their medication in order to purchase other drugs.

Chapter 19.

Post-Treatment Behavior Following Ambulatory Detoxification

Arthur D. Moffett,
Irving H. Soloway
Marcia X. Glick

THE ISSUE

The most popular model for viewing narcotic addiction is as a chronic relapsing disease. Although relapse is predictably high, the addict's "right" to medical care, the clinician's desire to "engage them in service" and the system's need for "crime control techniques" require detoxification services be available. We *know* we reduce the level of tolerance, e.g., reduce the addict's "habit." All other benefits must be inferred. How quickly the addict relapses after a detoxification service is not generally known to those who provide the service.

With the current heightening of public awareness concerning the epidemic proportions of drug abuse in this country and the fantastic toll in life and property this social epidemic takes, it has become critically necessary to evaluate the efforts of the various treatment modalities in terms of their respective potentials in treating drug abusers and to specifically examine the results of treatment by these various modalities. As more is learned about drug-dependent individuals and the various modalities of treatment, it is hoped that a particular addict can be assigned to a specific therapy geared to treat his individual problems. Follow-up studies are a crit-

215

ical part of this plan. This study was designed to follow a population of addicts provided an ambulatory detoxification service.

RESEARCH DESIGN

During 1969 the Narcotic Addiction Treatment Program of the West Philadelphia Community Mental Health Consortium offered two treatment modalities with the synthetic narcotic drug methadone. All patients were inducted into an ambulatory detoxification program and stabilized on low doses of substitute methadone. Following initial evaluation which included drug and social histories, employment evaluation, and clinical evaluation, the patient was assigned to a counselor for continual supportive therapy and the ambulatory withdrawal procedure was begun. The goal of the program was to assist the patient in becoming an individual who was not drug dependent. There was no stipulated detoxification schedule, treatment being fitted to the individual idiosyncrasies of the patient as reflected in his particular career of addiction. (The alternate treatment modality was high dose methadone maintenance. Inducted into this maintenance group during 1969 were persons who failed to successfully detoxify, and patients who were clinically evaluated as being potentially most successfully treated on a maintenance basis.)

Considering the experimental and currently controversial nature of Narcotic Substitution Therapy, the research staff clearly saw the necessity of an in depth and comprehensive examination of post-treatment behavior of persons who had been treated within the detoxification program and who had either successfully detoxified or left the program against medical advice.

During 1969, a group of 21 patients had been discharged as detoxified and ostensibly "drug free" as of their last visit to the clinic. This evaluation was validated by urinalysis as tested by the Department of Clinical Pharmacology and Toxicology at Philadelphia General Hospital. A second group selected for this study consisted of 34 patients who were discharged from treatment against medical advice (A.M.A.) during the months of October and November 1969. All of the second group had voluntarily dropped out of the program without completing the detoxification process.

During the summer and fall of 1970, all members of both samples were located, contacted, and interviewed. Two teams, each composed of an ex-addict street worker and a "square" member of the research staff, jointly completed a detailed questionnaire and tape-recorded the interviews on each subject. As a validating device, a urine sample was requested from each subject at the time the interview was conducted; the sample was analyzed at Philadelphia General Hospital laboratory. The urine was analyzed by thin layer chromatography for the presence or absence of the following substances: morphine, quinine, methadone, barbiturates, amphetamines. This laboratory analysis was supplemented by interviews with the subjects themselves and by collaborative statements from family, friends, and official agen-

Table 1.
Demographic Characteristics

	Detoxification N = 21	A.M.A. N = 34	Total N = 55
Age:			
range	18-51	20-46	18-51
mean	32.8	31.4	32.10
Race:			
White	19 (90.4)	25 (73.5)	44 (80.0)
Black	2 (9.6)	9 (26.5)	11 (20.0)
Sex:			
male	17 (81.0)	30 (88.2)	47 (85.45)
female	4 (19.0)	4 (11.8)	8 (14.55)
Education:			
range	7-17 years	7-16 years	7-17 years
mean	11.4 years	11.1 years	11.25 years
Marital Status			
single	5 (23.8)	12 (35.4)	17 (30.90)
married	13 (62.0)	16 (47.0)	29 (52.72)
divorced or separated	3 (14.2)	6 (17.6)	9 (16.36)

cies (i.e., probation officers, welfare workers, counselors) connected with and referred by the subject in question. The investigators found that in an overwhelming majority of cases, "soft" data generated from the interviews was validated by laboratory urinalysis results.

Description of the Population

The 55 subjects reported on in this study can be characterized as hard core criminal addicts, who typically had begun using heroin in their teens, had been using heroin for an average of 9.3 years and had been incarcerated several times. During this time, the only criteria for admission to the program was addiction to a narcotic drug and residence in one of three mental health catchment areas. Psychotic patients and patients with mixed addictions were not excluded from the program.

Of particular interest were the facts that 15 (71.9 per cent) of the detoxification group and 25 (75.6 per cent) of the against medical advice group (A.M.A.) had never been treated for their addiction problems in the past, excluding instances of involuntary withdrawals as a result

Table 2.
Addiction Characteristics

	Detoxification N = 21	A.M.A. N = 34	Total N = 55
Heroin Addicts	21 (100)	34 (100)	55 (100)
Years of use			
range	1-26	1-24	1-26
mean	9.8 years	8.8 years	9.3 years
	* T = .4500		
Prior formal treatment			
range	0-3	0-4	0-4
mean	1.7	1.6	1.65
	** T = .1127		

* Difference of means tests were T = .4500 (p = .05) No statistical difference was found between the two groups
** Difference of means tests were run T = .1127 No statistical difference was found between the two groups

of periodic jailing. Therefore, a total of 73.5 per cent of the combined total population had no prior treatment of any kind.

The following tables summarize data on the two groups.

As previously reported, the model patient was in his late 20's, had been addicted 9 years, had committed crimes, had been arrested and was from the lower socio-economic classes. He achieved a similar education as his non-drug abusing peers and tended to be immobile in relation to his living situation.

RESULTS

The results of the study will be presented as follows: 1. the status of patients at time of termination, and 2. the status of patients at time of follow-up.

At the time of discharge, the detoxification sample had spent a mean time of 5.7 months in the program as compared to a mean of 3.9 months for the A.M.A. group (Table 3). All of the detoxification patients tested at the time of discharge were methadone free at termination

Table 3.
Discharge Data (Summary)

	Detoxification N = 21	A.M.A. N = 34	Total N = 55
Months in Treatment			
range	1-15	1-24	1-24
mean	5.7	3.9	4.8
	* T = 1.3640		
Daily methadone dose			
range	-0-	10-80 mg	0-80
mean	—	30 mg	—
Required weekly clinic visits			
range	1-5	1-5	1-5
mean	2.7	2.2	2.45
	** T = 1.2297 (N.S.)		

* Difference of means tests were run T = 1.3640
** Difference of means tests were run T = 1.2297

Table 4.
Employment Status at Time of Discharge

Category	Detoxification N = 21	A.M.A. N = 34	Total N = 55
Employed	7 (33.3)	15 (44.1)	22 (40.0)
Not in Labor Force	2 (9.5)	10 (29.4)	12 (21.81)
Welfare	12 (57.1)	9 (26.5)	21 (38.18)
	21	34	55 (99.99)
	$x^2 = .6290$ (N.S.)		

whereas most of the A.M.A. group were still receiving methadone at their last clinic visit. Detoxification patients were being seen an average of 2.7 times a week and the A.M.A. patients were seen an average of 2.2 times per week (Table 3).

Legal employment at the time of termination was reported by 33.3 percent of the detoxification group and 44.1 percent of the A.M.A. sample. The percentage of patients with neither employment nor welfare status was 9.5 percent for the detoxification sample and 29.4 percent for the A.M.A. sample. A total of 38.2 percent were receiving welfare as their sole source of support (Table 4.).

During the follow-up interview it was found that 38.1 percent of the detoxification sample and 44.1 percent of the A.M.A. sample had been arrested at least once during treatment (Table 5.). This was a greater incidence of arrests than had been reported in previous studies of this treatment program. Although arrests have never excluded active patients from the program, the belief may

Table 5.
Arrest Since Beginning of Treatment

Arrests since beginning of treatment	Detoxification	A.M.A.	Total
Yes	8 (38.09)	15 (44.1)	23 (41.81)
No	13 (61.91)	19 (55.9)	32 (58.18)
Total	21	34	55

$x^2 = .1935$ (N.S.)

exist among patients that reporting an arrest to the counselor may jeopardize their treatment status. At the time of follow-up this factor would not be a concern to the subjects.

During the last month of treatment the incidence of cheating was significantly greater for the A.M.A. group than for the detoxified group (X^2=8.0769; P < .05). It was impossible to obtain a complete profile of the cheating history for both groups because urine testing was not begun until April 1969 and 13 of the subjects had left the program by that time (Table 6.).

Drug abuse for the detoxification group revealed that 2 (12.5 percent) were positive for heroin; 2 (12.5 percent) were positive for amphetamines and 2 (12.5 percent) were positive for barbiturates. For the A.M.A. group 16 (61.5 percent) were positive for heroin; 1 (3.8 percent) was positive for other opiates; 2 (7.7 percent) were positive for amphetamines, and 2 (7.7 percent) were positive for barbiturates.

FOLLOW-UP

The central question to which this study adressed itself was the rate of return to the habitual use of opiates and other illegal drugs following treatment from the methadone program at the Narcotic Addiction Rehabilitation Program. Of the 21 patients discharged as detoxified, 9.5 percent were drug free at the time of the follow-up interview. Of the 34 A.M.A. patients, 11.8 percent were not abusing drugs at the time of the interview. *The total relapse rate for the combined population was 89.1 percent(49 of the original 55 were back on drugs.)*

Table 6.
Drug Abuse During Last Month of Treatment

Category	Detoxification N = 16	A.M.A. N = 26	Total
Abuse	6	21	27
No abuse	10	5	18
Total	16	26	42
No Data	5	8	13

x^2 = 8.0769; p < .05

An issue of mounting concern is the increasing abuse of methadone obtained through illegal channels. A greater percentage of patients admitted abusing methadone than was expected. At the time of follow-up 19.0 percent of the detoxified sample and 38.2 percent of the A.M.A. sample were found positive for methadone. Of the entire relapsed population (49) 34.7 percent reported abusing methadone at the time of the interview. Of this combined relapsed population 8.2 percent maintained that they were using methadone as their sole drug of choice with no other opiate abuse. When queried as to their reasons for choosing methadone in preference to the more traditional heroin the subjects generally responded that methadone was cheaper ($35.00 for a "jug," i.e., a 20 cc vial of injectable methadone 10 mg. per cc). Methadone obtained "on the street" is seen as more reliable than heroin since it has not yet begun (at least in the injectable form) to be adulterated and "cut" by "dealers." Although, incidentally, there have been recent reports of counterfeit dolophines in circulation in the Philadelphia area and of 100 percent Tang orange drink being sold at $5.00 per ounce.

As expected, the rate of return to the use of opiates was greater for the A.M.A. group than the detoxification group. Statistical tests could not be performed to compare the two groups because the members in each cell were too small. Table 7 illustrates, however, that 88.2 percent of the A.M.A. group were abusing drugs at the time of discharge and continued their abuse to the time of follow-up. For the detoxification group 10 (47.6 percent) returned to the regular use of opiates within one month following discharge. The rest of the detoxified sample reported a return to the regular use of opiates as is illustrated in Table 7.

A comparison of legal employment reveals that 21 (38.2 percent) of the total populations were legally employed at time of follow-up. In addition, 24 (43.6 percent) were on public assistance and 10 (18.2 percent) were not in the labor force. Four of those N.L.F. were incarcerated. There was no significant differences between the two groups (Table 8.).

Table 7.
Rate of Return to Use of Opiates following Discharge

Time	Detoxification N = 21	A.M.A. N = 34	Total N = 55
Abusing when discharged	0	29 (88.2)	29 (52.7)
1-5 days	8 (38.1)	—	8 (14.5)
6-30 days	2 (9.5)	1	3 (5.5)
31-90 days	3 (14.3)	—	3 (5.5)
91-181 days	5 (23.8)	—	5 (9.1)
181 +	1 (4.8)	—	1 (1.8)
No Abuse	2 (9.5)	4 (11.7)	6 (10.9)
Total	21 (38.2)	34 (61.8)	55

In the detoxification group, 9 (42.8 percent) of those not employed were on welfare; 2 (9.5 percent) reported not working and not on welfare; and 1 (4.8 percent) was in jail. For the A.M.A. group, 15 (44.1 percent) were on welfare; 4 (11.8 percent reported not working and not on welfare; and 3 (8.8 percent) were in jail.

Arrest Status

In the period between the time of termination and the follow-up interview, 8 (38.1 percent) of the detoxification group and 18 (52.9 percent) of the A.M.A. group were arrested once. Although no subject was arrested more than once, four of the arrested received prison sentences following arrest (Table 9.)

Legal Status

Legal status at the time of follow-up revealed that 58.0 percent of the total population reported being free of any

Table 8.
Employment Status at Time of Follow-up

Employed	Detoxification N = 21	A.M.A. N = 34	Total N = 55
Employed	8	13	21 (38.2)
Not Employed	13	21	34
Total	21	34	55

$x^2 = .0440$ (N.S.)

Table 9.
Arrests Since Discharge

Arrests	Detoxification N = 21	A.M.A. N = 34	Total N = 55
Yes	8 (38.1)	18 (52.9)	26 (47.3)
No	13 (61.9)	16 (47.1)	29 (52.7)
Total	21 (38.2)	34 (61.8)	55 (100.0)

$x^2 = 1.1479$ (N.S.)

legal restrictions (Table 10). There appears to be more reported criminality in the A.M.A. group than the detoxification group.

For those in the detoxification group, 1 (4.8 percent) was on parole; 2 (9.5 percent) had cases pending; 1 (4.8 percent) was in jail; and 3 (14.3 percent) were on probation. For the A.M.A. group 3 (8.8 percent) were on parole; 1 (2.9 percent) had cases pending; 3 (8.8 percent) were in jail; and 9 (26.5 percent) were on probation.

DISCUSSION AND CONCLUSIONS

This study has demonstrated the need for all narcotic addiction treatment programs to conduct frequent and possibly, on-going follow-up studies. As previous follow-up studies have shown, this is the only positive vehicle for measuring the effectiveness of a treatment program. As with other reported follow-up studies a great deal was learned in terms of the methodology of the "field work." The research follow-up teams composed of an ex-addict and "square" professional, operated efficiently and each member of the team had his own "role of specialization" to play. The ex-addicts' knowledge of "the street" cannot

Table 10.
Legal Status at Follow-up

Legal Status	Detoxification	A.M.A.	Total
Yes	14	18	32
No	7	16	23
Total	21	34	45

$x^2 = 1.0051$ (N.S.)

be over-estimated and most of the subjects would not have been located if it were not for this "street" knowledge. The professional brought interviewing skills and structure to the team.

Once located, most of the subjects were cooperative and interested in the study. It was not an intention of the study to recruit the subjects back to treatment, but, as was expected, most of the subjects applied for readmission shortly after the interview was completed. Of the 19 relapsed subjects from the detoxified sample 12 (63.2 percent) have been readmitted to treatment. Of the 30 relapsed against medical advice (A.M.A.) subjects, 16 (53.3 percent) have been readmitted to treatment.

Most of the subjects understood the need for a urine sample. The authors had anticipated problems with this segment of the study, but most of the subjects gave the sample willingly. Since urine collection has always been an integral part of the treatment process at the N.A.R.P., this may have been a contributing factor to the subjects' acceptance of the request.

In all cases, once the subject had been located and interviewed, he was not interviewed again. Collaborative information was sought in all cases, but due to time some of the sources were not contacted. Because of this, the validity and reliability of the subjects' statements should be questioned. However, most of the subjects willingly gave a urine sample under direct observation and permitted the tape-recordings of the interviews. The authors, therefore, accepted the collected data acknowledging the limitations of the validity and reliability of the data.

For those subjects who terminated A.M.A. from this outpatient detoxification methadone program, legal involvement, incarcerations, family disorganization, multi-drug abuse and unemployment appeared to be the greatest risks. The outpatient modality offers less structure to the patient than an inpatient facility and premature termination must be recognized as a real problem to be coped with, especially when, as in a methadone detoxification regime, the dosage was constantly decreased. The evidence suggested that efforts must be intensified to set up structure within the program in an effort to decrease the premature terminations (A.M.A.).

Methadone programs with a detoxification component must continue to evaluate each new patient carefully as he begins treatment. The data indicated that many of the patients come for treatment just to obtain the medication and apparently have little motivation for detoxification. The staff must be aware of this reality and involve their unmotivated patient in a treatment regimen that will meet his needs. If the staff loses contact with the unmotivated patient during the treatment process, that patient will probably become discouraged with treatment as the methadone is decreased and will probably terminate.

For those patients in the study who terminated drug-free but failed to maintain this status in the community, problems similar to those of the A.M.A. group also occurred. The data indicated that the relapsed "detoxification" patient spent an average of 6.1 months in treatment while the patients who did not return to the use of drugs had been treated for an average of 2.8 months. While the number of cases reported on in this study were small, the results did favor a short term, highly structured detoxification schedule in contrast to a long term detoxification schedule. Detoxification is an anxious time for an opiate dependent individual. If the detoxification process is not structured to include unlimited supportive counseling, and a rigidly enforced short-term detoxification schedule, the patient will probably fail and terminate from the program. The role of the counselor becomes extremely important during this period and the patient should have access to counseling 24 hours a day. As indicated, outpatient methadone programs offer the patient a treatment service, but one that is less structured than the institutional treatment model. The patient receives treatment, but continues to live in the community, and treatment personnel need to be available 24 hours a day, especially when a patient is undergoing detoxification.

Of great concern to the authors was the abuse of methadone by the terminated patients. As more of the monetary resources and efforts are geared to chemical substitution therapy (i.e., methadone) programs the likelihood of abuse of this drug will increase. Programs must be administered with a high degree of efficiency. Programs must keep detailed records and maintain a high degree of knowledge about each patient. Quantitative and qualitative urine surveillance must be maintained as the only positive measure of the patients' abuse of drugs, including methadone. Law enforcement agencies must work together with treatment agencies to enforce the therapeutic use of methadone only. Unless we monitor the distribution of this drug, it may become a drug of "choice" for many as it was the drug of "choice" for some of the subjects reported on in this study.

PART FOUR

Methadone Versus Other Chemical Substitution Therapies

Chapter 20.
Comparison of Acetylmethadol and Methadone in the Treatment of Long-term Heroin Users*

Jerome H. Jaffe
Charles R. Schuster
Beth B. Smith
Paul H. Blachley

Treatment with high doses of methadone hydrochloride, administered orally, facilitates the social rehabilitation of long-term compulsive heroin users. However, the duration of action of orally administered methadone poses problems. In order to avoid withdrawal symptoms, patients must take methadone at least once every 24 hours. Some patients feel they must take it more frequently. Early in treatment when patients are unemployed or in need of emotional support it may be desirable to have them visit the clinic each day. Later, when patients are employed and have reassumed family obligations, it is taxing and possibly antitherapeutic to require them to travel to a clinic every day. The usual solution to this problem is to give reliable patients a supply of medication to take at home. However, in some cases this creates the possibility of illegal redistribution. It also creates the possibility of accidental ingestion by nonpatients, a potentially serious problem because of the high doses employed.

In 1952, Fraser and Isabell[1] reported that *dl-a*-acetylmethadol hydrochloride, a synthetic congener of methadone, can prevent withdrawal symptoms for more than

* Reprinted with permission from the *Journal of the American Medical Association,* **211,** 1834-1836, 1970.

72 hours. Its long duration of action caused problems when attempts were made to use it clinically as an analgesic,[213] and its use was soon abandoned. With the development of the methadone-maintenance concept of treating narcotic addicts, it seemed appropriate to reexamine the possibility that for this application dl-a-acetylmethadol might be as effective as methadone while obviating the need to dispense medication to patients for self-administration outside of the clinic.

METHOD

Twenty-one volunteer patients from the methadone clinics of the Illinois Department of Mental Health Drug Abuse Program were used in this study. All patients' conditions had been stabilized with a daily methadone hydrochloride dosage (range 20 to 90 mg) and the patients were judged to have good potential for rehabilitation. They were instructed that the study required their taking a new form of methadone to determine whether it had fewer side effects. The patients were not informed that the experimental drug (dl-a-acetylmethadol) had a longer duration of action. Of the 21 patients, 12 were randomly assigned to the experimental group and 9 to the control group.

Patients conditions were studied for seven weeks during which they were required to report to the clinic on

Comparison of Mean Baseline Scores (6 Tests Obtained Over Two Week Period) for dl-a-Acetylmethadol (N=8) and Methadone (N=8) Groups on Opiate Withdrawal Subscale of ARCI and Symptom Checklist*

Group	Mean	SD OPWL Scale	Test
dl-a-acetylmethadol	17.82	5.74	1.65 (N.S.)
Methadone	13.91	3.46	
		Symptom Checklist	
dl-a-acetylmethadol	2.36	2.47	0.30 (N.S.)
Methadone	2.74	2.64	

* SD signifies standard deviation. NS signifies not significant.

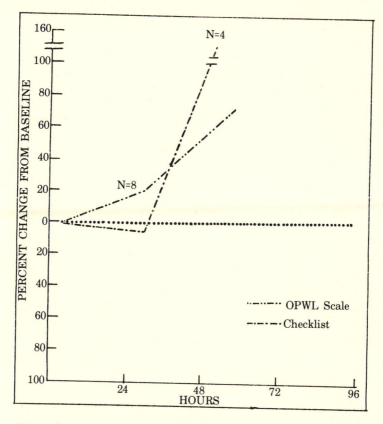

Fig 1. Patients receiving methadone orally: Percent change from baseline on opiate withdrawal (OPWL) scale and symptom checklist as function of time since last dose.

Monday, Wednesday, and Friday of each week. On each clinic visit patients gave a urine specimen for the detection of illicit opiate use. Patients were required to fill out the opiate withdrawal subscale of the Addiction Research Center Inventory (ARCI) as well as a symptom check list designed to measure the intensity of opiate withdrawal. Patients also participated in open-ended interviews with the staff.

The first two weeks of the study were used to obtain baseline measures of opiate symptoms and withdrawal symptoms while the patients' conditions were maintained with their usual regimen of daily methadone. Fol-

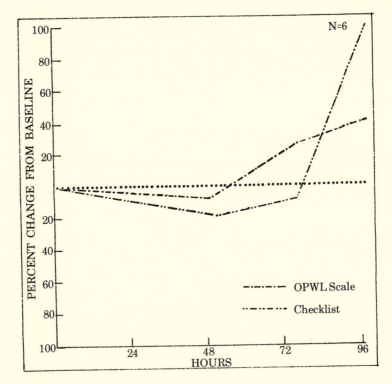

Fig 2. Patients receiving *dl-a*-acetylmethadol: Percent change from baseline on opiate withdrawal (OPWL) scale and symptom checklist as function of time since last dose.

lowing this baseline period, the flavor of the vehicle in which the medication was given was changed for all patients. Patients in the control group continued to receive their usual daily dosage of methadone. Patients assigned to the experimental group received *dl-a*-acetylmethadol on Monday, Wednesday, and Friday. The initial dose of *dl-a*-acetylmethadol was obtained by multiplying the patient's daily methadone hydrochloride dosage by 1.2. Thus a patient taking 50 mg of methadone hydrochloride each day would be given 60 mg of *dl-a*-acetylmethadol hydrochloride on Monday, Wednesday, and Friday. On intervening days the experimental patients received placebo medication matched for taste by the addition of 30 mg of dextromethorphan hydrobromide. In the case of two patients it was necessary to make slight increases in the dosage of *dl-a*-acetylmethadol over the first two weeks. For this reason, data are presented for the final three weeks of the study when all patients were receiving a stable drug dosage. During the final three weeks the average dosage of methadone hydrochloride was 37 mg/day (range 20 to 55 mg) and the average dose of *dl-a*-acetylmethadol hydrochloride was 50 mg given Monday, Wednesday, and Friday (range 24 to 66 mg).

On Monday of the seventh week a placebo was substituted for active medication in six control patients and six experimental patients. This allowed observation of the control patients 48 hours after the last dose of methadone, and of the experimental group 96 hours after the last dose of *dl-a*-acetylmethadol. Because we were not sure of how intense the methadone withdrawals would be, all patients had been provided with a single emergency dose of methadone. Two of the methadone patients complained that withdrawal symptoms were so severe 12 hours after the placebo (36 hours after their last dose of methadone) that they felt compelled to take the emergency medication (methadone). For simplicity of presentation the results of this portion of the study are based upon only those four subjects who did not take the emergency medication and rated their withdrawal symptoms at 48 hours after the last methadone dosage. Obviously the intensity of the withdrawal at 48 hours for the group of six would have been higher had no emergency medication been available.

RESULTS

Sixteen of the 21 volunteers completed the study. Four patients assigned to receive *dl-a*-acetylmethadol requested to be dropped from the study on the first day because of complaints of anxiety and nervousness. They were returned to their usual daily dosage of methadone. One patient in the control (methadone) group complained of abdominal pain in the third week of the study and requested to be returned to his usual methadone regimen. Thus, regular measurements were completed on eight patients in the experimental group and eight patients in the control group.

The table shows the mean scores for the experimental and control groups during the two-week baseline period on the various test measures. Neither the opiate withdrawal subscale of the ARCI nor the withdrawal symptom check-list showed any significant differences between the two groups.

Figure 1 shows the percentage change from baseline on the ARCI subscale and the opiate withdrawal symptom check list for the methadone group at 24 and 48 hours following the administration of methadone. With the 24-hour interval between doses neither the ARCI nor the symptom check list showed any change from that observed under baseline conditions. Of the six patients in whom a placebo was substituted two patients took their emergency medication after 36 hours because of intense withdrawal symptoms. The results shown are those of the four patients who completed the 48-hour deprivation period without any extra medication. All four patients showed dramatic increases in the intensity of withdrawal symptoms as measured by both the ARCI and the symptom checklist. However, interviews with the patients after the 48-hour interval revealed such obvious complaints that the checklists were hardly required. After 24-hour intervals between doses the patients expressed no withdrawal distress whereas after 48 hours without medication they complained of intense withdrawal distress.

Figure 2 shows the results of the percentage change from baseline of the ARCI and the opiate withdrawal symptom check-list for the *dl-a*-acetylmethadol group after 24-, 48-, 72-, and 96-hour intervals between administration of active medication. With the 24- and 48-hour intervals between doses, the ARCI and the symptom check-list showed no change from baseline conditions when the patients were receiving methadone daily. At the 72-hour interval there was a slight rise in the opiate withdrawal subscale of the ARCI. This was not accompanied by complaints of withdrawal either on the symptom check list or during the patients' interviews. At the 96-hour interval, however, there was a sharp (marked) rise in the intensity of withdrawal symptoms as evidenced by both the test results and patients' complaints during interviews.

An analysis of the general functioning of the two groups of patients (methadone and dl-a-acetylmethadol) revealed no significant differences between them in terms of number gainfully employed, the number showing illicit drug use (as measured by thin-layer chromatographic analysis of monitored urine specimens), and the number arrested or admitting to illegal activity.

COMMENT

The results of the present study corroborate the previous findings of Fraser and Isbell in showing that dl-a-acetylmethadol can effectively suppress opiate withdrawal symptoms for periods of up to 72 hours. More important was the observation that former compulsive heroin users who had made satisfactory social adjustments while receiving methadone orally continued to do as well while taking dl-a-acetylmethadol only three times each week. The fact that four of the 12 patients assigned to the dl-a-acetylmethadol groups dropped out of the study because of side effects requires further investigation. Based on some reports in the Fraser and Isbell communication,[1] it is conceivable that in high doses the d isomer has some tendency to produce anxiety and confusion. Although it is our suspicion that the anxiety reactions that occurred in the present study were largely psychogenic in origin, the possibility that these reactions are direct phamacological effects of the dl-a-acetylmethadol can not be ruled out. However, in contrast to the racemic mixture, the l-isomer may not induce such effects. (Studies with the l-isomer are now under way.) Those patients who did not experience such reactions reported being more comfortable receiving dl-a-acetylmethadol and expressed a reluctance to return to their regular methadone.

This preliminary study suggests that the a-acetylmethadols may have practical therapeutic advantages over methadone in the treatment of heroin addicts.

This investigation was supported by Public Health Service grants K2-MH-25, 393, and H17-MH-16409.

Norman David, MD, supplied the dl-a-acetylmethadol for this investigation.

REFERENCES

1. Fraser and Isbell: Actions and addiction liabilities of dl-alpha acetylmethadol, 1952.

2. David, et. al.: Control of chronic pain by dl-alpha acetylmethadol, 1956.

3. Keats & Beecher: Analgesic activity and toxic effects of acetylmethadol isomers in man, 1952.

Chapter 21.

Methadone and L-Methadyl Acetate: Use in Management of Narcotic Addicts

Jerome H. Jaffe
Edward C. Senay

In pilot work in ambulatory individuals previously stabilized with methadone hydrochloride, *dl*-methadyl acetate (*dl-a*-acetylmethadol) suppressed narcotic withdrawal syndrome for periods up to three days. As compared to subjects who were maintained on a regimen of methadone, individuals maintained on a regimen of *dl*-methadyl acetate had no serious toxic effects, and there were no statistically significant differences between the groups with respect to illicit drug use or subjective experiences.[1]

As in the case of methadone, which is a racemic mixture, there are substantial differences in analgesic and narcotic-withdrawal-syndrome suppressing properties between the *d* and *l* isomers of methadyl acetate; *l*-methadyl acetate is reported to be five times as potent in suppressing the narcotic withdrawal syndrome as the *d* isomer.[2] However, clinical experience with either isomer is limited. The study presented in this communication had two major objectives: to gain further clinical experience with *l*-methadyl acetate, and to determine if *l*-methadyl acetate could be interchanged repeatedly with methadone.

The potential advantages of a long-acting, methadone-like substance are at least twofold. First, patients at the beginning of treatment in most methadone maintenance

* Reprinted with permission from the *Journal of the American Medical Association,* **216**, 1303-1305, 1971.

237

programs must travel to a clinic for medication from five to seven days each week. Since methadyl acetate suppresses the narcotic withdrawal syndrome even when administered as infrequently as three times per week, the travel problems of patients just starting treatment are markedly decreased. Second, and of equal importance, is the possibility of reducing illicit redistribution of the maintenance medication. When patients come to clinics for methadone less frequently than every day, the clinics must permit them to take medication for use at home. In any large-scale program, it is inevitable that a few patients will abuse this opportunity and give away or sell their medication. In addition, there is a possibility that a patient's medication may be ingested by someone not tolerant to methadone, inducing serious toxic reactions. All of these problems are ameliorated by the use of a long-acting drug that reduces the amount of medication that a clinic must provide to patients for use at home. If necessary, a clinic can establish a policy that all patients will ingest medication under direct observation three times a week, thereby entirely eliminating problems of illicit redistribution or accidental ingestion.

Unfortunately, for the next year or two, it is unlikely that large amounts of methadyl acetate will be available for use in the treatment of the several thousand patients now treated with methadone. Therefore, it would be of both practical and theoretical interest if patients maintained on a regimen of methadone could be given methadyl acetate each weekend and placed back on a regimen of methadone each Monday without ill effect. Such a procedure would markedly extend the population with whom the limited supplies of methadyl acetate could be used. The drug used in this study was from a supply that had been previously synthesized and has now been exhausted.

METHOD

Male patients "stabilized" with methadone hydrochloride—i.e., taking between 30 and 100 mg/day, with no change in medication for three weeks prior to inclusion in the study—were asked to participate in the study of "a drug similar to methadone, but one which lasted longer." Patients were told that they might or might not receive this drug and that nothing in their treatment program would change except the medication they would receive. They were asked to fill out a symptom checklist that prior research had established as a useful measure of narcotic withdrawal symptoms.[1] Subjects filled out these checklists at the end of the week (Friday) and at the beginning of the week (Monday) just prior to receiving their medication.

Ten volunteer patients were randomly assigned to experimental (five patients) and control (five patients) groups. The mean methadone hydrochloride dose for the experimental group was 50 mg/day (range, 40 to 70 mg/day). The mean methadone hydrochloride dose for the control group was 68 mg/day (range, 30 to 100 mg/day). The groups were studied for three weekends. The first weekend began on a Saturday, with one half of the patients receiving *l*-methadyl acetate and a 30-mg dextromethorphan hydrobromide placebo which they were to take at home on Sunday. The control group received their usual dose of methadone on Saturday and a dose of methadone to consume at home on Sunday.

The initial procedure for determining a two-day dose of *l*-methadyl acetate was simply to substitute 1 mg of *l*-methadyl acetate for each milligram of methadone. Thus, a patient maintained on a regimen of 50 mg of methadone hydrochloride daily would be given 50 mg of *l*-methadyl acetate for the Saturday dose.

The initial conversion factor for computing a three-day dose of *l*-methadyl acetate was 1.2 mg. of *l*-methadyl acetate for 1 mg of methadone hydrochloride daily—e.g., a patient stabilized with 50 mg of methadone hydrochloride daily would be given 60 mg of *l*-methadyl acetate for the three-day period. The second and third study weekends extended for three days. Patients in the experimental group (*l*-methadyl acetate) were given active medication on Friday and 30-mg dextromethorphan hydrobromide placebos for home use on Saturday and Sunday. The control patients received their usual doses of methadone—one dose ingested at the clinic on Friday and two doses to be consumed at home.

Urine specimens were collected from each patient and tested for presence of narcotics. Clinical interviews were held on Monday and on Friday by an experimenter who was unaware of the medication being given to the particular patient. Clinical observations were recorded after each interview.

At the end of the study period patients were asked whether they believed that they had taken methadone or l-methadyl acetate. They were asked to describe the difference and to state whether they would or would not like to take l-methadyl acetate on a routine basis.

RESULTS

There was no significant difference between experimental-group and control-group checklist scores on Fridays or on Mondays. Table 1 gives the means and standard deviations for the experimental and control groups on the various study days, while Table 2 presents the analysis of variance for each of the study weekends.

Clinically nothing in the behavior or in the reports of patient provided the "blind" experimenter with any basis for determining who was taking experimental or control medication. Patients in both groups complained of sweating, but none reported problems with sweating that had not existed prior to the study. No other side

Table 1.

Means and Standard Deviations of Symptom Checklist Scores for l-Methadyl Acetate and Methadone Groups

Day	I-Methadyl Acetate		Methadone	
	Mean	SD	Mean	SD
1st Saturday	6.80	5.42	7.20	3.76
1st Monday	4.40	3.82	8.40	3.44
2nd Friday	6.00	4.69	8.60	4.41
2nd Monday	8.20	6.14	9.60	3.20
3rd Friday	4.60	4.70	7.20	2.20
3rd Monday	6.20	6.00	6.60	1.00

Table 2.
Analysis of Variance Comparing Symptom
Checklist Data of *l*-Methadyl Acetate
and Methadone Groups

1st Saturday and 1st Monday

Source	df	MS	F
Groups	1	24.20	0.67
Subjects within groups	8	36.00	—
Days	1	1.80	0.30
Groups × days	1	30.20	5.03
Days × subjects within groups	8	6.00	—

2nd Friday and 2nd Monday

Source	df	MS	F
Groups	1	20.00	0.40
Subjects within groups	8	49.72	—
Days	1	12.80	2.07
Groups × days	1	1.80	0.29
Days × subjects within groups	8	6.18	—

3rd Friday and 3rd Monday

Source	df	MS	F
Groups	1	11.25	0.34
Subjects within groups	8	33.10	—
Days	1	1.25	0.18
Groups × days	1	6.05	0.88
Days × subjects within groups	8	6.90	—

effects were reported by either group. The two groups did
not differ in rates of clinic attendance or in the frequency
of urine specimens positive for morphine (when tested by
modifications of the procedures described by Dole *et al*[3]).
There was one urine specimen positive for morphine in
each group each week.

With respect to the subjective experience of the
patients, the "set" was more powerful than drug differences; patients in the methadone group were as likely to
report spontaneously a feeling of receiving a new drug as
were patients taking *l*-methadyl acetate.

DOSE

Substituting 1 mg of *l*-methadyl acetate for 1 mg of methadone hydrochloride proved to be satisfactory for all patients for the 48-hour period. After the first 72-hour period, several patients in both groups requested to have their dosage of medication increased. When clinical judgement deemed an increase to be appropriate, the suggestion was transmitted to the investigator prescribing the medication. The intensity of complaints about withdrawal symptoms 72 hours after the administration of the dose of *l*-methadyl acetate was not great enough to permit the "blind" investigator to differentiate the patients treated with *l*-methadyl acetate from those receiving their usual doses of methadone. Nevertheless, the "1.2 factor" seemed inadequate for converting the daily methadone dose into a suitable 72-hour dose of *l*-methadyl acetate, since three of five patients in the *l*-methadyl acetate group complained of withdrawal symptoms in the 24-hour period preceding the interview—i.e., 48 to 72 hours after the administration of the dose of *l*-methadyl acetate. On the basis of the complaints after the first 72 hour period, the dosage of *l*-methadyl acetate was increased for the next weekend. In each instance, complaints of withdrawal symptoms disappeared following the adjustment. The average *l*-methadyl acetate conversion factor that proved to be satisfactory for the five patients was 1.3 mg (range, 1.2 to 1.5 mg) to 1 mg of methadone hydrochloride.

In spite of the need to adjust dosage, the groups did not differ with respect to frequency or intensity of requests for increases in medication over the period of the study.

We had expected that *l*-methadyl acetate would be approximately twice as potent as the racemic mixture. Yet, the dosage of the *l* isomer of methadyl acetate that was substituted for a given dose of methadone (conversion factor) in this study was similar to the dosage which we had previously found to be generally appropriate for the racemate.[1] This observation suggests that more systematic comparisons of the relative potencies of the *l*-form and of the racemate in suppressing opiate withdrawal symptoms are needed.

COMMENT

Clinical judgement, corroborated by scores on the withdrawal symptom checklist, demonstrated the feasibility of interchanging *l*-methadyl acetate with methadone. A physician blind to the experiment was not able to discriminate patients maintained on a regimen of methadone from patients given *l*-methadyl acetate. It is, therefore, possible to give *l*-methadyl acetate on weekends to patients taking methadone, thus decreasing the possibilities for illegal redistribution of medication while retaining the desirable effect of suppression of narcotic hunger.

An additional advantage of *l*-methadyl acetate is the freedom of the patient from the necessity to engage in drug-taking and drug-seeking behavior for longer periods than is the case with patients taking methadone. Such an effect is consistent with treatment goals of a program which seeks to de-emphasize the mystique of drugs and drug-taking while emphasizing activity and human relationships as sources of gratification.

The results of this pilot study suggest that further work should be carried out with *l*-methadyl acetate. Currently, a number of longer studies with larger groups are planned.

REFERENCES

1. Jaffe, *et. al.*: Comparison of acetylmethadol and methadone in the treatment of long-term heroin users, 1970.
2. Fraser and Isbell: Actions and addiction liabilities of alpha-acetylmethadols in man, 1952.
3. Dole, *et. al.*: Detection of narcotic drugs, tranquilizers, amphetamines and barbiturates in urine, 1966.

Chapter 22.

Methadone and the Antagonists: A Review of Program Experiences

James A. Inciardi

INTRODUCTION

In earlier chapters, the evolutionary and developmental aspects of methadone maintenance as a chemotherapeutic modality in the treatment of opiate addiction have been discussed, with special references to the relative effectiveness of its differential applications. As such, methadone tends to intervene in the pharmacological condition of the addict which has placed him in a state of functional disability, by partial or total inhibition of both euphoria and the abstinence syndrome. In this respect, the ideal typical intervention restrains the phenomenally untoward effects of morphine-like drugs *by substitution.* In more theoretical terms, the cross-tolerant quality of methadone causes the properly stabilized patient to become dependent upon the medication without the threat of escalation of dose, and experimentation with opiates during maintenance produces neither the seemingly anticipated state of euphoria, nor any other narcotic effects. (Yet as indicated in earlier chapters, this effected "blockade" can indeed be overcome by excessive dosages of a narcotic, and unauthorized supplementary doses of the substitute are not totally uncommon.)

An alternative chemotherapeutic approach which effects a *narcotic blockade* has been developed through the synthesis of *narcotic antagonists.* Pharmacologically, it has been hypothesized that such medication exhibits an affinity for morphine-receptor sites in the nervous

245

system, with little or no activity of its own at these sites.[22] When administered, the antagonist occupies the receptor site thus inhibiting the usual narcotic effects when a morphine-like drug is subsequently introduced; and when given subsequent to an ingestion of the narcotic, the antagonist will displace this narcotic from the receptor with a consequential termination of the narcotic effects.

Hundreds of narcotic antagonists have been synthesized and produced during the past few decades, and it is the purpose of this chapter to review the major contributions to this field of scientific inquiry, and to compare the effectiveness of both methadone and the antagonists as applied to the treatment of narcotic addiction.

NALORPHINE AND LEVALLORPHAN

The evolution and development of narcotic antagonists dates back to the latter part of the nineteenth century to the chemopharmacologic search for a non-addicting analgesic, and to the attempts to dissociate the pain-killing and the physical-dependence-producing properties of the morphine-like agents. Numerous manipulations of the morphine molecule had been undertaken, and in 1898, heroin was introduced as the first non-addicting analgesic.[11,60]

Heroin at that time was viewed by physicians as a drug of choice over morphine in that it relieved pain without the fear of severe respiratory depression and physical dependence.[6,59] This mistaken belief, that heroin was non-addicting, can perhaps be attributed to the ignorance of what is now known as cross-tolerance. Morel-Levalée (1900),[61] for example, had observed that the new drug was a safe and temporary substitute for morphine during withdrawal treatment for addiction since it did not precipitate a severe abstinence syndrome. Although heroin was indeed effectively substituting for morphine, *it was preventing the appearance of abstinence phenomena by the maintenance of physical dependence.* And since relief from the more obvious undesirable effects of morphine was apparent, the heroin was continued as physicians had little opportunity to observe that the same morphine dependence was being maintained. This process was further complicated by the fact that testing of the relative effectiveness of oral and intraveneous dosage administration was not undertaken; it was not known that dosages beyond the symptomatic need enhanced the development of physical dependence.

An important advance in the dissociation of analgesia and addictiveness came when Pohl (1914-15)[62] developed N-allylnorcodeine which antagonized the respiratory-depressant effect of morphine. N-allylnorcodeine was the first known morphine antagonist, but it was not until almost three decades later that significant advances in the development of antagonists began to appear.

During the early 1940's Weijlard and Erickson,[68] researchers with Merck & Co., produced the morphine analog N-allylnormorphine, or nalorphine (Nalline®-Merck, Sharp and Dohme), and the new drug was found to antagonize the narcotic effects of both morphine and morphine-like analgesics. Further confirmations as to nalorphine's antagonistic effects were offered almost immediately by Unna,[67] Hart,[32] and Hart and McCawley.[33]

By the 1950's, considerable testing had been undertaken with nalorphine, and its attributes, both negative and positive, were apparent. Eckenhoff, Elder and King[12] demonstrated that the drug was an effective antagonist even against the respiratory depression provoked by morphine overdosage in man. This antagonistic property was then extended to include the synthetic analgesics from which such poisoning could occur, including methadone,[23] dihydromorphinone and methorphinan,[5] meperidine,[12] and heroin.[64] In terms of intensifying the morphine abstinence syndrome, Wikler, Fraser and Isbell[73] reported both the provocation and intensification of such a syndrome when nalorphine was administered to patients during maintained addiction to morphine. Furthermore, while it was also observed as an effective analgesic in man, [48,46] nalorphine was not considered to be addictive in the same sense as was morphine.[36]

On the basis of numerous clinical observations,

Fraser[20] outlined the major pharmacological actions of nalorphine, each of which was dependent upon dosage of both the morphine (or morphine-like drugs) and the nalorphine, and upon whether the administration of the antagonist had been preceded by one dose, several doses, or an addictive dosage schedule of the narcotic.

"(a) In a dose of 10 mg. subcutaneously nalorphine depresses respiration and body temperature in a manner comparable to that of 10 to 30 mg. of morphine. It provokes dysphoria in many subjects and it moderately constricts the pupils. (b) When a single dose of 10 to 20 mg. of morphine is followed one hour later by 10 mg. of nalorphine, the latter will counteract to a considerable degree morphine-induced miotic effects and "morphine euphoria," but, under these conditions, it will not counteract morphine-induced respiratory depression. (c) If, however, the dose of morphine is sufficient to induce severe respiratory depression, then administration of 10 mg. of nalorphine promptly restores normal respiration. (d) If a patient is addicted to 120 mg. of morphine daily, administration of 10 mg. of nalorphine will provoke a violent abstinence syndrome."

Nalorphine is an analgesic in man, for when tested for relief of post-operative pain, data indicated that 15 mg. of nalorphine had the approximate analgesic potency of 10 mg. of morphine.[48] The side effects consequent to its administration as an analgesic or antagonist, however, have appeared to be too drastic to preclude widespread clinical use, and the intensity of such effects seem to be directly proportional to the size of the dosage. Single doses of nalorphine as small as 3 mg. administered subcutaneously have exerted subjective effects of dizziness, drowsiness, decreases in respiratory minute volume by 10 to 15%, declines in rectal temperature, and miosis.[22] An increase of such a dosage to 10 mg. also increases drowsiness and is accompanied by lethargy, dysphoria, and in many cases, nausea and vomiting, wierd dreams, pseudoptosis, perspiration and a rise in the pulse rate and blood pressure.[37,73]

With the dosage increased to 75 mg., patients often experienced vivid daydreams which they could suppress, and acute panic reactions have been known to develop.[73] In one experiment with ten subjects, nalorphine produced anxiety, and the refractory complications of a

peculiar dreamy state with vivid fantasies, miosis, pseudoptosis, sweating and diuresis.[70] After an increase to 75
mg., bradycardia was observed and some subjects experienced a numbness and heaviness in their limbs.

As an antagonist, nalorphine does not antagonize respiratory depression induced by a single therapeutic dose
of morphine,[45] but can if administered after the second
dose of morphine. Antagonism by nalorphine in the case
of chronic morphine intoxication can precipitate readily
observable abstinence syndromes. In the case of a patient dependent upon 300 mg. daily of morphine, for example, 30 mg. of nalorphine was administered subcutaneously five and one-half hours after the last dose of
morphine. Five minutes later he complained of chills, was
shaking all over, and manifested yawning, rhinorrhea,
lacrimation, dilated pupils, gooseflesh and vomiting.[20]

Nalorphine, then, is an effective narcotic antagonist in
that it antagonizes both respiratory and circulatory depression, and has the ability to precipitate an abstinence
syndrome. And although it does not produce physical dependence in the same sense as morphine (craving for the
drug), the accompanying sedation and psychotomimetic
effects tend to downgrade its usefulness in chemotherapy.

Subsequent to the development of nalorphine, the N-al-
lylmorphinan analog, levallorphan (Lorfan®—Roche),
was produced. Although it proved to have antagonistic
properties many times greater than those of nalorphine,
it too manifested unpropitious side effects which de-
tracted from its widespread clinical use.

As chemotherapeutic agents in the treatment of narcotic addiction, nalorphine and levallorphan have been
employed for their antagonistic effects when the drugs
are administered in small doses as a "secondary prevention." By injecting 3 mg. or less of nalorphine or 1½ mg.
of levallorphan, the presence of opiates can be detected
in a user by the dilation of the pupil. Several practitioners have discussed the positive effects of such "anti-drug
testing" as a means of self-induced rehabilitation in that
the threat of detection will allow, or perhaps force, the
addict to break his dependence cycle. Known as "Nalline®

testing," the procedure has been used extensively in California, but clinical and research findings have tended to be inconclusive.[1,4,35]

CYCLAZOCINE

The undesirable side effects of nalorphine and levallorphan led to the testing of additional compounds under the sponsorship of the Committee on Drug Addiction and Narcotics of the National Academy of Sciences–National Research Foundation.[66] Of the six preparations developed however, one had good analgesic effects but with morphine-like side effects with minimal antagonistic action, while the others were both analgesic and antagonistic but were like nalorphine with respect to side effects.

Profiting from previous demonstrations that the presence of the complete morphine molecule was not mandatory for morphine-like analgesic action and morphine antagonism, May and Eddy, in 1952, began the synthesis of the benzomorphan series and the development of phenozocine.[58] Phenozocine exhibited analgesic effectiveness reportedly ten times greater than and abstinence suppressant potency less than 1/5 that of morphine, which led to the suspicion of some dissociation of morphine-like properties, and finally to the preparation of the N-allyl-benzomorphan analog of nalorphine. Of the numerous compounds developed, pentazocine (Win 20, 228) appeared among them as a promising non-addicting analgesic, and cyclazocine (Win 2Q, 740) as a morphine antagonist.

Prior to the 1960's, and especially with respect to nalorphine and levallorphan the usefulness of the narcotic antagonists as "antagonists" was related to the relief of *respiratory depression*. *Respiratory depression* is known to appear following the administration of narcotic analgesics even in small therapeutic doses, and in this sense, refers to the disturbance of respiratory control mechanisms. In more contemporary applications in the chemotherapeutic treatment of addicts, narcotic antagonism has found its usefulness in its *blocking effects*, in that morphine-like euphoria, tolerance and dependence reduced or even totally prevented. Furthermore, the use of antagonists in this context has been based to some extent upon a series of theoretical and clinical foundations.

Martin,[52] for example, in a recent discussion of the possible utility of opiate antagonists, outlined two accepted overviews of the addictive process. The causes of addiction on the one hand have been viewed in terms of some underlying psychopathology. The addictive state in this sense is objectively given, and may be the result and outgrowth of some disorder intrinsic to the psychosocial construction of the individual. Alternatively, addiction has been viewed as a disease process which can be subjectively problematic in that drug use itself can give rise to anti-social behavior. Both views look to adequate social adjustment as the successful response to treatment, a process which seeks to suppress both the drug-taking and anti-social behavior. Such suppression, however, through abstinence, may not necessarily cope with or alter any underlying pathological state, and indeed may even reinforce and strengthen it.

Yet further, in addition to or in spite of any pathological motivation, the addictive state as a disease process can involve a state of physical dependence to which the abstinent patient may relapse should the period of recovery be of only short duration. Himmelsbach[34] offered evidence suggesting that this period of physical recovery may be as long as six months, and later studies presented additional support for this hypothesis.[57,72,74]

With the view that opiate addiction, then, may involve a pathological state combined with a physical dependency which would require long-term detoxification, Wikler's hypothesis of *conditional abstinence* offered a further refinement to a developing theoretical construct.[71] He suggested that drug-seeking behavior may be constantly reinforced by the relief of the abstinence syndrome provided by narcotic injections. Furthermore, such symptoms might also be precipitated through conditioning by the environmental and interpersonal stimuli that have become associated with the drug-seeking activity of the addict. This latter notion was based on the observations of Wikler and others that many addicts who have been drug free for long periods often suddenly experience acute symptoms of the abstinence syndrome when they return to their old neighborhoods.

According to these hypotheses, patients receiving regular doses of a narcotic antagonist, after initial detoxification, could be protected from relapse in the home environment if experimentation with heroin failed to relieve the "conditioned" symptoms of the abstinence syndrome; and ultimately, this conditioned dependency and its complement of drug-seeking behavior could be mitigated. Furthermore, in that total relief of physical dependency may indeed take as long as six months as Himmelsbach has suggested, the initially detoxified patient who maintains a regular dose of the antagonist could be further protected should glimpses of the abstinence syndrome reappear. Finally, if the view that the addictive state may ultimately be rooted in a psychopathological disorder is correct, effective treatment might encompass alternative efforts in addition and incidental to this chemotherapeutic approach without threat of program disruption due to relapse or drug-seeking behavior. While this general thesis has received little empirical substantiation, it has, in part, represented a framework within which many of the recent experimental programs with narcotic antagonists have been undertaken.

Cyclazocine, a benzomorphan-derived compound, was first introduced into the treatment of opiate dependence in 1965. In the first clinical studies undertaken with the new drug, [21,55] cyclazocine was shown to effectively block the narcotic effects of morphine, while the patient was also able to develop tolerance to the same side effects found concomitant with the use of nalorphine. These findings led to further speculation and experimentation on the basis that:

> "(1) If an ambulatory abstinent addict who is protected with cyclazocine for one reason or another becomes involved in drug-seeking activity, perhaps in response to an unpleasant and stressful environmental circumstance, he would not have to prolong his spree because physical dependence had developed. (2) It is possible that subjects on

cyclazocine who experiment with narcotics may actually, as a consequence of their experimentation, extinguish conditioned abstinence and conditioned drug-seeking behavior. (3) If protracted abstinence is a slowly reversible phenomenon, then it may be possible to prevent subjects from reestablishing dependence during the time that protracted abstinence is decreasing to an insignificant level."[51]

Pharmacologically, cyclazocine has a high affinity for the hypothetical morphine receptor sites in the nervous system and will prevent the morphine-like drugs from producing their effects by occupying the receptor site, or by displacing the morphine-like drug from the receptor site. Furthermore, in the patient physically dependent upon a morphine-like drug, the administration of cyclazocine will not only terminate the narcotic effect but also precipitate the abstinence syndrome.

When administered on a daily basis, cyclazocine will prevent the physical dependence associated with repeated dosages of morphine-like drugs. Martin, *et. al.,*[55] for example, pointed out that 60 mg. of morphine given four times daily for several weeks produced only minimal physical dependence in subjects stabilized on as little as 2 mg. of cyclazocine twice daily. This, in turn, has led to the suggestion that when a patient is protected with cyclazocine, it would be almost impossible for him to take a lethal overdose of heroin or morphine.[52]

In common with nalorphine, cyclazocine produces a series of psychotomimetic effects, including sensory distortions, mental clouding, weird thoughts, and altered states of consciousness. Furthermore, it can produce respiratory depression, miosis, constipation, irritability, and somnolence. Research has indicated, however, that tolerance develops to many of these subjective changes and *tolerance does not develop to its antagonist properties.*[55,56]

Also as in the case of nalorphine, cyclazocine can produce a variety of physical dependence, yet such dependence is qualitatively different from that produced by morphine.[52,53,54,55] In analyzing this dependence, the following should be noted:

1. in the individual dependent upon a morphine-like

drug, both nalorphine and cyclazocine precipitate abstinence;

2. subjects highly tolerant to the subjective effects of
morphine do not evidence cross-tolerance to the dysphoric
effects of cyclazocine;

3. subjects tolerant to cyclazocine or nalorphine are
cross-tolerant to nalorphine or cyclazocine respectively,
and are refractory to the effects of morphine;

4. when subjects dependent on cyclazocine or nalorphine are withdrawn, hyperthermia and mydriosis are
more marked than in the morphine abstinence syndrome,
yet hypertension and hyperpnea are less conspicuous;

5. subjects undergoing cyclazocine withdrawal report a
sensation of lightheadedness or "electric shocks," which
appear between 20 and 48 hours subsequent to the last
dosage; other signs of withdrawal, while not severe, have
included lacrimation, runny nose, dilated pupils, perspiration, fatigue, inability to sleep, headache, nausea, loose
bowels, back pains, and sudden brief episodes of weakness;
and

6. most characteristic of nalorphine and cyclazocine dependence is that the abstinence syndromes do not give rise
to drug craving and hence, drug-seeking behavior.

Cyclazocine also has demonstrable analgesic action,
for when given in moderate doses, it produces analgesia
equivalent to 10 mg. of morphine.

Although objectively similar, the use of cyclazocine for
narcotic addicts should be distinguished from antabuse,
the chemical aversion therapy used with alcoholics. The
patient using antabuse must avoid all contact with alcohol since its use in such a therapeutic orientation will
produce serious toxic effects. Cyclazocine, on the other
hand, produces no such effects but renders the morphine-
like drug ineffective. As suggested by Laskowitz, Brill
and Jaffe,[50] antabuse is an "adversive stimulus," while
the antagonist is a "negative reinforcer" which blocks
the incentive value of heroin. As such, the negative reinforcement function of cyclazocine enables the clinician
"to buy time" as he controls the pharmacological deter-
minants of drug-seeking behavior.

In an attempt to control the drug-seeking behavior of
opiate dependent individuals, numerous clinical efforts
have been undertaken, and the results, while inconclusive, appear promising.

Jaffe and Brill [38,39] initiated a pilot study of 27
patients, essentially middle class with low arrest rates

and stable employment histories, who voluntarily sought treatment. The patients were withdrawn from narcotics with methadone, and were challenged with nalorphine 48 to 72 hours subsequent to the last dose of methadone. If abstinence was not precipitated, cyclazocine (0.25mg.) was administered orally twice daily. The dosage was then increased by 0.25 mg./day until the patients were receiving, after two weeks of hospitalization, between 2.0 and 3.0 mg. of the antagonist per day. Of the 27 patients, 33% (9 cases) had remained on cyclazocine for over nine months; two patients had remained totally abstinent (a physician and a student), and several converted to weekend or spree use of other drugs, continuing cyclazocine between sprees. A total of 11 patients or 40% had withdrawn from the project at the time of the evaluation. The authors concluded, however, that the majority of the patients "did extremely well" in that they were abstinent or reduced drug intake to a weekend basis.

Freedman, et. al.[25] have used cyclazocine in two patient cohorts. In the first group, 51 patients who were part of a developing therapeutic community volunteered for cyclazocine treatment. It was apparent, however, that the structure and processes of the therapeutic community represented a polar antithesis to successful chemotherapy. Many of the patients, discharged from the therapeutic community for rule infractions, were unable to continue on cyclazocine. Conversely, the long residential stay provided little opportunity for "drug testing," and hence, many discontinued the use of the antagonist. In the second study,[26] 60 patients from 17 to 64 years of age with addiction histories of 2 to 15 years were hospitalized for treatment. Of these 60 cases, 58 completed the cyclazocine induction period. Various induction periods ranging from 10 to 30 days were studied. Induction was defined as achieving a daily therapeutic dose of 4.0 mg. of cyclazocine subsequent to detoxification and a drug free period of one week. The 20 and 30-day induction periods were well tolerated, and in a narcotic challenge of 15 mg. of heroin administered intravenously in the cyclazocine-stabilized patients, over 80% experienced little or no narcotic effects. Those who did experience euphoria received an increased dosage of cyclazocine which provided an effective blockade.

Following stabilization and challenge, patients were discharged and instructed to return to the clinic three times weekly for medication. Of these 58 patients, 47% (27 cases) remained in treatment for at least two months, and 33% (19 cases) failed to return to the clinic. Of the remaining 20%, 3 cases discontinued the chemotherapy as trips to the clinic interfered with their jobs, 5 were arrested and incarcerated for narcotic violations, and 4 were discharged for irregular program participation. The researchers' clinical impressions suggested that among the patients studied, anxiety was relieved, criminality declined, and interest in vocational activity was increased; and furthermore, it was hypothesized that the high dropout rate was the result of a lack of an intensive rehabilitation program combined with the need for an inordinate number of visits to the clinic.

In a more recent study,[63] cyclazocine was administered to 31 chronic male addicts, ages 19 to 43, who volunteered for treatment at a community general hospital in New York City. Prerequisites for treatment included New York City residence, two or more unsuccessful hospital treatments for addiction, absence of any psychoses, physical illness, current addiction to a non-narcotic substance, or pending court case, and all subjects were required to sign a consent for experimental drug treatment.

After detoxification by decreasing dosages of methadone, a drug-free period of one to two weeks followed. The subsequent induction to cyclazocine involved dosages increasing to 4 mg. daily over a 20-day period. Patients were divided into two groups: those for which heroin acted as a "normalizer" and increased their capacity to function; and those for whom drug-seeking behavior was related to environmental factors and in whom the feeling of an inability to function did not predominate. During the period of hospitalization which ranged from two to four months, job placement and/or training was made available, and a narcotic challenge was introduced. Subsequent to discharge, patients were asked to return to a clinic two to three times weekly for medication.

The follow-up evaluation indicated that 50% of the patients remained in treatment (as of January, 1969). The duration of outpatient treatment ranged from 4 to 33 months with a mean of 20 months, and the mean age of this group was 31.6 years with a range of 22 to 44 years. Marital status best differentiated the two groups in that married patients less often discontinued treatment. Neither age, duration of addiction, nor lengths of times abstinent from drug use were discriminating factors. Of the two addict types outlined by the researchers, the relative success of one group over another did not appear significant.

Clinical trials suggest, then, that cyclazocine, which can reliably block narcotic effects, may be useful in the treatment of addiction in a voluntary hospital program. Cyclazocine eases the transition from addiction to treatment and represents a catalyst in that its use motivates the patient to continue seeing the therapist, if only for the sake of securing more medication. A patient stabilized on 4 to 6 mg. of cyclazocine per day would probably be unable to recognize the effects of 60 mg. of morphine or 20 mg. of heroin within the first 18-20 hours subsequent to the introduction of the antagonist. Furthermore, while cyclazocine can produce hallucinations and amphetamine-like or barbiturate-like effects in some subjects, tolerance develops to these pharmacological effects without altering the blocking effect.

NALOXONE

Naloxone (N-allyl-noroxymorphone) is a derivative of the synthetic narcotic analgesic oxymorphone hydrochloride (Numorphan®-Endo), a compound found to be eight to ten times more potent than morphine.[7,13]

As an opiate antagonist, naloxone has been found to be more potent than either nalorphine or levallorphan.[2,3,8,16,17,18,19,25,42,49,65] It will precipitate an abstinence syndrome in narcotic-dependent subjects, and does not produce respiratory depression when given alone.

Extensive clinical studies have shown that cyclazocine, like the shorter-acting antagonists nalorphine and levallorphan, causes numerous disturbing side effects, and abrupt cessation of cyclazocine may produce a variety of abstinence syndrome. Neither adverse effects nor an abstinence syndrome have been apparent upon abrupt withdrawal of naloxone, and tolerance to the antagonistic properties of the drug does not develop during long-term administration. In that naloxone does not produce morphine-like subjective effects, will not produce physical dependence, and will precipitate an abstinence syndrome in morphine-dependent individuals, it can be concluded that it does not possess an abuse-potential of the morphine type and hence, might represent an even more effective narcotic antagonism therapy for opiate dependence.

In testing the chemotherapeutic potential of naloxone, Fink et. al.[15] initiated a pilot study with seven patients. The subjects ranged in age from 26 to 37 years with a mean of 30.9 years. Each had been using narcotics on a daily basis for a period of 3 to 13 months immediately preceding admission to the hospital, and narcotic histories ranged from 4 to 17 years with a mean of 11 years. Of the 7 cases, 3 were Puerto Rican, 3 black and 1 white; 6 had criminal histories.

Following detoxification and a 5-day drug free period, the 7 patients received oral naloxone on a long term basis. Five patients were started on a daily dose of 20 mg., and 3 of these received increments of 20 mg. per day; 2 patients received an initial dose of 40 mg. per day with daily increments of 40 mg. The patients were maintained at either 100 or 120 mg. per day until their initial heroin challenge. The challenge of 20 mg. produced feelings ranging from relaxation to mild euphoria in some cases, but with an increased dosage of naloxone to 200 mg. per day, the narcotic blockade was effective and complete. The abrupt cessation of naloxone produced no discomfort and hence, no abstinence syndrome.

In short-term administration of heroin followed by naloxone, the euphoric effects of the narcotic were abolished within ½ to 2 minutes subsequent to dosages of the antagonist, even at a lower limit of 0.7 mg. administered parenterally. The duration of naloxone antagonism, however, was found to be shorter than the action of heroin in that for 13 of 29 trials, the subjects reported the recurrence of the narcotic effects 3 to 5 hours later, ranging from relaxation and feelings of well-being to full-scale heroin euphoria. The research suggested, however, that naloxone was an "ideal clinical agent" in that its use was not accompanied by systemic effects or changes in visual analysis, and it was estimated that 1 mg. of intraveneous naloxone would effectively block 40 mg. of heroin.

In a subsequent effort, naloxone was administered to nine subjects in order to determine whether increases in the oral dosage levels of the drug would prolong the duration of heroin antagonism to a degree sufficient for providing the basis for a more extended clinical trial.[75] Naloxone was administered in single, daily oral doses ranging as high as 3,000 mg., and persistent antagonism to 25 mg. and 50 mg. heroin challenges for periods of 24 hours and without secondary effects was demonstrated.

A more recent assessment of the effectiveness of naloxone was undertaken by Kurland and Kerman[47] with 20 subjects who had been paroled from correctional institutions in the State of Maryland. The parolees were divided into two equal groups, the first including direct admissions to the naloxone program immediately subsequent to their release from prison, with the other composed of "failures" in an alternative abstinence program. The naloxone was administered during the evening hours, and was packaged in small envelopes containing four drug and placebo tablets. This deployment pattern thus provided the opportunity to manipulate the dosage from 0 to 800 mg. in increments of 200 mg. without the subjects' awareness of any changes. Continuence in the program was one of the conditions of the subjects' parole, and arrangements were made to maintain daily urine surveillance and weekly group therapy.

Six of the ten subjects in the "direct admission" group remained in the program for a year or longer, while four of the ten "transfers" were reinforced sufficiently to reach their parole expiration dates while still in a program status as contrasted with the alternative of being returned to prison for parole violation. While these results were not dramatic, the research effort did demonstrate that the administration of naloxone on a maintenance basis was reatively non-hazardous, nor was it dependency producing. It was further indicated that the dosages could be rapidly manipulated to provide additional support for subjects who were becoming increasingly vulnerable to opiate usage, with a more frugal use of the drug employed during periods when the maintenance of high levels of abstinence were apparent.

In spite of the merit attributed to naloxone by the initial investigative research probes, a series of limitations continue to beset its widespread clinical use. Its effective antagonism was found to be shorter than that of cyclazocine, and the studies suggest that since the medication tends to be poorly absorbed, an 18-hour blockage against 25 and 50 mg. of heroin would not be possible until a dose of 1500 mg. or more of naloxone was administered. Perhaps an even more severe limitation on the use of naloxone is its excessive cost. The pilot study of 7 patients by Fink, et. al.[15] had to be interrupted after only three months due to a shortage of the drug, brought about by the high cost of *thebaine*, a convulsant morphine analog, which represents the raw material from which naloxone is manufactured.

NALBUPHINE

Nalbuphine, the most recently developed of the antagonists, is structurally related to oxymorphone, a potent analgesic, and to naloxone. Clinical trials have indicated that nalbuphine produces pupillary constriction, and will precipitate abstinence in subjects dependent upon 60 mg. of morphine per day. [41,43] These initial studies have indicated, however, that clinical applications of nalbuphine appear to be undesirable at this time. With a potency only 1/4th that of nalorphine, the medication will produce marked agonistic effects at dose levels achieved during chronic administration, and may produce some degree of morphine-type euphoria and an abstinence syndrome characterized by compulsive drug-seeking behavior.

THE ANTAGONISTS COMPARED

The foregoing discussion of narcotic antagonists has suggested that each has positive and negative attributes. Nalorphine and levallorphan were first introduced and although they manifested strong antagonistic properties, the relatively short duration of action and the hallucinogenic potential precluded widespread clinical use. The development of cyclazocine, with its longer duration combined with the patients' potential for developing tolerance to the side effects, led to a test of Wikler's conditioning theory of opiate dependence. The relative degree of success in the use of cyclazocine for the addicted state led to further clinical trials with other antagonists, notably naloxone. Naloxone was found to be an antagonist with little or no agonistic opiate actions and to which no tolerance and dependence developed. Its action was found, however, to be of short duration and its cost prohibitive.

In Table I, the major properties of these antagonists can be more readily compared. The "desirable" effects of antagonism, of respiratory and circulatory depression, and ability to precipitate abstinence, are those directly concerned with antagonistic activity. All of these compounds indicate positive antagonistic properties. (While there seems to be some differences of opinion apparent in the literature regarding the relative potency of the antagonists on a mg./kg. basis, the figures in this table reflect a broad and general consensus of research findings.) The "undesirable" effects, however, have tended to preclude the clinical use of nalorphine and levallorphan. Naloxone has no undesirable properties.

Some distinctions, however, are discernible with respect to nalorphine, levallorphan and cyclazocine. While all exhibit psychotomimetic effects, the patient is able to develop tolerance of those of cyclazocine. The physical dependence, as indicated earlier, is of a physiological nature and does not bring about drug-seeking behavior. Naloxone, then, would appear to be the antagonist of choice, but its short duration and high cost tend to detract from its clinical adoptability. Cyclazocine, therefore, with its longer action and lack of lasting undesir-

Table 1.
The Desirable and Undesirable Properties of the Narcotic Antagonists

Properties	Nalor-phine	Leval-lorphan	Cycla-zocine	Nalox-one
Desirable				
1. antagonism of respiratory depression	1*	5	3	30
2. antagonism of circulatory depression	1	5	3	30
3. ability to precipitate abstinence	1	2	1	7
Undesirable				
1. psychotomimetic effects	Yes	Yes	Yes	No
2. sedation	Yes	Yes	Yes	No
3. pupillary constriction	Yes	Yes	Yes	No
4. physical dependence	Yes	?	Yes	No
5. alteration of general systemic functions	Yes	Yes	Yes	No

* Relative potency on a mg./kg. basis

able side effects, would appear to be the choice of antagonists in the treatment of narcotic addiction at the present
time.

METHADONE AND THE ANTAGONISTS

A comparison of methadone with cyclazocine or any
other narcotic antagonist would be difficult in that pharmacologically, the two compounds have separate and divergent actions. Methadone maintenance is *substitution
therapy* while cyclazocine and naloxone programs antagonize the effects of the opiates. In common, however,
each approach effect a variety of "narcotic blockade"
and within this framework, these chemotherapeutic
programs can be analyzed and compared.

To have any pragmatic value for the treatment of addiction to morphine-like drugs, the ideal-typical medication employed, whether it be a drug substitute or a drug
antagonist, must:

1. eliminate the euphoric appeal of heroin;
2. preclude abstinence symptoms;
3. produce no toxic or dysphoric effects;
4. be orally effective;
5. have long duration;
6. be medically safe;
7. be of moderate cost; and
8. be compatible with normal social roles.

Neither the substitutes nor the antagonists eliminate
the euphoric appeal of heroin or other morphine-like
drugs. The ability of the opiates to produce an euphoro-
genic effect upon the patient properly stabilized on methadone or cyclazocine, however, tends to be restrained. In
most cases, while the *appeal per se* may still exist, the
noumenal and phenomenal effects are prevented either
partially or totally. The characteristic of methadone's
cross-tolerance for morphine-like drugs as well as the antagonists' blocking effects prevent the onset of the abstinence syndrome when the approved clinical directives
are adheared to. Furthermore, both drugs are medically
safe and the patient properly stabilized on methadone or
cyclazocine will not be exposed to any toxicity or dyspho-

ria. The duration of action, oral effectiveness and compatibility of the two latter drugs with normal social roles are somewhat similar, but these seemingly interrelated contingencies have presented an arena for problematic encounters within a variety of therapeutic applications.

As discussed in earlier chapters, methadone maintenance patients have been found to both supplement their prescribed daily dosage as well as "cheat" by the simultaneous use of heroin and other opiates, amphetamines, barbiturates and sedatives, and cocaine, as well as overcome the blockades effected by the substitute. This possibility of abuse then, may tend to alter the desirable compatibility of the use of the medication with normal social roles. Furthermore, since methadone is legally and pharmacologically a narcotic, it has an intrinsic abuse potential, and a monetary value in the illicit narcotics trade. By contrast, cyclazocine has a considerably lower abuse potential in that it has no market value. Such factors would suggest that the ways in which methadone is to be distributed should be structured to reduce to a minimum its illicit diversion. Greater freedom can be exercised with the dispensation of cyclazocine which, in turn, extends greater freedom to the patient.

Abuse patterns are also not unknown to cyclazocine patients. [38,39,50] Though it tends to block the effects of the opiates, cyclazocine does not satisfy "drug craving." Unlike the narcotics which the patient has been taking regularly, the antagonist does not produce any pleasurable effects in itself causing much frustration, and efforts to circumvent the narcotic blockade occur. Patients learn that the duration of cyclazocine's action ranges little beyond 20 hours with a peak effectiveness only 8 hours subsequent to administration. As this shielding ability diminishes and approaches its low point, experimentation with heroin often takes place. An additional shortcoming exists in that cyclazocine's effective narcotic blockade permits the intake of large doses of heroin without the anticipatory anxiety of physical dependence. Yet the danger of overdose exists for those who experiment in such a manner after having become accustomed to the "protection" afforded by the antagonist, by omitting, either by choice or oversight, their daily oral dose.

A cursory glance of the statistical comparisons of the relative effectiveness of methadone and antagonist programs might initially suggest that a greater degree of success has been exhibited by substitution therapy. This would be a premature judgement, however, and a violation of the canons of scientific research. The programs cannot be compared as such since the very structure, process and history of each program has precluded the generation of data of a comparative nature.

Attrition rates in the cyclazocine programs have been reported as high as 83%.[50] An overview of the methadone maintenance studies on the other hand, indicates that the majority of patients remain in the programs. As the mean length of maintenance increases, employment rates also increase while arrest rates severely decrease. The substitution of methadone has shown success with criminal addicts, with one study reporting 94% of the cases ending such behavior.[10] While overall success rates in methadone maintenance programs have ranged upward from a lower limit in excess of 50%, those cases who remain in the programs are usually older, long-term addicts, with histories of criminal involvement.[9,28-31,40,44,69]

In regard to the non-comparability of data, each type of program requires divergent forms of motivation and commitment. Methadone relieves drug craving, yet since cyclazocine *blocks* the effects of heroin, it does not relieve this chronic need as well as the physical and mental side effects brought about by the loss of the narcotic's role as an adaptive mechanism. Secondly, substitution therapy has had more widespread experimental use, while a comparable number of patients have not yet been exposed to treatment with antagonists. Thirdly, the two chemotherapeutic approaches have been directed toward different segments of the population, and in this respect, some initial parameters of success are beginning to emerge. Older long-term addicts with a criminal history have been successfully maintained by narcotic substitution, and studies have shown that middle class addicts, as well as addicts with stable marital relationships have been successful cyclazocine patients.[50,63]

The suggested strategy for the further development of the usefulness of each chemotherapeutic approach would involve extensive experimentation for the purpose of determining which approach would be most effective for varying types of addicts. The recent pilot project described by Laskowitz, Brill and Jaffe,[50] undertaken with a collaborative arrangement between New York City's Bronx State Hospital and Lincoln Hospital's Department of Psychiatry, points to the continuing evolution and refinement of the use of narcotic antagonists in the treatment of opiate addiction. With more rigorous screening devices with rehabilitative efforts concomitant with chemotherapy, a greater degree of success has been apparent.

The future direction of antagonist research is not centered upon the rehabilitative value of the modality, for clinical experiences have demonstrated its usefulness for a specific segment of the population. But rather, research priorities must be directed to the identification of those addict-patients who will profit most from this type of treatment and under what circumstances, to the development of an antagonist with longer chemopharmacological duration, and to the selection of the specific forms of social/psychotherapeutic and other chemotherapeutic approaches that ought to be used in conjunction with this treatment venture.

REFERENCES

1. Bailey: Nalline control of addict-probationers, 1968.
2. Blumberg, et. al.: Narcotic antagonist activity of naloxone, 1965.
3. Blumberg, et al.: Use of writhing test for evaluating analgesic activity of narcotic antagonists, 1965.
4. Brown: Narcotics and nalline: Six years of testing, 1963.
5. Chase, et. al.: 1952.
6. Daly: A clinical study of heroin, 1900.
7. De Kornfeld: Clinical laboratory study of hydroxydihydromorphinone (Numorphan HCL), 1961.
8. Devine, et. al.: The effect of simultaneously administered N-allyl-noroxymorphone on the respiratory depression induced by oxymorphone, 1964.
9. Dole and Nyswander: The use of methadone for narcotic blockade, 1966.

10. Dole, *et. al.*: Successful treatment of 750 criminal addicts, 1968.

11. Dreser: Uber die Wirkung einiger Derivate des Morphins auf die Athmung, 1898.

12. Eckenhoff, *et. al.*: N-allyl-normorphine in the treatment of morphine or Demerol narcosis, 1952.

13. Eddy and Lee: Analgesic equivalence to morphine and relative side action liability of oxymorphone (14-hydroxydihydromorphinone), 1959.

14. Fink, *et. al.*: Narcotic antagonists and substitutes in opiate dependence, 1968.

15. Fink, *et. al.*: Naloxone in heroin dependence, 1968.

16. Fiut, *et. al.*: Antagonism of convulsive and lethal effects induced by propoxyphine, 1966.

17. Foldes, *et. al.*: Comparison of the respiratory and circulatory effects of narcotic antagonists, 1964.

18. Foldes, *et. al.*: The respiratory, circulatory, and analgesic effects of naloxone-narcotic mixtures in anesthetized subjects, 1965.

19. Foldes, *et. al.*: Studies on the specificity of narcotic antagonists, 1965.

20. Fraser: Human pharmacology and clinical uses of nalorphine (N-allyl-normorphine), 1957.

21. Fraser and Rosenberg: Comparative effects of (i) chronic administration of cyclazocine, (ii) substitution of nalorphine for cyclazocine, and (iii) chronic administration of morphine. Pilot crossover study, 1966.

22. Fraser, *et. al.*: Studies on N-allylnormorphine in man: Antagonism to morphine and heroin and effects of mixtures of N-allylnormorphine, 1956.

23. Fraser, *et. al.*: Use of N-allyl-normorphine in treatment of methadone poisoning in man. Report of two cases, 1952.

24. Freedman: Drug addiction: an eclectic view, 1966.

25. Freedman, *et. al.*: Cyclazocine and methadone in narcotic addiction, 1967.

26. Freedman, *et. al.*: Clinical studies of cyclazocine in the treatment of narcotic addiction, 1968.

27. Freedman and Fink: Basic concepts and use of cyclazocine in the treatment of narcotic addiction, 1968.

28. Gearing: Progress report of evaluation of methadone maintenance treatment program use of March 31, 1968, 1968.

29. Gearing: Evaluation of methadone maintenance treatment program progress report through October 3, 1968, (mimeographed).

30. Gearing: Evaluation of methadone maintenance program: program progress report through March 31, 1969, (mimeographed).

31. Gearing: Methadone maintenance treatment program progress report of evaluation through March 31, 1970, (mimeographed).

32. Hart: N-allyl-norcodeine and N-allyl-normorphine, two antagonists to morphine, 1941.

33. Hart and McCawley: The pharmacology of N-allylnormorphine as compared with morphine, 1944.

34. Himmelsbach: Clinical studies of drug addiction. Physical dependence, withdrawal and recovery, 1942.

35. Hurley: Anti-narcotic testing: A physicians' point of view, 1963.

36. Isbell: Attempted addiction to nalorphine, 1956.

37. Isbell: Nalline—A specific narcotic antagonist. Clinical and pharmacologic observations, 1953.

38. Jaffe and Brill: Cyclazocine, a long acting narcotic antagonist: its voluntary acceptance as a treatment modality by narcotics abusers, 1966.

39. Jaffe and Brill: Cyclazocine, a long acting narcotic antagonist: I. Its voluntary acceptance as a treatment modality by narcotic abusers; and II. A three-month progress report. Unpublished observations reported to the Committee on Problems of Drug Dependence, 1966.

40. Jaffe, et. al.: Experience with use of methadone in a multimodality program for the treatment of narcotics users, 1969.

41. Jasinski and Mansky: The subjective effects of GPA-2087 and nalbuphine (EN-2234A), 1970.

42. Jasinski, et. al.: The human pharmacology and abuse potential of N-allylnoroxymorphone (naloxone), 1967.

43. Jasinski, et. al.: Progress report on the assessment of the antagonists nalbuphine and GPA-2087 for abuse potential and studies of the effects of dextromethorphan in man, 1971.

44. Joseph and Dole: Methadone patients on probation and parole, 1970.

45. Keats and Mithoefer: Nature of antagonism of nalorphine to respiratory depression induced by morphine in man, 1955.

46. Keats and Telford: Nalorphine, a patent analgesic in man, 1956.

47. Kurland and Kerman: N-allyl-14-hydroxydihydronormorphinone (Naloxone) in the management of the narcotic abuser: a pilot study, 1971.

48. Lasagna: Nalorphine (N-allylnormorphine) practical and theoretical considerations, 1954.

49. Lasagna: Drug interaction in the field of analgesic drugs, 1965.

50. Laskowitz, et. al.: Cyclazocine intervention in the treatment of narcotic addiction: another look, 1971.

51. Martin: Pharmacologic factors in relapse and the possible use of the narcotic antagonists in treatment, 1966.

52. Martin: The basis and possible utility of opioid antagonists in the ambulatory treatment of the addict, 1968.

53. Martin and Gorodetzky: Demonstration of Tolerance to and physical dependence on N-allylnormorphine (nalorphine), 1965.

54. Martin and Gorodetzky: Cyclazocine, an adjunct in the treatment of narcotic addiction, 1967.

55. Martin, et. al.: An experimental study in the treatment of narcotic addicts with cyclazocine, 1966.

56. Martin and Sloan: The pathophysiology of morphine dependence and its treatment with opioid antagonists, 1968.

57. Martin, et. al.: Tolerance to and physical dependence on morphine in rats, 1963.

58. May and Eddy: Synthetic analgesics: Part II, B. 6, 7-Benzomorphans, 1963.

59. Medea: L'impiego terapeutico dell-heroina, 1899.

60. Mering: Physiological and therapeutical investigations on the action of some morphine derivatives, 1898.

61. Morel-Levalée: La morphine remplacé par l'heroine pas d'euphorie, plus de toxicomanes traitment heroique de la morphinemanie, 1900.

62. Pohl: Uber das N-allylnorcodeine, einen antagonisten des morphins, 1915.

63. Resnick, et. al.: A cyclazocine typology in opiate dependence, 1970.

64. Strober: Treatment of acute heroin intoxication with nalorphine (nalline hydrochloride), 1954.

65. Sadove, *et. al.*: Study of a narcotic antagonist—N-allylnoroxymorphone, 1963.

66. Telford, *et. al.*: Studies of analgesic drugs: VII morphine antagonists as analgesics, 1961.

67. Unna: Antagonistic effect of N-allyl-normorphine upon morphine, 1943.

68. Weijlard and Erickson: N-allylnormorphine, 1942.

69. Wieland and Chambers: Methadone maintenance: a comparison of two stabilization techniques, 1970.

70. Wikler: Clinical and electroencephalographic studies on the effects of mescaline, N-allylnormorphine and morphine in man, 1954.

71. Wikler: Conditioning factors in opiate addiction and relapse, 1965.

72. Wikler: Interaction of physical dependence and classical operant conditioning in the genesis of relapse, 1968.

73. Wikler, *et. al.*: N-allylnormorphine: effects of single doses and precipitation of acute "abstinence syndromes" during addiction to morphine, methadone or heroin in man (post-addicts), 1953.

74. Wikler and Pescor: Factors disposing to "relapse" in rats previously addicted to morphine, 1965.

75. Zaks, *et. al.*: Naloxone treatment of opiate dependence: a progress report, 1971.

PART FIVE
Innovative Programs

Chapter 23.

A Review of Innovative Approaches and Techniques

Leon Brill

The number of innovative methadone programs has proliferated in various parts of the United States, building on the Dole-Nyswander model yet adding elements which, it is believed, improve on the model and deal more effectively with specific addict populations. Some of the changes formerly deemed innovative are, in fact, rapidly becoming "standard operating procedure"—as in the use of ambulatory rather than inpatient stabilization techniques and the treatment of younger patients with a lesser narcotic addiction history.

The programs to be discussed here cover different areas of the United States, and are interesting in terms of their variations in approach based on geography, population served, differing conceptualizations and treatment rationales. Among the programs to be discussed are the Chicago program, which includes a variety of modalities, the Bellevue program for psychiatric patients, and Van Etten for chest conditions, the Vera Institute program, which is experimenting with random assignment of patients and dose manipulation; the Blachly self-supporting program in Oregon, using sensitization and aversive therapy techniques, a black program in Pittsburg and others.

THE VAN ETTEN METHADONE PROGRAM FOR ADDICTS WITH CHEST AND CARDIOVASCULAR DISEASES

This program combines the treatment of hard-core

heroin addicts with the needs of a municipal hospital chest disease service. Increasing attention had been devoted to the medical problems of heroin addicts, and it was discovered that several types of respiratory diseases were common among them. One of these was tuberculosis, which has a greater incidence among New York heroin addicts than among the general population. Treatment of tuberculosis, cardiovascular and other diseases has been generally unsatisfactory in these patients.

In June 1966, a methadone unit was begun in the Chest Service of the Van Etten Hospital for inpatients with tuberculosis who were known to be hard-core heroin addicts. Subsequently, the scope of the Methadone Chest Disease Program (MCDP) was expanded to include hard-core heroin addicts who had any chronic disease of the heart or lungs, whether they were inpatients or outpatients.[1]

Structure of the Program

The program is divided into four phases: (1) in the "Medical Inpatient" phase, the goal is to remove those immediate problems that prevent the addict from remaining in the hospital as long as medically indicated for the adequate initial treatment of his chest disease; (2) in the "Medical Outpatient" phase, the goal is to have the patient take all the medicine prescribed for his chest disease and report for medical examinations and x-ray films. Patients whose chest disease does not require hospitalization begin the program in Phase II; (3) The "Social Rehabilitation" phase is the area into which most of the MCDP's energy is placed. The initial attitude towards each patient is that if he is physically able, he should be working full-time or be in training. In the case of certain patients, usually the heavy drinkers, this goal may be revised downward, and part-time employment or maintenance on welfare accepted as the best possible degree of rehabilitation (4). The "Cured" phase is reserved for patients who have completed medical treatment for their chest disease and are also rehabilitated to the point where they no longer feel the need for methadone. Their methadone dose will be tapered off and stopped, but they will continue to be seen by their counselors who will observe them closely to detect any evidence of the recrudescence of the urge for drugs.

Patient Material

The 63 patients first studied had used heroin for an average of 16 years. They were between 23 and 52 years of age, with a mean age of 38 years. Seventy-five percent of them were men, 25% women. Fifty-three percent were born in New York City, 71% did not complete their high school education. Seventy-five percent of the patients had tuberculosis and 11% had non-tuberculous chest disease (emphysema, endocarditis, empyema, pulmonary hypertension, etc). The 14% who had no chest disease qualified for admission because they were the spouses of patients already in MCDP. Five percent of the patients had debilitating alcoholism, but 23% were considered to have some degree of an alcohol problem.

Results

Inpatient Chest Disease Treatment—Phase I. Prior to June 1966, at which time MCDP was begun, 49% of the heroin addicts who entered the chest service in Van Etten Hospital left with irregular discharges, while the irregular discharge rate for the general hospital population was 16%. For the period June 1966 to March 1969, the irregular discharge rate for the general hospital population dropped to 11%, or a decrease of 90% from the addict discharge rate in the prior period.

There have been three relapses of tuberculosis, two of them in-patients with far advanced cavitary disease. Both patients were detected early, were rehospitalized, had lobectomies, and are doing well. The third patient was a primary drug treatment failure who also was detected early, rehospitalized, and is doing well on a new drug regimen. Other patients have been rehospitalized, several for exacerbations of chronic obstructive pulmonary disease and others because they had suffered general deterioration associated with alcoholism.

Social Rehabilitation—Phase III

Change in Life Style. Of patients currently in the program, 40% are either working or in training, 10% are homemakers, 10% are physically disabled or presently hospitalized, and 40% are unemployed. Only three of the 63 members were conviction-free prior to joining the program. Since being on the program, 62 have been conviction-free.

Most MCDP patients appear to have given up the use of addictive drugs. At the time of writing, ten patients had completed the active treatment of their chest disease. Staff began decreasing the methadone dose in three patients who had been in the program for two to three years and showed excellent progress. Of the 127 patients interested in joining MCDP, 19 (14.9%) were rejected. Of the 93 taken into the program, 24 were lost, with a loss rate of 26%.

LINCOLN HOSPITAL—IN THE SOUTH BRONX, NEW YORK CITY

The Lincoln Hospital devised an interesting innovation in methadone stabilization and treatment based on a specific community problem. The Hospital's Drug Abuse Unit had earlier arranged a collaborative methadone program with the Bronx State Hospital, with the latter offering inpatient stabilization services and Lincoln Hospital providing the outpatient (Phase II) methadone outpatient clinic. It was soon observed that a large number of narcotic addicts were being admitted to the Surgical Ward with traumatic knife and gunshot wounds. To facilitate the recuperation period, these patients were maintained on methadone to avoid the additional shock of withdrawal while they were being treated for their injuries and repairs made. It was decided that this could constitute a natural transition into the existing methadone program for those addicts who met the usual criteria for admission to the program and evidenced an interest in participating. These patients were then screened by representatives from the program and, if accepted, were admitted into the program after they had recovered.

HARLEM HOSPITAL IN NEW YORK CITY

Harlem Hospital, apart from its regular methadone program, has an Ambulatory Detoxification Unit and a "methadone-therapeutic community." After a preliminary physical workup, the patient receives a detoxification schedule and a time is assigned by the counselor for him to come for his medication. The medication is administered twice daily in a schedule based on the patient's responsibilities: if a patient is working or attending school, special schedule adjustments are made. The usual procedure is b.i.d. morning and evening. The detoxification schedule calls for oral administration of methadone in gradually decreasing doses for a period of 12-14 days, starting with approximately 50 mg. The referring agency must assume responsibility for counseling. Twice weekly, starting 4 days after admission, patients submit urine specimens to test for possible drug abuse. For recidivists, readmission is permitted 30 days after discharge. Admission is open to narcotic addicts of all ages and both sexes. The detoxification unit is closely tied in with the day care unit and therapeutic community, where more intensive help is offered if needed.[2]

A novel feature of the program is a "methadone-therapeutic community" where residents are maintained on a stabilization dose of methadone ranging from 80-150 mg. After the addict has been on methadone for 3 months, he may decide to become drug-free. He has this option every three months. After twelve months, he is automatically detoxified over a period of six weeks. If the addict chooses to detoxify himself, he has further options: to remain in the "methadone therapeutic community," transfer to a total drug-free therapeutic community or other drug-free program component or simply leave the program.

BELLEVUE HOSPITAL— NEW YORK CITY

Addicts with Severe Psychiatric Problems

This program proposed to study the effects of methadone treatment on a population of heroin addicts with coexistent psychiatric illness. Almost all prior studies had screened out such cases from their populations.[3] The population is unselected, in the order of their admission to the hospital. Additional cases can be drawn from outpatient referrals. There are three criteria for inclusion:

> 1. Heroin addiction without alcoholism or other drug abuse
> 2. Co-existing psychiatric disorder and
> 3. The determination that the patient does not require state hospitalization and can be discharged back to the community from Bellevue.

On discharge, the patient is assigned to a therapy group. Each group contains between 8–10 members and meets twice weekly, under the leadership of a member of the professional study staff plus an ex-addict. Each patient also receives vocational counseling, social service assistance with situational problems and psychiatric treatment as indicated. Methadone is administered and periodic spot urine checks are done. It is planned to study a total population of 100 cases. Four to five months will be required for this purpose.

THE VERA PROGRAM—
THE ADDICTION RESEARCH
AND TREATMENT CORPORATION

The Vera Institute designed a proposal in 1968 which has since been implemented by the Narcotic Addiction Research and Treatment Corporation in the Bedford-Stuyvesant area of Brooklyn under Dr. Beny Primm, with plans for further expansion in the Bronx. It has been the goal of the program to eliminate what they felt were a number of research and treatment deficiencies in the Dole-Nyswander program. They therefore designed a research program in which "numerous separate investigations might be conducted at different centers through-out the city. [4,5]

Possible Variations in Treatment Techniques to be Authenticated

Ambulatory Heroin Detoxification with Methadone Support. This method would have total drug abstinence as a treatment goal. The addict would report regularly to an outpatient clinic for the medication and would receive counseling.

Ambulatory Methadone Sustenance. In this program, patients would report regularly on out-patient status and receive dosages of 30-40 mg. daily, which would not have the "blockage" effect to other narcotics. Patients would receive social service counseling, training and job placement. Contact groups would be established and de-toxified from methadone sustenance after a period of suc-cessful social adjustment.

Ambulatory Methadone Maintenance. Patients would be stabilized at the normal blocking dosages of 80-120 mgs. daily.

Pre-treatment with Methadone Support. The research plan seeks to compare the efficacy of methadone on a local spectrum of patients: —self-selected volunteer patients from waiting lists, "addict-criminals" inducted at every stage of the criminal cycle (prior to commission of a crime, after arrest but before conviction, after convic-tion, but before release). Matched groups of patients would undergo different kinds of methadone treatment and the results would be compared with findings for control groups. Later phases of treatment could be ad-ministered through the City's District Health Clinics.

METHADONE MAINTENANCE IN A PROBATION SETTING— THE NEW YORK CITY

Office of Probation of the Courts of the City of New

York in conjunction with the Beth Israel Medical Center established its own methadone program, using probation officers and other court personnel (psychiatrist, physician, and psychologist). Twenty patients were accepted from February-October 1970 and, of these, two were discharged because of rearrest. All patients had tried and failed in other methods geared to abstinence. Probationers entered the program voluntarily, and they were not penalized if they wished to withdraw. The advantages of the program are: the ease with which it could be reproduced in other court and probation and parole settings, the economical use of existing personnel and avoidance of "expensive treatment bureaucracies."[6]

THE ILLINOIS DRUG ABUSE PROGRAM

Jaffee and colleagues have reported on their use of methadone in a multi-modality program for the treatment of narcotics users in Chicago. They proceeded from the assumption that there are different kinds of addicts, and a variety of treatment approaches therefore need to be provided. The patient group was composed of a random sample of individuals who were not excluded on the basis of previous treatment failures, other drug problems, physical or psychiatric disorders or legal entanglements. Sixty patients were taken at random from a waiting list of chronic users who had volunteered for treatment.

Methadone was used in two distinct ways: (1) in high blocking doses after the Dole-Nyswander model, and (2) lower doses (less than 45 mg. daily), with the explicit statement that they might remain on this medication for only a limited period of time and it was only a stop-gap measure. When other programs became operational, they could be asked to switch to any one of them (detoxification, group therapy, cyclazocine). No patients were admitted to a hospital, and stabilization was on an outpatient basis. The procedures used thus differed from the Dole-Nyswander model in three ways: (1) stabilization was entirely ambulatory; (2) patients with current legal problems or history of psychosis, alcoholism or non-opiate abuse were not screened out; and (3) dosage was distinctly lower and probably below the level required to produce a high degree of cross-tolerance (blockade).

Results

Of sixty patients, only 7 were placed on high-dosage methadone maintenance, the remainder on low "support" dosage. The sample was predominantly black male over 30, with 9 using narcotics for more than 17 years.

From July 15 to August 15, 1968, 49 (75%) were still in active treatment and 12 were not. Only 8 of the 12 could appropriately be viewed as "treatment failures." The drop in the use of illegal drugs and rate of incarcerations was the most dramatic aspect of the patients' progress. There was a significant increase in employment, but this was due in part to their employment by the Drug Abuse Program. "The findings were clear: There is more than one way to use methadone. Most of the patients on low-dose methadone did well without a prolonged period of in-patient treatment." Another finding was that many of the low-dose methadone patients had no desire to switch to the high-dose program, but expressed a wish to be withdrawn, or participate in group therapy, cyclazocine or other abstinence-oriented programs. Results were good, also, though this was an essentially unselected group. Seven months after initiating the study, 75% of the patients were still in treatment, and making good progress; 75% of these were working and only 15% were still using drugs illicitly.

Dr. Jaffe's program was the first to use methadone maintenance in a "holding" or "pre-treatment" approach. As a means of coping with their waiting list and retaining patients for the program, 70% of the patients were thus held until they could be admitted to a regular treatment program. Drug use was reduced, but other areas did not change since no other services were offered.[7]

PHILADELPHIA

Wieland and Chambers, in the Narcotic Addict Reha-

bilitation Program in Philadelphia instituted a methadone maintenance program to replicate the Dole-
Nyswander model in New York City. Techniques of initiation and stabilization on an ambulatory bases were
demonstrated.[8]

DR. DUPONT AND THE
NARCOTICS TREATMENT
ADMINISTRATION
OF WASHINGTON, D.C.

Introduction and Overview

In the Washington program, methadone treatment is
seen as only one part of the NTA treatment program. Abstinence is encouraged for all patients. It is felt that no
drug other than methadone should be prescribed for
treatment of heroin addiction, except for occasional tranquilizers.[9]

For all NTA treated patients receiving methadone
maintenance treatment, the physician should attempt to
give a "blocking" dose of 80 to 120 milligrams a day. It is
believed that lower doses are associated with significantly higher failure rates and that lower doses do not
produce any advantage to the patient.

Outpatient methadone withdrawal (or "detox") is tried
with any patient who has a history of addiction to heroin
of less than two years, who is under 18 years of age, or
who requests this treatment. Methadone withdrawal
should begin by "catching" the addict's habit, usually
with doses in the range of twenty to fifty mg. per day.
This holding dose should then be reduced very gradually
over a four-to twelve-week period. Regular urine testing
and monitoring of the patient's taking his doses should
be followed as in the methadone maintenance program.

If a patient fails at outpatient withdrawal even if he
has used heroin for less than two years or is less than
eighteen years old, he may be considered for methadone
maintenance if he volunteers for this treatment. How-

ever, under these circumstances, written approval must be obtained from the Director of the NTA.

The procedure is for methadone detoxification not to be prolonged for more than three months. A patient on detoxification should not receive more than 50 mg. a day at any time. The physician in charge of the patient's treatment should establish a schedule for gradually decreasing doses, with abstinence to be achieved between two weeks and three months after the start of methadone detoxification.

Urine Testing

Every patient will submit a monitored urine specimen at least twice a week. After the patient has three consecutive months of clean urines, the urine testing frequency should be reduced to once a week. If there is renewed evidence of illicit drug use, then the patient should be returned to twice a week schedule until he has three more months of clean urines.

DR. BLACHLY'S OREGON PROGRAM

Self-Supporting Methadone Program

This self-supporting program of outpatient methadone maintenance, initiated in April 1969 under State University sponsorship, reported 209 patients enrolled in the program at the end of the first 50 weeks, with 39 failures and a waiting list of 95 applications. Staff agreed from the start to accept anyone who applied, with some age exceptions. A therapeutic trial was thought to be the best way to distinguish between those who would benefit from the program and those who wouldn't. Staff was subsequently pleasantly surprised by "impossible" candidates who did well, and disappointed by "good" candidates who failed.

To avoid the complications of hiring their own pharmacist to dispense methadone, the treatment team arranged for a private pharmacist to dispense oral doses and be responsible for their consumption in his presence. Patients also paid the pharmacist directly at the rate of $1.00 per dose. In addition to the daily methadone costs, the patient was charged $3 per urinalysis; 25¢ per visit to the clinic for the first 3 months, $2 for the next 9 months, and $5 per visit thereafter. Analysis for barbiturates and amphetamines was performed at $5 each only when there was clinical evidence to suspect thei use, but the patient denied it.

Dr. Blachly asserts that this type of "pure" drug treatment program, "which relies on the patients using existing community agencies for social, vocational, and financial assistance seems to be producing results indistinguishable from those having comprehensive services, and is much less expensive. However, 50 weeks of operation is undoubtedly too brief a period to assess long-term effects."[10]

PITTSBURGH, PENNSYLVANIA

In the predominantly black Manchester area of Pittsburgh, Dr. Charles Burks described his Methadone Maintenance Clinic operated by the Black Action Inc. Drug Abuse Program as "conceived and implemented by the black citizens of Manchester, responding to an urgent need and desire to save and, hopefully better our community."[11]

The drug abuse program was started in August 1968, with two physicians and two staff members, volunteering their services until funds were secured from the state of Pennsylvania, which regards drug addiction as a mental health problem. Methadone did not become an official part of the program until June 1969.

The average Black Action patient comes to the center at the age of 22 and carrying a $25 a day drug habit. His first step toward admission is an "intake interview" with one or more members of Black Action's eight-man counseling staff.

Dr. Burks makes it clear that he regards methadone not as an end in itself, but as a means of approaching the elimination of all drug addiction. "An addict on methadone is not cured of his addiction, but he is able to function as a normal human being without the pressure of satisfying a monstrous habit." For some young addicts, this may mean being able to have a job for the first time; for others, week-end trips and vacations without worry about where to find an out-of-town "fix."

Members of the Black Action staff are quick to recognize that the methadone program is not suitable for all addicts. Counselor Larry Turner states that "To me, methadone is the last shot. A youngster, if caught in time, should have the privilege of trying another way." Says Dr. Burks, "We need more time to do research to find out which patients can do without methadone and then develop a program for them." And, " ... while the search for a cure is of obvious importance, as this search is taking place, proper attention must be given to dealing with the immediate social and personal dilemmas of the addict. It is an accepted fact that all addicts, black and white, need look no further that the ghetto to find heroin."

CALIFORNIA DEPARTMENT OF CORRECTIONS

Legislation was enacted in California, effective November 1, 1970, removing previously restrictive legislation in regard to setting up methadone programs. The California Dept. of Corrections instituted a methadone program as part of its Civil Commitment Program. The new project is intended to explore the use of methadone as an adjunct to the rehabilitative efforts of the Parole and Community Services Division in the management of drug addicts for a period of one year.

The program will involve a maximum of 200 adult parolees and outpatients: 150 will be from the Felon Program and 50 will be from the Civil Addict Program. Both will include an appropriately representative number of female participants.

The following Selection Criteria are to be used:

(a) That all candidates be under active parole supervision and in the community at the time of application;

(b) That the parolee or out-patient be 21 years of age or older;

(c) That the participant have a history of opiate drug use of at least five years duration;

(d) That the program participant should have had a history of at least one prior detoxification and narcotic treatment failure;

(e) That the parolees' and out-patients' participation in this program be voluntary.[12]

SANTA CLARA, CALIFORNIA

The Santa Clara County Methadone Program (San Jose, California) authorized by the State of California Research Advisory Panel had been in operation for about a year at the time of writing, and two hundred patients admitted. The main research aim initially was to conduct blind dosage schedules. Random urine testing and a special questionnaire administered periodically and processed by computer were the sources of data about heroin use, side effects, and social rehabilitation.[13] This study is summarized in the chapter on the "Comparison of High and Low-Dose Techniques in Methadone Treatment."

PROGRAM FOR ADOLESCENT HEROIN ABUSERS IN NEW YORK CITY

The interesting paper by Millman and Nyswander[14] describing their program for adolescent heroin addicts in New York City (actually a low-dose maintenance program) is similarly described elsewhere in this volume.

THE MIAMI PROGRAM

The Miami Program can be considered "innovative" only in the sense of serving as a caveat or object lesson on how not to institute a methadone program. In brief, pressure was exerted to establish, immediately, a structured program in an area where methadone had been freely prescribed and dispensed by local physicians and pharmacists, and by loosely-organized "programs". In one such program, approximately 600 people were receiving regular methadone prescriptions ranging between 400-600 mg. daily as well as other narcotics and a variety of sleeping medications.[15]

Miami became aware of its "methadone problem" through admissions to the Medical School's Psychiatric Hospital emergency room and evaluations in jail. Increasing numbers of patients were discovered to be taking methadone either regularly or sporadically when heroin was unavailable, or to be involved in illegal traffic in methadone. Most frightening was the fact that the incidence was highest in the 16-25 year-old group. Its ready availability not only led to methadone diversion and addiction, but opened avenues to heroin addiction as well: —youngsters could sell the methadone tablets prescribed or use them for intravenous injection after grinding and dissolving them in water.

While the existence of a problem was thus recognized for some time, county representatives and medical school officials were reluctant to assume responsibility for action. The situation came to a head with the death in 1969 of three adolescents, allegedly of methadone overdose. The largest source of methadone dispensing and prescribing, a clinic sponsored by the Catholic Welfare Bureau, was closed after Federal officials insisted that only a well-controlled program would be tolerated. The precipitous closing of the clinic left a number of bona fide patients without medication or other help.

Under this crisis, representatives of Dade County, the Medical Association, University of Miami Medical School, United Health Foundation and others planned a clinic to be operated jointly by the County and Medical School at the Jackson Memorial Hospital. For a time, the emergency room of the hospital was flooded with patients in a panic because their supply had been cut off. Because of these bad experiences, the Medical School at first planned not to recreate a methadone maintenance program, only a detoxification center, but this proved not feasible.

The methadone center was opened in August 1969 on a shaky financial basis and staffed largely by inexperienced volunteers. Volunteer doctors were easily conned into increasing dosages and prescribing more than a day's supply at a time. Staff was also aware that some of the methadone was being sold illicitly, that the clinic was not reaching the black community and that methadone was still being prescribed by several physicians in Miami in large amounts and dosages. After a year, the clinic has been established on a far firmer basis today and approximates the programs operating effectively in other areas.

GENERAL DISCUSSION

A New York Times article dated July 26, 1970, offers a broad picture of the status of methadone maintenance programming nationally: it is described as gaining powerful foothold in dozens of cities throughout the country. More than 60 methadone centers had filed applications with the Federal Government to use methadone at that time. "Many of the centers, public and private, have chosen methadone maintenance hurriedly in the last several months amid rising public alarm over addiction and, according to recent independent studies, confirm the dramatic successes attributed by the New York program in keeping addicts off drugs and out of jail.[16]

"At the same time, there are indications of growing abuse of the drug. BNADD guidelines require that methadone, which is as addicting as heroin, be given only under conditions of close medical supervision and scientific evaluation.

"The only city in which legal opposition to methadone has been raised is Fort Worth, where Dr. Peter J. Carter, a private physician is fighting an attempt by the State Board of Medical Examiners to censure him and cancel his medical license for prescribing methadone.

"Private physicians are particularly unhappy about the new Federal regulations. One doctor in the Washington area says he has treated more than 2,500 addicts in the last two years. But the new guidelines, which require frequent urine tests and other controls, make it very difficult for the individual practitioner to continue such a high patient load.

... In New York City, Dr. Beny Primm reported on the work of the Addiction Treatment and Research Corporation in the Bedford Stuyvesant section of Brooklyn. He stated that he had 301 addicts taking methadone, 36 of whom were on methadone without other supportive services. By October 1, 1970, Dr. Primm hopes to have 350 addicts of a projected total patient population of about 650 receiving methadone under these conditions. Dr. Primm's program is experimenting with a variety of ways of using methadone. He has been using somewhat lower doses than Dole-Nyswander and actively encouraging addicts towards eventual drug freedom.

... Milton J. Luger, Chairman of the New York State Narcotic Addiction Control Commission, which helps to finance the Beth Israel Medical Center program and others, said that, just on the basis of programs already started, about 13,000 addicts would be on methadone by the end of the year. But at the rate new programs are starting, the number could easily approximate the 20,000 Governor Rockefeller said he wanted earlier this year when the Legislature approved a $15 million expansion of methadone programs in New York.[11]

Dole has stressed the problems to be anticipated in the next few years in relation to this vast proliferation of methadone programs—which poses serious administrative and treatment problems. He is concerned about the use of methadone for "criminal addicts" and about the possible role of private physicians in maintenance; believes leadership must remain in the hands of the medical profession to "head off Government interference."[17]

Comments

This chapter has attempted to describe a representative cross-section of innovative methadone programs in the United States for which data were available at the time of writing. As the *Times* article emphasized, there has been a vast proliferation of programs, some replicating the classic Dole-Nyswander model, others modifying or building on it in line with the particular demographic characteristics and social needs of the area; though often also deriving their particular coloration and rationale from the personalities and conceptualizations of the individual program directors. The numerous programs thus offer a unique opportunity for learning and innovation, based on the individual experiences and expertise accumulated. Research is underway in relation to such questions as optimal dosage for different kinds of patients, the role of urinalysis and ancillary services, reasons for continued "cheating" of certain patients even after lengthy stabilization on methadone, development of longer-acting forms such as acetyl-methodol and others.

Apparently, the astonishing expansion of methadone programming offers continuing testimony to its effectiveness in the treatment of hard-core addicts. Beyond this, however, the existence of so many variegated programs here and abroad should insure that paralysis never sets in; and simultaneously afford a remarkable opportunity for further learning about the nature and treatment of opiate addiction.

REFERENCES

1. Hoffman: A methadone program for addicts with chest diseases, 1970.

2. Wesley: Program description of Harlem Hospital narcotic program, mimeographed, 1969.

3. Bellevue Hospital: New York City methadone proposal for patients with severe psychiatric problems, 1970.

4. Primm: Ancillary services in methadone treatment in the Bedford-Stuyvesant experience, Proceedings Third National Methadone Conference, 1970.

5. Riordan: Progress Report of Addiction Research and Treatment Corporation Evaluation Team, Report submitted to Department of Law Enforcement Assistance Administration, unpublished, mimeographed, 1970.

6. Joseph: Court services and methadone treatment, Proceedings Third National Methadone Conference, 1970.

7. Jaffe, et. al.: Experience with the use of methadone in a multimodality program for the treatment of narcotics users, 1969.

8. Chambers: Drug abuse in Philadelphia, 1971.

9. Dupont: Personal Communication and program materials for Narcotic Treatment Administration of Washington, D.C., 1970.

10. Blachly: Report on Oregon program described in Narcotic Research Information Exchange Newsletter, 1970.

11. Ebony: The methadone method, magazine article, Report on Black Action program, 1970.

12. California Department of Correction: Proposal for methadone program, 1970.

13. Goldstein: Uniform dosage of methadone hydrochloride, described in Narcotic Research Information Exchange, 1970.

14. Millman and Nyswander: Slow detoxification of adolescent heroin addicts in New York City, Proceedings Third National Methadone Conference, New York City, 1970.

15. Hoogerbetts: Methadone in Miami, 1970.

16. Reinhold: *New York Times* article entitled "Methadone for drug addicts is gaining in popularity," 1970.

17. Dole: The future of a medical institution, Proceedings Third National Methadone Conference, New York City, 1970.

Chapter 24.

The Rationale and Design for a Multi-modality

Leon Brill
Carl D. Chambers

Methadone maintenance programs have been subjected to a good deal of criticism because of the impression conveyed that they entail a lifelong dependency or, at the very least, maintenance for an indefinite though very prolonged period of time. It may be well to recall that such a view of methadone is relatively recent: for many years now methadone has been the drug of choice for detoxifying addicts from opiates. Originally developed by the Germans in World War II, it was used thereafter in the standard "substitution withdrawal" procedure in which addicts were switched from opiates to methadone, and then gradually withdrawn from the methadone to minimize the withdrawal symptoms. This procedure was deemed practicable only in a "drug-free environment"—i.e., an institution or hospital—in line with the only treatment goal felt indicated—total immediate abstinence.

This goal was subsequently questioned from the standpoint that nothing very worthwhile had been accomplished if an addict was deprived of his defenses, but remained too incapacitated to function in the community in a socially productive manner. The idea of methadone maintenance was associated with the concept that social rehabilitation of an individual is a worthwhile goal in

* The original version of this paper appeared in Social Work, 16(3), 39-51, 1971. Reprinted by permission.

itself, even irrespective of the achievement of total abstinence. This rehabilitation concept was reinforced by use
in recent years of the major tranquilizers to help psychotic patients leave State hospitals and return to the community; and the fact that many individuals were leading socially useful lives and functioning adequately with the
help of medication—as in the use of insulin for diabetics
and Dilantin® (Parke-Davis) for epileptics.

Some critics of methadone maintenance have urged
that more emphasis be placed on methadone *therapy* -
i.e., on the use of methadone as an intervening support.
With intensive counseling and group therapy services
built in, it might be possible to help a number of patients
be rehabilitated or "cured" and give up the prop of methadone as well in time.[1] Pioneers in the field spoke only of
methadone *maintenance*, which would be required indefinitely, if not forever, because of a "metobolic deficiency"-
either existing previously, or else consequent to sustained opiate abuse. They de-emphasized the idea of prior
psychological problems and, therefore, the need for intensive psychotherapeutic services. They have nevertheless
engaged in some experimentation to learn whether
selected patients could function without methadone after
a suitable interval.

In their previous writings, the authors proposed a
multi-modality approach to the problem of opiate abuse,
emanating from the belief that there is no such universal
as "the addict," but rather a variety of addicts with different social and psychological characteristics, varying
ages, ethnic and class backgrounds, stages of involvement in the addiction system and states of readiness for
help. By building in evaluation to determine what characteristics lent themselves to help under particular treatment modalities, it was hoped to develop effective objective criteria for the screening and treatment of patients.
Thus, after an initial interview, patients could be
referred to the modality best equipped to help
them—whether a residential center, religious approach,
the narcotics-antagonist cyclazocine, methadone or
another program or even combination of
programs—either to reinforce treatment or cover different stages of treatment.

More recently, the thought of developing a multi-modality approach within methadone treatment itself arose. Although the classic pioneering approach has been that of Dole-Nyswander in New York City, much experience has been accumulated already in developing variations and innovations on methadone maintenance—as in utilizing ambulatory stabilization for selected patients, instead of a six-weeks' impatient phase. This approach would answer some of the criticisms levelled against methadone maintenance as the "substitution of one opiate for another"—or as a "lifelong crutch"—first because the approaches using methadone would have the same goal as other treatment approaches—i.e., the achievement of abstinence as quickly as possible. In all the methadone approaches to be discussed, even that of variable dose, high-level methadone maintenance, the goal visualized was abstinence as a first possibility—though simultaneously building in research and treatment services to learn which patients can get off in time and which may indeed need to be maintained indefinitely.

The multi-modality concept of methadone treatment thus comprises a gradient or continuum of two elements:

> (1) initial attempts geared to abstinence and ranging from low to regular high-dose methadone if the initial efforts fail; and
> (2) building in increasing chemical support and increasingly intensive services with more resistive or difficult patients.

The gradient would, concretely, include the following steps:

(1) *Inpatient or ambulatory detoxification*—This would have the clear goal of helping addicts get off heroin or other opiates on either an inpatient or ambulatory basis. The period of effort could cover from weeks to months until the goal of abstinence is achieved. Psychological help in the way of concrete services and supportive assistance could be offered simultaneously towards this end, though more intensive services could be provided if required.

(2) *Low-dose methadone*—If patients do not succeed in

the inpatient or ambulatory detoxification, the next step of low-dose methadone maintenance at about 40-50 mg. daily can be attempted. The express goal here is still abstinence as soon as possible. It would be recognized that this group requires some degree of chemical support analogous to tranquilizers, to help them cope with anxiety, stress or depression. Psychological services would be built similar to those in Group 1. The maintenance would be geared to a longer period of support, ranging from several months to about a year.

(3) If this group (2) did not respond, we could then go on to high-dose methadone support. As we can see, each step has thus far served not only to help those addicts who can respond at the level of (1) or (2), but also to screen out those who cannot and thus prepare them for the next step.

Even in group (3), it is hoped that by providing intensive individual counseling and group therapy, we may be able to sift out those who can get off high-dose methadone, 80-120 mg. or more in time, from those who may indeed need to be maintained indefinitely.

(4) Combined residential centers plus methadone maintenance—Some methadone patients have been described as so "weak" or "psychopathic" that they cannot make it in the community even with the help of methadone maintenance plus counseling or other services. For them, a combined residential center plus methadone is suggested since they may require a period of removal from the community, and an experience of socialized living and therapy. Methadone could serve additionally, as a bridge in making the subsequent transition back to the community.

It would be useful to present, at this point, more detailed descriptions of how the various methadone approaches have worked in practice. This section will cover a discussion of:

    I. The Inpatient Detoxification of Narcotic Addicts with Methadone
   II. The Ambulatory Detoxification of Narcotic Addicts with Methadone
     1. Short-Term Detoxification
     2. Long-Term Detoxification

THE INPATIENT DETOXIFICATION OF NARCOTIC ADDICTS WITH METHADONE

The use of methadone during the gradual withdrawal from an opiate was pioneered by Isbell in 1949 at the U.S. Public Health Service Hospital at Lexington, Kentucky. Isbell administered the drug subcutaneously in a dose of 1 mg of methadone for 4 mg of morphine. This regimen was repeated twice a day.

The Lexington facility, now an N.I.M.H. Clinical Research Center, currently detoxifies narcotic addicts with oral doses of methadone two to four times a day and in ranges from 5 mg to 20 mg, depending in both instances on the severity of the withdrawal signs. The detoxification progresses with a reduction in the methadone at the rate of 5 mg to 10 mg per day. Following this regimen, withdrawal can normally be completed within seven to ten days.

One must remember, however, that the detoxification accomplished in the above manner represents only a *primary* stage of withdrawal. A *secondary* stage of withdrawal not characterized by marked physical discomfort for the addict-patient, but with discernible physical symptoms appears to last for another two or three weeks. These symptoms, usually high blood pressure, rapid pulse rate and a high body temperature, will not normally require medical attention. Concurrent symptoms of depression or anxiety are quite frequent during this stage of withdrawal and, in most cases, do require a chemotherapeutic regimen. The *terminal* stage of withdrawal apparently begins approximately nine weeks after the *primary* stage of withdrawal, and lasts up to 30 weeks. Martin and Jasinski, scientists at the Addiction Research Center in Lexington, Kentucky, first reported this prolonged physical dependence in 1968.[2] Their findings indicated that addict-patients during this *terminal* stage of withdrawal exhibit lower than normal blood pressure, pulse rate and body temperature. These symptoms as well as a marked decrease in the respiratory center's sensivity to carbon dioxide and elevated levels of epinephrine in the urine - possibly indicating hyper-responsivity to stress - have been documented several months after the initial detoxification associated with the *primary* stage of withdrawal.

Of marked significance to clinicians who utilize only short-period inpatient detoxification regimens is the probability that drug hunger will be ever-present in their abstinent addict-patients for up to seven months. Coupling their findings with human test subjects with earlier animal studies, Martin and Jasinski suggest that dependence on the opiates may cause changes in the central nervous system and produce altered physiological functions, an altered psyche and increased drug-seeking behavior.[2]

In view of the above, it would appear that the inpatient detoxification of narcotic addicts with methadone will be less than adequate for preventing relapse in most addicts if it encompasses only treatment and follow-up during the *primary* stage of detoxification.

THE AMBULATORY DETOXIFICATION OF NARCOTIC ADDICTS WITH METHADONE

It has been well documented that ambulatory detoxification can be an effective treatment modality for some, but not all narcotic addicts.[3,4] Quite obviously, this modality is most effective with those addict-clients who are either well integrated and highly motivated to give up their addiction or with those addict-clients who had become addicted only recently. The Narcotic Addict Rehabilitation Clinic located at the Philadelphia General Hospital pioneered in the development of this modality, and it is from their experience with ambulatory detoxification regimens that the following descriptions were generated.

Addict-clients come to the outpatient clinic voluntarily after having been on a waiting list for up to six months. They are usually self-referred, having heard of the program from their peers. The only criteria for admission are addiction to a narcotic drug and residence in one of three mental health catchment areas. Experience has shown that psychotic patients and mixed addictions need not be excluded from treatment. Psychiatric or medical admissions to a hospital can be arranged when indicated by the clinical conditions. This occurs, however, in less than 10 percent of the cases.

Most addicts can begin treatment of 40 mg of methadone per day, either 20 mg b.i.d. or 10 mg q.i.d. Those with small habits (1-3 bags per day) may only require 20 to 30 mg per day, and those with large habits (over 7 bags per day) may require initial doses of 50 to 80 mg per day. Addict-clients must be seen every day during the initial phase of treatment; the original dose may be adjusted when necessary, although such adjustments would be the exception.

The 10 mg *tablets* of methadone have been used in the Philadelphia program for several reasons: (1) Low doses of methadone, if taken in a single dose, are *only effective* for 6-12 hours, and tablets provide a convenient way to prescribe divided dosage; (2) addict-clients can space their dose as they perceive withdrawal distress, which may vary from patient to patient or from day to day; (3) addict-clients know exactly how much methadone they are getting, which reduces suspiciousness and mistrust. Liquid methadone could, of course, also be used but the division and spacing of doses would make it impractical with any large number of patients. The possibility of the illicit diversion of medication must be a major concern among those who use pills. Illicit diversion of medication cannot occur if only small numbers of tablets are dispensed at frequent intervals, preferably on a daily basis and if the addict-patients ingest portions of their medication while being observed in the clinic.

On each daily visit, the addict-patient must see his counselor, who should be a social worker or trained ex-addict, for a 20- to 30-minute session. The main therapeutic emphasis should be on supportive counseling on present and future behavior, including such areas as drug abuse, employment, domestic relations, interpersonal relations, and general attitudes. The work role, being a major index of male normality, should be strongly encouraged and assisted, when indicated, by job counseling or vocational training. After the counseling session, the patient receives a day's supply of methadone and leaves a urine specmen, which is analyzed for methadone, morphine, quinine, barbiturates, amphetamines, and cocaine. This urine surveillance is a primary component within any detoxification program, but is most significant in an ambulatory program.

Since there is no selection process, each addict-patient must be evaluated by a psychiatrist before beginning treatment. The psychiatrist can assist the counselor in devising an individualized treatment plan and managing any psychiatric complications, such as schizophrenia and severe depression. The psychiatrist must also be available for frequent consultation with the counselors.

Ideally, when the addict-client has ceased "cheating" with heroin or other drugs, and has shown some progress toward emotional and social rehabilitation, the daily dose of methadone will be decreased by 10 mg. If he is working, the frequency of clinic visits should also be reduced to 2 or 3 times per week. With further progress, the daily dose can again be reduced by 10 mg and the frequency of clinic visits may also be reduced to once a week. In the event of emotional or behavioral relapse, either the dosage or the number of visits or both can again be increased until restabilization occurs. The process of reducing the dose begins again when the clinical condition warrants it.

Certain aspects of this ambulatory treatment can be viewed as a reward-punishment system. These include the variations in the frequency of clinic visits, the adjustments in dosage, the possibility of temporary suspension from treatment, and the verbal responses of the counselor. Recalcitrant patients may be required to accomplish some task in a given time period (e.g., obtain a job, cease cheating, etc.) or face suspension for a period of time (usually 30 days). This reward-punishment system provides a concrete frame of reference for both the patient and his counselor to judge overall progress.

If there is a persistent failure to respond effectively to detoxification treatment, two alternatives are available at the Philadelphia clinic:—transfer to methadone maintenance or suspension from treatment. It would, of course, be preferable if other modalities of treatment were available, e.g., inpatient detoxification facilities, halfway houses, etc.

Detoxification regimens accomplished in outpatient clinics must be highly individualized. Detoxification can be accomplished with some addict-clients in a matter of a few days. In others, however, this process may span several months. Central to this modality must be the philosophy that addicts have the right to become drug-free, *but* the quest for this goal depends primarily upon the addict-client's perception of his ability to function satisfactorily within various social roles in an abstinent state.

Short-Term Detoxification - A Case Example

At the time of acceptance for treatment, this 41-year-old black male was living with his legally married spouse. The subject had first used drugs at age 15 and had undergone a total of 7 formal detoxifications. He admitted to a total of 7 arrests, of which 4 were drug-related. He had been incarcerated a total of 15 years.

Immediately prior to this current addiction, the subject had remained abstinent voluntarily for nine years. During these years, he worked steadily, sometimes holding two full-time jobs during the normal workweek while working part-time as an entertainer on weekends. Although the precise reason for returning to drugs is unknown, his contact with other musicians, some of whom used drugs, was at least a factor. He began "snorting" cocaine and eventually returned to "shooting" heroin. He had been readdicted to heroin 4 months when the detoxification began.

His detoxification began at 40 mg daily. He remained on this daily dose for ten days. At his request, on the eleventh day he was reduced to 30 mg which was continued for three days. At this time, he reduced himself to 20 mg for two days and 10 mg for one day. At the end of 16 days, he declared himself detoxified and requested termination of the medication.

At last contact, the subject had remained abstinent for approximately three months. During that time, however, he continued to return to the clinic once a week for a group therapy session and for a one-to-one encounter with a supportive counselor. He credited these two activities with assisting him in remaining abstinent.

Case Example of a Long-Term Detoxification

At the time of acceptance for treatment, this 24-year-old black female was separated from her legal spouse and was living alone. She supported herself and 2 children through "hustling" and through welfare grants. The subject had first used drugs at age 18 and had never undergone a formal detoxification. She had never been arrested.

This female subject typifies those addict-clients who will spend considerable time trying to manipulate a detoxification program into providing them with an "easy habit." They will take their methadone so they are never "sick," but when drugs are readily available will skip their medicine or "shoot over it." It is to their advantage to prolong the detoxification process as long as possible. Several factors combined to allow this particular subject to extend her regimen with little effort at detoxification for a full five months. She was young, attractive, and rather skillful in using a slight limp, the aftermath of a polio attack, to portray herself as a helpless individual who needed to be sheltered and given preferential treatment. Not only were most of the male addict-clients interceding in her behalf; she was able to seduce, literally, one of the staff who in turn interfered with the normal progression of the detoxification process. Her own individual counselor was also easily manipulated during the initial weeks of treatment.

After three months of little or no progress, however,

very severe limits were placed on her behavior, e.g., increased frequency of clinic visits to pick up her methadone, increased contacts with her supportive counselor, and punishment by the withholding of medication for all of the rule infractions from "heroin cheating" to being late for appointments. Once she came to realize this structuring was because people had faith she could become detoxified and abstinent if she would seriously exert herself, her detoxification became possible.

This subject spent one month on a daily dose of 40 mg, two months on 30 mg, 1.5 months on 20 mg and two weeks on 10 mg.

At last contact, she had been abstinent for three months and, although she was still receiving welfare, was living within the confines of her grant, having ceased "hustling."

As indicated earlier, not every addict is capable of, or willing to become abstinent. A two-year evaluation of the Philadelphia experience indicated only approximately 25 percent of those attempting a detoxification were capable of, or willing to complete it. An additional 25 percent, while incapable of becoming abstinent, were willing to remain in treatment. Fortunately, the Philadelphia clinic also provided a methadone maintenance program which could meet these addict-clients' needs. The remaining 50 percent of the addict-clients who attempted detoxification, but neither completed that program nor began a maintenance program, terminated the treatment process against the advice of the staff, were incarcerated, moved away from the city or were suspended for rule infractions.

It is apparent that a large number of addicts will "use" this type of program in various ways. For example, those who come along only once or twice quite probably only want the methadone to hold them over until they can secure heroin. This problem is eliminated by having a waiting period before dispensing medicine. A second large group who "use" such a program consists of those who want only to reduce their habit or to have an easy habit combining methadone and heroin. Some systemic benefit is derived from the first since the addict does not have to steal as much to support his habit. The latter must be discovered and either terminated or transferred to a maintenance program where he will be unable to receive the euphoric effects of the heroin. Urinalysis is the most effective tool in isolating the persons who only want an easy habit.

In spite of the inherent problems associated with this type of program, there are a number of theoretical and practical considerations in favor of outpatient detoxification. Of primary clinical importance is the fact that the rehabilitation occurs in the community with all of its normal stresses and temptations. The ability to cope with these problems has much greater poignancy and relevance to patients than the limited environment of an institution or the somewhat artificial projections of what will happen after discharge. Furthermore, certain types of behavior can occur in the community which would be intolerable in an institution, including sexual intercourse, aggression and drug abuse. In most hospitals or therapeutic communities, any of these behaviors are grounds for immediate discharge and termination of treatment. By contrast, in an outpatient clinic, these behaviors become topics for therapeutic discussion; and, in fact, may represent essential learning experiences for both the patients and the staff. Treatment does *not* have to be terminated and the deviancy can be resolved rather than a solution imposed.

Secondly, outpatient treatment avoids the difficulties of re-entry into the community. After extended institutionalization, re-entry is traumatic and often results in relapse to drugs. Recognizing this, the Philadelphia clinic has provided supportive counseling and non-medicine follow-up therapy for ex-addicts during their re-entry phase from other institutions. Even well-planned reintegration is difficult for the ex-addict returning to his drug-using environment.

Thirdly, some addicts do not seek treatment for fear of jeopardizing their jobs, their school attendance, or their maternal roles. They will, however, accept treatment in an outpatient clinic where they can continue their normal activities. Experience has shown this group to have an excellent prognosis for successful treatment.

Those attempting to detoxify narcotic addicts in these outpatient clinics quite rightly believe that the 25 percent who do achieve abstinence represent sufficient justification for requiring all addict-clients to attempt the process. Related to this belief, however, is the availability of other methadone programs to service those who could not or would not detoxify. As such, a detoxification attempt should become the pre-treatment phase for methadone maintenance programs.

THE MAINTENANCE OF NARCOTIC ADDICTS WITH METHADONE

The clinical basis typically utilized in justifying methadone maintenance programs is that in *sufficient* doses, methadone will produce a blockade to other narcotics while producing few side effects, and will markedly reduce drug-craving in stabilized patients. Sufficient daily doses to accomplish this have been reported as low as 40 mg but normally exceed 60 mg with a mean of 110 mg.[5] Daily doses at these levels, however, must be considered as representing only the "high-dose maintenance" modality. There is a smaller group of addict-clients who will stabilize themselves on very low daily doses of methadone, e.g., 10 to 30 mg.

Low-dose methadone maintenance appears to be a treatment of choice for certain addict-clients who *do not* require a cross-tolerance or blockade as a deterrent for further heroin abuse. Drug-craving for these persons is suppressed at these low-dose levels and they appear to "use" the methadone as a form of tranquilizer or antidepressant while they reconstruct or indeed, in some cases, construct their lives. In short, methadone is being used as a stabilizing drug, which offers an extended period of time for rehabilitation to occur without any of the withdrawal problems associated with normal maintenance level doses. Used in this manner, it permits outpatient treatment without the usual institutional restraints in much the same way as the various psychotropic drugs have permitted the outpatient treatment of psychiatric patients.

Low-Dose Maintenance—A Case Example

At the time of acceptance into treatment as a detoxification patient, this 37-year-old black female had been using drugs for 18 years and had undergone 6 formal cures. She was divorced and, during a recent two-year prison term, her four children had been placed in separate foster homes. This subject's background included 8 arrests, one prison term and one extended stay in a mental hospital for an undisclosed psychosis. Most of the subject's adult life had revolved around drugs, lesbian "marriages" and affairs with much older men who had fathered her four children. She supported her drug habit through manipulating her lesbian partners and older "tricks."

The addict-client was initiated into treatment as a detoxification at 40 mg daily. On this dose she was able to begin work as a practical nurse and cease her lesbian activities. She was able to secure custody of her four children. One child, her oldest, resisted returning to her mother so the subject quit working and went on welfare to be able to spend more time with the children. With a limited amount of concurrent psychotropic medication and extensive supportive counseling, her daily methadone dose was reduced to 15 mg. After six months at this dose, it became apparent she was unwilling or unable to detoxify or to even reduce this daily dose. Attempts to enforce such a reduction were consistently countered with inappropriate clinical symptoms and behavior.

At this stabilized daily dose of 15 mg of methadone (and she is, of course, aware this is her daily dose), she does not "cheat," experiences no drug hunger, is not involved in any illegal activity, and engages in neither homosexual nor "unhealthy" heterosexual relations with older men. Until the time all these roles become habitual and inculcated, no attempt will be made to force total detoxification upon her.

Most addict-clients who are unable or unwilling to detoxify will require high-dose maintenance. While the Philadelphia experiences must be viewed as inconclusive, probably less than 20 percent of those addict-clients requiring maintenance will be capable of profiting from a low-dose regimen.

High-dose methadone maintenance will be the treatment or choice for those addict-clients who *do* require a cross-tolerance or blockade as a deterrent to further heroin abuse. Drug-craving for these persons is suppressed only with high doses of methadone and almost universally reappears when the daily dose is reduced below 40 mg.

In the high-dose maintenance programs, addict-clients are initiated at the 40-60 mg dose per day level, with gradual increases until individual stabilization occurs, usually in the 80-100 mg range. Most programs require up to six weeks on an inpatient basis to accomplish this stabilization. Experience at the Philadelphia clinic indicates this stabilization can also be accomplished on an ambulatory basis.[6]

High-Dose Maintenance—A Case Example

This 37-year-old married black male with a 16-year history of drug abuse, typifies the rather large group of addict-patients who are either unwilling or incapable of detoxifying. Rather than suspend these persons or to carry them indefinitely in a treatment program which is quite obviously inappropriate, they should be transferred to another modality, e.g., methadone maintenance. Although this subject had successfully detoxified on an earlier treatment admission, he had relapsed shortly after becoming abstinent, ostensibly because of the distress of being cut across the face with a razor over an $8.00 debt. On the basis of the apparently successful first treatment, his reinstatement into treatment was for a second detoxification.

During approximately six months of treatment at a daily dose of 40 mg, the subject continued to use heroin daily. This daily "cheating" occurred in spite of several punitive measures taken. He was made to come to the clinic daily for his medicine, was required to meet with his supportive counselor for at least three sessions a week and underwent several encounters with supervising therapists. When all of these failed, a temporary suspension of two weeks was imposed. Detoxification was reinstated at 40 mg and arbitrarily reduced to 30 mg after a month. He continued to use heroin daily. It was at this time that the addict-client was counseled concerning the implications of high-dose methadone maintenance and, with his permission, he was transferred.

This subject stabilized in three weeks at a daily dose of 100 mg. At this dose level, he reported his drug craving was stemmed and he ceased attempting to "shoot over" his medicine. This was confirmed through urinalysis. During six months of high-dose maintenance, the subject had engaged in only occasional "cheating" with heroin. Two factors appear related to this cheating. First, he seemed determined to test the medication to see if it was still "working" and second, he maintained an attitude that since he was employed and wasn't causing any problems, he owed himself an occasional bag of heroin as a "treat." It was anticipated that personality or character reformation sufficient to alleviate these attitudes would require long-term treatment.

The value of an outpatient stabilization technique is seen in two factors of this subject's history. First, he was able to maintain his work role as a dental laboratory technician during the entire process. His employer was, and remains unaware that the subject used drugs. This buffering might not have been possible if an inpatient phase of treatment were required. A hidden addict was able to remain hidden. Second, the counselor who knew most about this subject's history was able to use this knowledge in adjusting the addict-client to the new modality.

COMBINED METHADONE
RESIDENTIAL CENTER FACILITY

This facility is visualized as a further intensive rehabilitative approach for addicts who have failed either in the residential center or methadone treatment program; as well as those who have never had any real experience of community embeddedness in terms of close family ties, jobs and interpersonal relationships, and have therefore suffered serious lacunae in the socialization or "habilitation" process.

According to the Gearing and other studies,[7,8] a number of methadone patients needed to be discharged because of behavioral or "sociopathic" features, which made it impossible for them to relate to the program, especially with the limited psychotherapeutic services offered. A number went on to other forms of drug abuse, continued to engage in criminal activities or selling of methadone and gave other evidence of being unable to shed their addictive life style. In the Lincoln Hospital methadone program, for example, a number of addicts were located who were homeless, had severed all family ties, were "catting" it on the street and occupying abandoned buildings in the South Bronx "jungle," and strongly needed some period of stable living where they could benefit from a group experience.

By the same token, available statistics from Synanon and prototype facilities point to very large numbers of dropouts, 50% in the first few weeks and ranging up to 72% thereafter. The focus in these facilities, moreover, has been on the intramural stay, with less emphasis placed on their "re-entry" to the community (Phase III). Synanon maintains very close ties with its residents and apparently never lets go. Graduates, after a number of years, may live outside the residence, but still remain in close proximity. In fact, what is advocated by Synanon is not a return of residents to society, but rather a reverse movement of squares into Synanon, "the only sane society." While residents gain greatly in self-awareness and knowledge of program goals, there appears to be little correlation between this understanding and an ability to return substantial numbers to the community. Those residents who cannot tolerate an indefinite, if not permanent stay and finally break away, relapse to drugs for the most part. It is these "failures" or dropouts, who may, with the help of methadone, be enabled to effect a transition to the community and obtain enough support until they can function independently of both methadone and the residential center.

Rationale for Residential Center

While we cannot enter into any elaborate analysis of the structure and functions of a residential center, we would like to indicate some of the important underlying assumptions. The addict who enters one of these facilities finds himself in an entirely new world in which his addict patterns of behavior and values are rather vehemently rejected. The rejection comes from a source close to him, namely, ex-addicts who have become abstinent for the most part by going through the same residential experience themselves. The concept of a communal organization or a community whose members share daily experiences is of vital importance in this setting. The closeness achieved has been described in terms of the "extended family," and banishment from the family group represents a most drastic punishment, which is used as a lever for social control. Characteristic also, is an achievable status system, with ex-addict leaders serving as successful role models. The new resident is visualized as an underdeveloped, inmature personality, who has never grown up. He can become part of the group by increasingly accepting responsibility and the community's standards and values. The rewards for conforming are upward social mobility since you can become a professional ex-addict and also cast aside the use of drugs and addictive life style. Violations of norms are treated as an attack upon the entire group. There are serious punishments for transgressions—"haircuts," silent treatment, ridicule and, of course, banishment if the transgression is serious enough. Through encounters and longer face-to-face sessions, "stews" and marathons, residents are forced to put aside resistances, lower defenses and face themselves in powerful direct confrontations with free expression of feeling.

Methadone Dropouts

In the experience with methadone maintenance treatment, it was found that some 20% left the program for a variety of reasons. The Gearing Progress Report evaluating the Dole-Nyswander program through March 31, 1970, indicates that "reasons for leaving the program continue to be the same as in previous reports."[7] Voluntarily withdrawals and discharge for medical and behavioral reasons have accounted for the majority of dropouts in the early months. Abuse of alcohol and chronic abuse of amphetamines or barbiturates were the major causes of discharge in the second or third year. Alcohol was the major reason for discharge among black patients; drug abuse a more prominent cause among white and Puerto Rican patients.

The authors' own experience in methadone programs confirms that there is a hard-core of patients who do not respond to the program, continue to act out antisocially or move to other forms of drug abuse, are unable to shed the addict life style or develop more conventional social patterns of functioning. These are the patients who sooner or later drop out of the program. In follow-up studies,[7,8] these dropouts returned to their former "junkie" existence. Where more intensive therapeutic efforts have failed to short-circuit this drift to other forms of drug abuse and continued antisocial behavior, it is hoped the combination of methadone treatment within a residential center, removed from the community, and an experience of socialized living can prove effective in reaching these "dropouts" from both modalities.

Residential—Methadone Treatment

Residents should remain in the center for varying periods of time, ranging from several months to a year or more, depending on their progress and readiness to return to the community while still leaning on methadone as a bridge and support. As in other prototype residential centers, they can be assigned a series of duties, starting with routine tasks, but increasing in responsibility and complexity as they show themselves able to take on additional assignments. As in other centers, also, a system of rewards and punishments prevails, based on the residents' response to the total program. Through their participation in frequent encounters, marathons, and seminars, they are helped to confront their problems and gain in awareness, thereby facilitating the socialization process.

As they become increasingly involved, the first steps to reentry into the community can be initiated, as in preparing for schooling, training and return to work. An important component of the residential center "concept" is the idea of offering incentives in the form of training residents to be part of the "system" by becoming staff and eventually rehabilitating others. From the standpoint of the sociological theory of "differential association," helping others becomes a most important dynamic in helping oneself, by reinforcing one's own adjustment and experience of success in the conventional world.

As residents indicate in a variety of ways, through attitudes elicited in the encounters and through behavioral changes, their ability to assume increasing responsibility, they move into the "reentry phase." This phase offers increased latitude in terms of leaving the residential center without supervision to attend outside schools, obtain training and gradually work as staff in other components of the drug program. The methadone can serve as a strong reinforcement at this time in permitting them to avoid temptation and relapse or other acting-out behavior. At this stage, the residents' situation corresponds to that of the regular methadone treatment program's "Phase II" in that they are largely or totally in the community, but coming to the outpatient clinic to pick up their methadone. Urine checks (TLC) should continue to be done to obviate the possibility of further drug abuse. More intensive therapy in the form of individual counseling and/or group therapy can be built in if this is indicated; or the patient could continue to participate in the residential center encounters, preferably as a leader with newer residents.

The staff for this combined facility should comprise ex-addicts who have experienced both modalities and can therefore bring their experience from both approaches to the facility. Specifically, dropouts from various therapeutic communities who later entered methadone programs could staff the key position. For lesser positions, staff from either modality could be used, though they would need to be screened and trained carefully to eliminate the serious prejudices and rancorous feelings which have existed until now between the various treatment approaches, especially between those geared to an abstinence, and those to a chemotherapy approach. Staff should also either have had experience, or receive training in group therapy. Professionals can be brought in to fill in the staffing pattern for assistance with screening, work with families and community agencies, and participation in the individual counseling and group therapy.

Residential Center—Methadone Maintenance— A Case Example

Since the combined residential center—methadone maintenance facility described here has nowhere yet, to our knowledge, been established.* It may be helpful to describe a prototype patient who we believe would benefit from such a residential experience.

The subject is a 29-year-old white male, very boyish looking, narcissistic individual of Italian extraction. His father was close to being a chronic alcoholic for many years, but grew out of it in his 40's. The mother was over-indulgent, catering to his whims and providing him with extravagantly expensive clothing even as a boy so that he is still very clothes-conscious, spending inordinate amounts of money on his dress and fussing over his physical appearance as well. He was the youngest of 3 boys: the oldest was a paratrooper, killed in battle, a vastly romanticized figure. The second brother, also a paratrooper in service, came very close to being a chronic alcoholic and was dependent on various women for support for many years.

There was a large age gap between the subject and his elder brothers: he always felt himself a child and dwarf in comparison with them and believed he could never measure up to them. Though he served in the Army

* Several have been established in the last two years in the Chicago Program and at the Bronx State Hospital.

himself, he considered himself a failure because he had never dared join the Paratroop Division. He impregnated a girl while still in service and was forced to marry her; had a son by her and subsequently divorced her. This family is on welfare and he has never supported them though experiencing some guilt about it.

After leaving service, he became a musician, playing the horn and singing. According to the subject, at the point of succeeding, he became frightened, "copped out" and increasingly became involved with drugs—first cocaine, then heroin. He has never revealed his full story. but there are intimations of extensive selling of drugs, involvement with the Mafia and international adventures, and it is not clear how much is real and how much fantasy. He has been living off a girl who masochistically supports him and stoically tolerates his abuse of her and rather continuous acting-out behavior and outbursts of rage.

A turning point came when the subject suffered a severe attack of hepatitis and his girl threatened to leave him. He came for private therapy at her urging and was also admitted into a methadone program. The subject continued to come in for therapy and use it as a means of protection against being expelled from the methadone program. For a long time, he used therapy as a safety device whenever he violated the program's rules or needed to con to gain his own impulsive ends. He discovered all sorts of interesting ways of overcoming the methadone blockade through barbiturates and manipulation of the dosage, and imparted this knowledge to other patients in the program.

In this therapy session, he revealed himself to be a very infantile person, barely socialized and frightened of responsibility and independence. He saw the world as a huge breast, obligated to feed him. He lived in fantasy a great deal, distorted reality and confabulated automatically so that he could concoct several different versions of an occurrence or explanations for his behavior, all within a short period of time. He was fearful of testing himself in the real world and veered between terror and grandiose dreams of success.

Therapy was characterized by severe testing out on a number of levels. For many months, he found it impossible to adhere to the treatment schedule, coming late or not at all. Since he is intelligent, he could conjure up an amazing number of explanations and rationalizations, which it was difficult to break through. Though "stabilized" on methadone, he could not satisfy his craving in spite of frequent dosage adjustments and periodically needed to abuse heroin and other drugs—cocaine, barbiturates, tranquilizers, valium and librium, even the laxative given him for constipation. He arranged deals with doctors and pharmacies in which he obtained large amounts of barbiturates and tranquilizers, and it was not clear that he might not also be selling pills as well as using them himself. He explained that his craving frequently became so overwhelming that he could not cope with it and needed to shoot up 4-5 bags and borrow the "works" although frightened of a recurrence of his hepatitis. Several times he wrecked cars, one of them his own, and others belonging to relatives. He kept the methadone staff busy, claiming either that the dosage was not adequate, or that he had lost his medication, or that it had been stolen. At other times, he reported he had regurgitated it and needed more. There were strong rumors about his occasionally selling his methadone to "take off" on heroin. He was on bad terms with his family who suspected him, and got involved in physical brawls with his brother. He struck his girlfriend whenever she pointed out realities to him—then felt penitent and worthless since he had feeling for her, though mixed with hostility over his dependency on her.

This listing of evidence of the subject's being unable to cope with his problems in the community and move towards productive social functioning and employment could be extended indefinitely. Though the methadone was gradually making itself felt and giving him increased support, he was still having too much difficulty remaining on an even keel and frequently came within a hair's breath of being expelled from the program. It was sufficiently clear that he had experienced some very basic failures in his socialization process, and that many gaps needed to be filled in in his impulse control, reality testing, and ego as well as superego development (to use the Freudian topology) before he could be trusted to function outside an institution. For him, it was felt, the combined methadone-residential center facility could serve as an important "habilitating" experience until he could realize himself more fully as a separate person who could function independently of others.

CONCLUSION

This paper has attempted to conceptualize a multi-modality approach to methadone treatment which builds on the classic Dole-Nyswander model. The new conceptualization views methadone as a chemical support, though within the wider framework of a more comprehensive medical and psychotherapeutic continuum geared primarily to the goal of abstinence and based on the assumption that there are preexisting psychological and social problems which may require more intensive therapeutic intervention for selected patients.

As described in the paper, this multi-modality concept entails the use of a gradient of services and levels of intensity, both of chemical and psychotherapeutic supports, ranging in time also from weeks to years, comprised of two essential elements:

(1) *Chemical supports*—initially methadone is offered in low doses, geared to rapid abstinence within a matter of weeks or months, and lasting for years or indefinitely in the high "variable-dose" methadone modality.

(2) *Therapeutic intervention*—in each modality, intensive individual counseling, group therapy and any other reinforcements indicated such as the use of "rational authority" can be offered individual patients. The "ultimate" approach described is the combined residential center—methadone treatment facility for the "failures" in either modality, or for individuals in the methadone program who clearly cannot meet the program's requirements in the community, and need a period of communal living or socialization away from their old haunts. Methadone can also serve here to bridge the gap back to the

community in time. Some of the steps in this continuum could be skipped if there were clear clinical indication that a patient could respond best to a particular modality—say high-dose methadone. By building in evaluation procedures, it should be possible, in time, to develop objective criteria for screening and treatment.

While we have focused all approaches towards the goal of abstinence, it is recognized that not all patients will be able to relinquish the prop of methadone support and may need to rely on it indefinitely. From the standpoint of rehabilitation, this too would be considered a worthwhile goal since the individual would have given up his addictive life style and would be functioning in a socially productive manner in the community. His reliance on methadone would be not too different from the dependence of psychotic patients on the major tranquilizers, of diabetics on insulin and epileptics on dilantin.

This paper has discussed, in some detail, the various modalities included—namely, the inpatient and outpatient detoxification of narcotic addicts with methadone, low-dose and high-dose methadone treatment and the combined residential center–methadone treatment facility. Case discussions for each approach were also offered.

REFERENCES

1. Brill and Lieberman: Authority and Addiction, 1969.
2. Martin and Jasinski: Physiological parameters of morphine dependence in man tolerance, early abstinence, protracted abstinence, 1968.
3. Chambers: The detoxification of narcotic addicts in outpatient clinics, 1971.
4. Wieland and Chambers: Narcotic substitution therapy, 1970.
5. Wieland and Chambers: Outpatient detoxification of narcotic addiction, Proceedings 32nd Annual Meeting of Committee on Problems of Drug Dependence, World National Research Council, 1970.
6. Wieland and Chambers: Methadone maintenance—a comparison of two stabilization techniques, 1970.
7. Gearing: Methadone maintenance treatment program, Progress report of evaluation through March 31, 1970, Report submitted to New York State Narcotic Addiction Control Commission, mimeographed, 1970.
8. Perkins and Bloch: A study of some failures in methadone treatment, Paper presented at 123rd Annual Meeting of American Psychiatric Association, San Francisco, 1969.

PART SIX

Chapter 25.

Opposition to Methadone Maintenance Therapy: A Study of Recent Sources of Criticism

Leon Brill

Opposition to methadone maintenance derives from a variety of sources as diverse as medical societies and law enforcement agencies, abstinence-oriented narcotics-treatment approaches, public and private agencies and black militant and Puerto Rican indigenous community groups—among a host of others. While some of the resistance is based on considered and rational criticism, much is related to stereotyped attitudes such as the long-prevailing concept that only total, immediate abstinence constitutes a worthwhile goal of treatment; or a continued clinging to such hopefully outmoded beliefs as that a "drug-free environment" must be the starting point and *sine qua non* of all rehabilitation—by which is meant institutionalizing and quarantining addicts to protect them and the community from a purportedly infectious disease.

Other stances derive from moralistic and judgmental feelings associated with the "Puritan ethic"; namely, that the use of any chemical is a sin, which violates our society's shibboleths and precepts, and must be curbed by all means, including—usually preferably—punishment. Black militant and Puerto Rican hostility to opiates and methadone goes with the belief that drugs are forms of "genocide" and enslavement deliberately fostered by white society as a means of holding minority populations in thrall and avoiding challenge to the "Establishment."

In the following sections, we shall examine more closely some different sources of criticism and the specific arguments used.

Recent criticisms of the methadone maintenance modality appear to fall into two distinct "camps"—those who are pro-methadone but express concern about any widespread noncontrolled application of this "experimental technique" and those who are anti-methadone for a variety of personal, philosophical, religious, etc. reasons. Statements by Eddy and Martin represent the first "camp" with Tabor and Allan representing the second.

A. *Statement prepared by Nathan B. Eddy for Bureau of Narcotics and Dangerous Drugs, Department of Justice (Eddy, 1969)*. In a detailed paper, Eddy offers a number of comments on methadone maintenance. He first summarizes the recommendations of the Committee on Problems of Drug Dependency, National Academy of Sciences, National Research Council which, in 1967 agreed that there "continued to be a need for controlled studies to establish the conditions, potentialities and essential restrictions of a program of management of drug-dependent persons by continuing administration of methadone, that this procedure remained a research undertaking, and that it could not be considered an established treatment."

"The National Research Council Committee urged that a number of control procedures be instituted: First, that a large number of addicts be screened to determine those who were and those who were not acceptable to the Dole-Nyswander program. Selection would then be made from both populations using one as a control for the other. As a further means of control comparison, selected patients from both populations would be referred to other treatment modalities. Further research would include attempted maintenance at different dose levels to determine what sufficed and what was optimal; and withdrawal from maintenance after a suitable interval."

The Sixteenth Report of the WHO Expert Committee indicates their belief that "methadone maintenance for drug dependence of the morphine type remains experimental . . . and has not yet been adequately evaluated. The techniques of well-designed clinical drug trials including scientifically controlled series and/or companion groups are required on these trials. It is important that the influence of factors other than methadone itself be evaluated . . . To date, patients involved have, in the main, been highly motivated, carefully selected and provided with organized aftercare arranged so as to develop a supportive group process. Furthermore, these patients have not been shown to be a representative sample of the drug-dependent population in other respects: e.g., age, ethnic grouping and educational level. Finally, it must not be forgotten that methadone itself is a drug of dependence and that persons taking it regularly in the methadone program continue to have a drug dependence of morphine type. . . . It will, therefore, be necessary to keep in view the question of final withdrawal of methadone from the patients."

Eddy next summarizes the report of the "Methadone Maintenance Evaluation Committee of Columbia University School of Public Health" under the Chairmanship of Henry Brill, as of March 31, 1968, to the New York State NACC, covering approximately four years of operation of the program. The Committee concluded that "For patients selected and treated as described, this program can be considered a success. It does appear that those who remain in the program have on the whole become productive members of society, in contrast to their previous experience . . . . It should be emphasized that these are volunteers, who are older than the average street addict and may be more highly motivated. Consequently, generalizations of the results of the program in this population to the general addict population probably are not justified." The Committee offers a number of recommendations for further controls, including the use of other groups, different criteria for admission such as younger patients or prison populations and variations in technique such as induction on an ambulatory basis.

Eddy concludes that "for a particularly selected group of persistent heroin abusers, methadone maintenance has brought about significant social and economic gain at relatively low cost compared to the loss to the individual and to society in these patients' previous experience. It must be emphasized, however, that until the recommended control studies have been instituted and evaluated, conclusions cannot be drawn in respect to general applicability, nor plans formulated for broad expansion of the program as an established treatment modality. Until such controls are carried out and their evaluation is at hand, the program is one of research only."

He suggests the following precautions:

> (1) Strict control of the amount and form of drug administration, designed to prevent accumulation or diversion, or recovery of methadone in injectable form.
> (2) Adequate and uniform record keeping for meaningful analysis of the patient's history, condition at the beginning and progress in treatment.
> (3) Constant monitoring by urinalysis to determine not only narcotic consumption but also resort to other drugs of abuse.
> (4) Such help as is indicated for vocational training, job placement, living adjustment and interpersonal relationships.
> (5) Eventual withdrawal of methadone maintenance must be kept in mind but insistence upon it should be left in abeyance at present.

Eddy finally summarizes what he believes are the two key issues:

> (1) "Is this a treatment modality to be recommended and sponsored as an established procedure? No. It is an experimental effort (research) in spite of any claimed or admitted success at least until the recommendations which have been made in respect to it are implemented and evaluated.
> (2) "Is this a treatment modality which can be employed by the individual, private physician in the course of his office practice? No.

B. *Commentary on the Second National Conference on Methadone Treatment* by Dr. William Martin, Director of the NIMH Addiction Research Center at the Lexington, Kentucky P.H.S. Hospital.

(1) In regard to medical aspects, the Addiction Research Center learned that chronic administration of narcotics creates a physiological disorder that persists

for many months after the narcotic withdrawn—termed "protracted abstinence." Animal studies show this is associated with relapse. Studies should be initiated to learn whether relapse rates and social adjustment are adversely affected by methadone maintenance.

(2) A methodological question relates to the extent to which results thus far obtained with methadone can be extrapolated to the addict population at large. Patients hitherto accepted for methadone maintenance have not been representative of the addict population. None of the treatment results reports have been statistically compared to an appropriate control group.

(3) Like morphine, methadone in all probability produces long lasting physiological and psychological abnormalities. It should therefore be used cautiously and as a last resort in treating narcotic dependency.

(4) The definitive assessment of the efficacy of methadone will require the clear identification of therapeutic goals and the development of valid methods for assessing the effect of methadone on these goals. Further, it will be necessary to have appropriate control groups for experimental variables that may also affect therapeutic outcome to allow the clear identification of those effects that are attributable to methadone maintenance. Systematic studies should be undertaken to assess potential and known undesirable effects of methadone maintenance, as well as its desirable actions, to assist in a social judgment that will have to be made at some future time as to whether the advantages of methadone maintenance do or do not outweigh the disadvantages.

C. *Other Sources of Criticism of methadone maintenance* have been the various narcotics rehabilitation approaches. These include:

Synanon and prototype ex-addict-directed therapeutic communities such as Daytop Village, Phoenix House, Odyssey and others. One of the obvious sources of disagreement clearly stems from the total abstinence orientation of these communities. The introduction of any "chemical" into the residence is grounds for expulsion. The methadone maintenance philosophy puts primary emphasis on the addicts' social rehabilitation, regardless of the achievement of total abstinence. They do not see patients on methadone maintenance as any better off than heroin addicts since they are still dependent and "stoned"; no one can be said to be rehabilitated unless he is completely off all drugs.

Religious approaches such as the Pentacostal Fundamentalist churches exemplified by the former Christian Damascus Church in the South Bronx, and the Addict Rehabilitation Center in Manhattan as well, see all chemicals as "sin." One overcomes this sin by embracing Christ and the Church and being redeemed. Some graduates of this modality have been tolerant to the point of supporting methadone treatment if this is the only way an addict can be saved.

An important base for opposition stems from society's "Puritan ethic" which has been a focal source of criticism. Many diverse groups have repeatedly criticized methadone maintenance on the grounds that it creates "euphoria" and merely "substitutes one drug for another." It is well established, however, that after the initial stabilization, if at all, no such euphoria is experienced.

Black militants have attacked methadone maintenance as "genocide," "narcotization of the blacks" and "honkie's way of making zombies of us and keeping us down." They feel methadone maintenance dilutes the militant attitudes of blacks, interferes with their rebellion against the Establishment and battle for equal rights (Tabor, 1970).

An example of combined religious—black militant—indigenous attitudes about methadone maintenance in a community program can be observed in an editorial from the February 1969 issue of *New Life*, a monthly paper of the Addiction Rehabilitation Center of Rev. James Allen, a minister and former addict.

METHADONE MAINTENANCE WILL BE A GREAT CONTRIBUTION TO OUR SOCIETY

Methadone is a crutch that transfers the addict from one drug to another. It does not put him back into the mainstream of life. It does not prevent or control the spread of addiction. It only controls and directs addicts to do what the dispensing agency mandates. It can "program" the addict population (50,000 strong) to "influence, work, vote" for whoever and whatever agency responsible for maintaining their supply of dope. Maintenance will not teach addicts to respect ethical, moral or spiritual values. Methadone can only "maintain" with no hope of a cure.

Methadone endangers social progress. Society progresses when people face and solve their problems. All forms of addiction—methadone maintenance included—takes away the opportunity to face and solve problems. Methadone does not curb the alarming increase in incident of addiction. Methadone maintenance is "psychological endorsement of addiction for an increasing number of adolescents who become addicts each year. We cannot afford to "maintain" these children at the development stage" of their lives. How can "maintenance" train adolescents to become responsible citizens in "tomorrow's world?"

Methadone maintenance is a "cure-hoax" that is being imposed upon our American Society at a time when we are plagued by bad foreign relations and critical internal problems. In our "zeal" to eliminate the drug problem, we have become ignorant to what has befell other nations when they surrender themselves to any form of drug induced existence. Any addict will tell you that he became addicted because he thought, "It can't happen to me." Are we going to experiment with the youth of our entire nation while thinking: "It can't happen to America?"

Methadone takes a sick dope fiend at a time when he is incapable of thinking for himself and turns him into a "maintained" robot, with no claim of a cure. Programs like Addicts Rehabilitation Center are curing addicts, not maintaining them!" If your son was a drug victim, would you send him to an agency that could "maintain" him or to an agency that could cure him?

HOW WILL METHADONE MAINTENANCE AFFECT THE DEVELOPMENT OF THE BLACK MAN

Heroin addiction is spawned among the ghetto problems of the Black Man. Dope is "always there", offering him a false escape from problems that are hard to live with. Black People make up half of all recorded drug victims. The reduction in the price of heroin from $10 to $2 a bag makes it "conveniently available" to thousands of little Black Children seeking an "escape." This makes methadone more of an "endorsement" rather than an effort to prevent or curb ghetto addiction.

I submit that as addiction increases in the ghetto, Black People will be reduced to the status of "Maintained Black Slaves." Black People are one tenth of the American population and one half of the addict population. At a one to one ratio, Black People could all become addicted with only a tenth percent loss to White America. I would not allow my child to be maintained on methadone. I will use my energy and money to educate and teach him to assume an equal position in the world. A methadone maintained person will never be thought of as equal. I would want my son cured and I know that he can be cured. I know some addicts who were cured. I'm an addict and I was cured. Some of my best friends were addicts and they are cured. Methadone is a waste of time, energy, intelligence, and money unless we're trying slowly to kill off Black People!

REFERENCES

1. Eddy: Methadone maintenance for the management of persons with drug dependence of morphine type, 1969.

2. Martin: Commentary on the Second National Conference on Methadone Treatment, 1971.

3. Tabor: Capitalism plus dope equals genocide, 1970.

4. Allen: New Life Editorial, 1969.

PART SEVEN

Chapter 26.

The International Experience: A Survey of Maintenance Programs

Leon Brill

From the original tiny groups of some 25 methadone patients of Dole-Nyswander, the nine patients of Jaffe and Brill at the Albert Einstein College of Medicine and the small program at Metropolitan Hospital, methadone maintenance has proliferated widely, burgeoning into ever larger numbers of "satellite clinics" in Manhattan clustered around the Morris Bernstein Institute and Beth Israel Medical Center, then gaining momentum under city and later state auspices and, most recently, under the Health Services Administration. From New York, the programs have spread to other parts of the country, Philadelphia, Boston, Chicago, New Haven, Miami, New Orleans, Denver, Oregon, California and abroad—first to Toronto and British Columbia. With the changing "British System," methadone programs have been established in England and appear to be ranging to the "far-flung corners of the world"—Sweden and other countries. Still others, like Hong Kong, are investigating the feasibility of establishing methadone programs in their areas.

This chapter will attempt to cover as many as possible of the international programs for which data were available at the time of writing. It thus constitutes an extension of the prior chapter on national programs in describing the specific elaborations and colorations methadone programs receive from their different geographical, social, political and cultural situations as well as from the individuals directing them. It may be recalled that the initial successes reported for the New York City program were attributed to the "charisma" of Dr. Nyswander, and it required replication before observers agreed it might be the program itself that was helping. A number of additional questions about these programs have since presented themselves in relation to such aspects as: the philosophical and conceptual underpinnings, role of urine-testing and ancillary services, the need for structure, proper cut-off points for "intractable" behavior, the place of low-dose as against high-does stabilization and others.

CANADIAN PROGRAMS

British Columbia

The most elaborate report of an international methadone treatment program is that provided by the Narcotic Addiction Foundation of British Columbia. The low- and high-dose methadone programs were part of a multi-modality approach including detoxification, cyclazocine and drug-free programs for the different patients able to respond to these individual approaches.

Low Methadone Maintenance Program. The Narcotic Addiction Foundation of British Columbia interestingly began with low-dose rather than the "classical" high-dose methadone, Dole-Nyswander model. Their designation for this, when they first began in February, 1963, was "The Prolonged Methadone Withdrawal Treatment Programme," first of its kind in North America. This was the only maintenance program offered by the NAF until 1968, when the "Massive Dosage Treatment Program," which focused on the establishment of a heroin blockade by using high-dose methadone was instituted. In 1969, these two programs were re-named the *Low-Methadone Maintenance Programme (LMMP)* and the *High-Methadone Maintenance Programme (HMMP)* respectively, in accordance with international usage.

The LMMP was first introduced because of the observation that routine (short-term) out-patient and in-patient withdrawal programs, though successful in withdrawing addicts from physical dependency on heroin, did not prevent subsequent drug use. Although the amount of methadone prescribed varies with the apparent need of the patient, a blockade is not effected in this program, but the goal is rather to stabilize the patient on a minimum dosage of methadone. If the patient remains in treatment, but stabilization is not possible without effecting a heroin blockade, then the patient can be transferred to the High-Methadone Maintenance Program.

Caseload—At the end of 1969, the caseload included 106 patients, an increase partly due to changes in treatment policy regarding withdrawals. In the extended withdrawal period (one month), patients who continued to abuse heroin were encouraged to seek maintenance. In all, 246 patients were thus treated in the LMMP in 1969. Forty-six patients in the LMMP were transferred to the HMMP during the year because of continued drug abuse. Patients who dropped out totaled 94, about 50% of the admissions for 1969. As a monthly average, dropouts represented 80% of the total caseload. Because of lack of follow-up, information on why patients dropped out was not available for 70% of the patients who left voluntarily in 1969.

Time in Treatment—Part of the success in treatment by the LMMP is attributed to the length of time patients are involved. From their experience, they concluded that the longer the patient stays in treatment, the better is his chance for stabilization.

Age and Sex—The prevailing ratio of males to females under the LMMP was three to one: of the 246 patients in treatment, 179 were males and 65 females. The percentage steadily increased, from the younger to the older age group:—8% were in their 20's, 11% in their 30's, 14% in their forties and fifties and 17% over 60. No patient under 21 remained in the program over two months.

Conclusions—"The LMMP continues to be an effective form of treatment for a substantial number of heroin addicts. Very few patients who have remained stabilized in the program for over a year have become re-addicted to heroin. Many have become productive members of society as measured by steady employment. They also demonstrate less antisocial behavior as illustrated by records of arrest when contrasted with prior criminal records after addiction.

"The LMMP population consists of a diversified group of addicts, from old-timers to young experimenters, from hard-core to new users and from pure heroin addicts to multi-drug users. It does not appear at present that a classification in terms of use or criminal activities is sufficient to predetermine who will be benefitted by this program."

The High Methadone Maintenance Program.   Early in 1968, the NAF initiated its study on HMMP. Its two major research purposes included: testing the flexibility of Dole's methadone blockade with a more severely addicted group who had assumed more extensive criminal activities and who indicated that they were more institutionalized due to longer periods of incarceration.

Patient Selection—Addicts selected for the HMMP included mainly ex-patients of the NAF, failures in other programs or applicants with a very extensive criminal record and severe heroin dependency as well as lengthy drug history. Addicts ranging from 20-55 years were admissible. Most of the addicts considered hopeless and not amenable to treatment by other NAF programs were offered a trial in the HMMP.

Dosage Levels—ranged from 70 mg. to 150 mg. daily.

Treatment—The program was divided into six phases. Each phase marked the patient's progress towards integration into a "square John" or non-user society. The achievement of each phase meant gaining more privileges in terms of lesser frequency of medication pick-up and leaving of supervised urine specimens for monitoring.

HMMP Caseload—In 1969, the caseload was 95-105 patients. A total of 218 candidates was considered for the program. Of these, 102 were actually in treatment and 66 discontinued treatment before completing a two-month's stabilization phase. Treatment retention rate was thus at a 46% level for the entire HMMP population and 56% for the patient group who completed the qualifying two months' outpatient stabilization phase. In general, the patients who discontinued treatment tended to be younger.

Effectiveness of the HMMP—Seventy-two percent discontinued HMMP before completing five months of treatment; 66 who had been in treatment two months or longer were dropped.

Conclusions—"The program data indicate a fairly substantial degree of success in treating individuals with long histories of heroin use. Many of the patients are employed, the majority are using heroin either infrequently or not at all: and a large percentage are less involved in criminal activities."

Toronto

In a personal communication received from Mr. A. Milligan, Program Director of the Addiction Research Foundation, Toronto, Ontario, the following program description was furnished for their methadone treatment:

The Agency. The Addiction Research Foundation of Ontario (Executive Director, Mr. H. D. Archibald) is an agency sponsored and supported by the Provincial Government of Ontario. The Narcotic Addiction Research Unit (Director, Mr. Milligan) is a clinical unit designed to formulate and test modalities of treatment for Narcotic Addiction.

Epidemiology. In 1968, it was estimated by the Department of National Health and Welfare, Ottawa, that there were 3,804 narcotic addicts in Canada.

The Methadone Maintenance Program. The method is essentially that established by Dole and Nyswander in terms of selection criteria and induction procedures.

The project is one of research and was designed to cover a period of two years; evaluation to commence eighteen months after induction. It was anticipated that the basic sample would be obtained during the first six months of the project's operation.

Chief evaluation methods to be used were questionnaires with independent confirmation of employment and criminal records. The Minnesota Multiphasic Personality Inventory was used and drug abuse was determined by laboratory analysis. Experimentation with various antagonists and longer acting methadone forms was also indicated.

Overview

An interesting overview of problems created by methadone programming in Canada is offered in a personal communication from Mr. R. O. Hammond, Chief, Division of Narcotic Control, Ontario. The letter is quoted at some length since it spells out very clearly some of the problems related to methadone programming.

Your letter has arrived at the time when developments in the use of Methadone in the treatment and management of opiate addiction here in Canada are causing the Division considerable concern. Information is reaching us from various parts of Canada and particularly the Western Provinces, indicating there is growing misuse developing in respect to this drug.

Approximately three years ago, the Narcotic Addiction Foundation in Vancouver, British Columbia, embarked upon a clinical programme using Methadone. Two approaches were followed—one, a minimum maintenance dose provided to selected addict-patients and the other a maximum maintenance dose. I might mention that most, if not all of the individuals concerned, had a history of heroin addiction and in addition, evidence of anti-social activities prior to their drug problem developing.

At any rate, as time passed, it was apparent a considerable number of individuals seeking help from the Foundation and through the medium of obtaining Methadone, were not able to remain within the terms of the requirements of the programme. As a consequence, they dropped out and sought Methadone or other drugs from different sources, including physicians. This resulted in many physicians being contacted and the suggestion made to them that Methadone be prescribed. Problems in this area have developed in British Columbia, and now have spread to Alberta, Saskatchewan and, to some degree, Ontario.

Broadly speaking, this is what occurs: when Methadone is made available by a physician as a result of issuing a prescription, the would-be patient may be satisfied with the euphoria obtained for a short period of time. Oral tablets are prescribed in Canada. In a great many cases, the tablets are dissolved by the addict-patients and the resulting solution injected. This in itself, as you know, creates medical problems. Even with the injection of the Methadone, many of the addicts are not satisfied with the dosage they receive from a physician—consequently, they contact different physicians in an effort to supplement their dosage. Various aliases are used to conceal their identity. Indeed, we know some addicts are recruiting non-addict associates, schooling them in the method of approaching physicians to obtain prescriptions for this drug; and, if and when successful, the prescription or actual medication is turned over to addicts. All this has resulted in medical supplies of Methadone now being available in the illicit traffic. In some areas of Canada at the present time a tablet of Methadone is selling for $5.00.

There is another angle which should be mentioned; we find that many addicts who are obtaining Methadone through medical treatment will seeek additional medication for euphoria and they obtain prescriptions for short-acting barbiturates. In other words, some physicians may be prescribing Methadone for the individual and other physicians are consulted for short-acting barbiturates. This, of course, creates a dual-addiction.

Reverting to the programme in operation at the Narcotic Addiction Foundation in Vancouver, we have established in the past that a considerable number of the patients involved, even though they are meeting the conditions of the programme, will contact outside physicians and obtain additional medication. This may carry on for some time until the situation is detected by the clinical staff of the Foundation.

Perhaps I should give you an indication of how we have been able to collect our information concerning the abuse of Methadone. In this Division, we maintain purchase records for all physicians and pharmacists throughout the country. If, therefore, a doctor or pharmacist buys Narcotic or Controlled Drug medication (barbiturates and amphetamines) from licensed pharmaceutical manufacturers or distributors, such commitments are recorded on individual purchase cards. Licensed dealers must submit monthly reports to the Division. In addition, approximately 5,000 retail pharmacies operating in Canada are required to forward to this Division, regularly at four-month intervals, duplicate sheets of a drug register which they are required to maintain showing the quantities of Narcotics and Controlled Drugs as such which are dispensed. These purchase cards and pharmacists' reports are screened regularly and pertinent information extracted.

As an example, the attached statistical sheet sets forth

details of the number of prescriptions for Methadone which were issued in Western Canada and reported by retail pharmacists in that area covering the four month period ending January 31st, 1970. It will be noted that in one City in the Province of Saskatchewan, 28 different individuals obtained a total of 216 prescriptions for Methadone as a result of ten different physicians becoming involved. I might say that the quantities of Methadone Tablets involved in these prescriptions would vary from approximately 12 to 100. In many cases, individuals would have obtained prescriptions from more than one physician.

From the details we have received and are continuing to receive, it is quite apparent that the demand on physicians to prescribe Methadone throughout our country is increasing and with this development, there is an increase in abuse. Our experience has been that, if the use of this synthetic narcotic has any value in the treatment of addiction, it is only when the programmes are carried out in a clinical setting and medication is not provided to the addict-patient for self-administration or consumption. Incidentally, we have also had misuse of Methadone solution which has emanated from a clinical programme.

Some other limited programmes of this type have been initiated in Central Canada yet not to the same extent as has occurred in Vancouver. Actually, the Province of British Columbia has always been the major problem area from the standpoint of Heroin addiction. As a result of the situation mentioned, the abuse of Methadone in Ontario and Quebec has not developed as in Western Canada. In spite of this, and within the last six months, there is increasing interest on the part of some physicians and social workers to embark upon methadone programmes in these two provinces—in some cases, clinics would be associated with hospitals.

Other than at the Narcotic Addiction Foundation in Vancouver, there are no major programmes. The Alcoholism and Drug Addiction Research Foundation in Toronto at the present time is making plans to commence such a programme. Incidentally, approximately three years ago this organization was involved in a limited way with such a plan but apparently decided to drop it through lack of facilities or results, or in fact, perhaps a combination of both.

There is one other centre where methadone is being used to a limited extent—it is at the Jewish General Hospital in Montreal, Quebec. A clinic has been in operation there for some time but again on a very limited scale as compared to the one at the Foundation in Vancouver . . . .

Finally, I would like to make it very clear that any comments I have made are not intended to question the sincerity of the individuals operating these programmes—in fact, it is just the opposite. They have cooperated with the Division in every respect. Problems which may arise through methadone treatment do not necessarily develop at a treatment center. Rather, through a lack of knowledge

on the part of private physicians as to the actual pharmacological properties of the drug and the conditions under
which it should be made available. In this connection we
are now encountering some cases of youth (who have been
using marijuana and hashish) seeking medical treatment
for drug dependence and methadone prescribed.

PROGRAMS IN GREAT BRITAIN

A General Overview

Edgar May commenting on the British scene in the
July 1971 issue of *Harper's Magazine* estimates that
there are fewer than 3,000 narcotic addicts in England
today, as compared to over 200,000 in America. The rate
of increase of heroin addicts has dropped sharply in the
last year and it is expected to show a reversal soon. Three
years ago, the Government limited heroin prescriptions
to special treatment centers in regional hospitals, thus
continuing to avoid the criminal definition prevalent in
America. There are 14 clinics in London, which holds
4/5ths of the country's addicts; and elsewhere there are
13 special facilities as well as services at some 42 hospital outpatient departments.

The clinic services vary since some have hospital beds
for withdrawal, others emphasize psychiatric services,
still others employment, etc. Almost all clinics permit
addicts to inject drugs away from the premises though at
least two insist that a nurse administer them twice daily.
Before admission to a program, a patient must be
checked against the Home Office records, be interviewed
by staff, and submit one or more urines to confirm drug
use. Once admitted, the patient receives his drugs from
his neighborhood druggist on a daily basis. All but a few
hundred addicts have gradually been converted to using
only methadone or partly methadone. Unlike America,
3/4ths of English addicts mainline their methadone like
heroin. Patients fall into roughly 4 groups: those who
inject heroin only; those who inject both heroin and methadone; those who inject methadone only, and those who
drink methadone. Although most addicts report weekly
to the clinic, there is seldom enough staff to provide inten-

sive social counseling. Most English workers do not believe even the most intensive psychological assistance will get a patient off drugs unless he has made the decision himself. (May, 1971.)

It has been difficult for clinics to hold their clients to the prescribed drug diet. Many abuse more than one drug while others sell, lend or exchange some of their own medication. It is felt this traffic would be reduced if the drugs were administered directly through the clinics, a practice most doctors do not favor. While there are no overall statistics on clinic performance, many doctors are encouraged by their initial successes with stabilized patients. Dr. Philip Connell, clinic director, expressed himself as pleased that the curve of heroin addiction had levelled off, but disturbed that methadone and barbiturates had risen. He also deplored the lack of research underway at the clinics. Thus, London clinics reported a large increase in employment, reduction of drug abuse and criminality.

Individual Programs

1. The National Addiction and Research Institute of Britain, under the name of *Cure,* offered the following report of their third year's work in a personal communication:

> ... During our first year's work, we had to show that it was possible to manage drug addicts against a very disturbed background created by the epidemic spread of the disease. We accomplished this and were able to bring a number of patients to think about treatment.
>
> In 1968, we started working seriously on our methadone (physeptone) maintenance programme and had ceased prescribing methedrine before the banning of this product. Last year, we continued to prescribe oral methadone and were able to make a long-term relationship with a number of our patients, a certain number of whom attended our Center on a daily basis. For this year we planned to aim at an "off-Physeptone" year and our efforts have been directed towards this end. We have had 152 patients under treatment of whom four died. One was a suicide, leaving a suicidal note following the rupture of a long-term relationship.

Present Drug State

Of the 132 patients under prolonged treatment with *Cure* 140 were narcotic addicts; 106 of these were prescribed oral methadone by the program, and a further 22 came off methadone in the course of the year. It should be emphasized here that there were a large number of patients who were reducing their oral methadone and are not shown in this figure. Of these 140 narcotic addicts, there were a group of 12 who were transients and did not come into a treatment programme.

Work Situation

It is difficult to give a clear picture here because, although 53 patients were in regular employment at the time of the report, there were a number of others who had worked sporadically during the year, but were classified as in prison, hospital, abroad or as transient. The main unemployed and unsatisfactorily employed group consisted of 20/30 patients. "Cure" has not been capable of influencing this group substantially.

One of the most encouraging aspects of the report was the figure of 20 who became full-time students or resumed full-time studies. Many of these would have been unable to do this without considerable help and had, until their contact with *Cure*, led vagrant or very unstable lives. *Cure* programmers are well aware of the fact that to start in full-time education is one thing and to finish it is another. They recognize these patients pose many unsolved problems but a number, at the comparatively easy level at which they began their studies, have received excellent reports.

General State of Improvement

For the purposes of an overall assessment, improvement was considered by *Cure* not only as an improvement in drug dosage, but also as an improvement in the life style, i.e., holding down a regular job, taking up full-time education, a more stable personal life, e.g. supporting a family, etc.

47 improved (or improvement maintained)
65 no change
12 deteriorated
 4 dead
24 don't know (in jail, prisons, lost to contact, etc.)

152

... Our therapeutic community needs strengthening and developing, and we are hoping to see an increasing number of patients in our off-narcotics—even off everything—programme, although it is already clear that prolonged follow-up is necessary. For example, we have two relapses this year in patients who had been off all narcotics for two years or more.

2. Dr. H. Dale Beckett, C.P.M., Consultant Psychiatrist at the Cane Hill Hospital Management Committee, Surrey, England, reports in a personal communication:

... When the Salter Unit was operating at this hospital, we tried various means of treatment. For a while, we tried intravenous injection of methadone, but found that this resulted in an addiction to methadone which was even more difficult to treat than the original addiction to heroin. As a result, when treating heroin addicts in my out-patient department I have, wherever possible, avoided prescribing ampoules of methadone, and prescribed it orally. Because of the desire on the part of the treatment centers to wean addicts off heroin at any cost, they have been prescribing relatively large quantities of methadone ampoules in replacement and as a result more and more kids are turning up at the centers with a primary addiction to methadone instead of to heroin. It is impossible at this stage to say whether this is to be welcomed or not. Certainly one does find that these patients are not injecting non-sterile solutions as was the case with so many heroin addicts.

In Salter, we developed a mixture of methadone which proved to be acceptable, and I have since been using it routinely in my out-patient department. At a recent meeting at the Department of Health of the clinicians who run treatment centers, this formulation was accepted and recommended for use as a standard preparation in all the treatment centers (with, however, orange or lemon syrup substituted for blackcurrent syrup).

Addicts attending my clinic are prescribed methadone mixture in quantities ranging from one day to one month at a time, depending upon the individual's progress and reliability.

After withdrawal from heroin, in my experience, a patient needs to be kept on a steady high-dose of methadone (100 mg. a day) for many months before he can begin to tolerate a progressive reduction.

Heroin Addicts and Methadone

1. Methadone may be used in three ways in dealing with heroin addicts. It may be given in progressively increasing doses during a withdrawal course of heroin so that eventually the patient is on methadone alone, beginning after a while to reduce the dose of methadone in its turn. He may be maintained on methadone without reduction. He may be prescribed methadone in addition to heroin so as to reduce his enjoyment of the latter and thus motivate him towards a cure.

2. In arriving at a suitable concentration of methadone in a mixture, one must recognize that an addict, if he is to receive enough methadone to last him for a week or a fortnight, will be required to handle comparatively large volumes of liquid. Above a certain volume, this becomes more and more difficult. On the other hand, if the methadone is given in too concentrated a form so that one small bottle will hold a whole week's supply there is considerable danger of his taking an incorrect dose. Also, because of the difficulty in measuring them accurately, a series of too-large doses will empty the bottle prematurely and the

addict will find himself unprotected—a common reason for buying heroin or methadone on the black market. A compromise must be reached between the two conflicting needs and a concentration of 1 mg. per ml. of base seems to be a useful one. In this way, an addict given a prescription for a fortnight's supply of mixture at a dose of 50 mg. b.d. collects from the chemist a bottle or bottles containing a total of 1.4 litres.

3. But a mixture consisting of methadone hydrochloride powder dissolved in water alone is one which can easily be mainlined and detracts from the advantage of giving an oral preparation. Consequently, additional ingredients need to be incorporated so as to discourage intravenous injection. Gum tragacanth is successfully used in this way by the Chelsea Addiction Center and by Dr. Christie in Portsmouth, but I use as the base chloroform water which causes some pain, but no damage when it is injected. Also I flavor the mixture with blackcurrent syrup, which produces an elegant preparation. The formulation which I use is as follows:—Methadone hydrochloride 50 mg., syrup rib. nig. 20 mls. aqua chloroformis to 50 mls. The dose of this mixture can be changed according to the prevailing clinical need, the patient having been advised to obtain a medicine measuring glass from the chemist in order to measure his dose out accurately.

3. Dr. Weir, Consulting Psychiatrist at St. Mary's Drug Dependency Center in Paddington describes methadone as used primarily for withdrawal purposes:

. . . I do apologize for the delay in answering your letter of May 4th, inquiring about the existence of methadone maintenance programmes in this country. We have consulted other London clinics and as might be expected, none of them have a methadone maintenance programme. I think the main use of methadone in this country is as a stepping stone to coming off heroin. The patient is persuaded to move gradually from intravenous methadone to oral methadone. (Some people have the intermediate step of subcutaneous methadone.) Finally, a gradual tailing off of oral methadone. This is not entirely wishful thinking: we have enticed patients through this whole procedure. As we discussed on your visit to our clinic, it would be impossible with our present laws and practices in this country to introduce ambulatory detoxification such as you have introduced in New York. If, say, we at St. Mary's were to offer this or nothing, our clients would move to some other clinic. The transfer of patients from one clinic to another is discouraged, but is occasionally allowed—from one London clinic to another, and if the patient failed to have his request to be transferred to another London clinic, he could move to some other city in the country to a drug prescription more to his liking.

4. A detoxification program which overlaps with a low-dose methadone over a period of months is described in a communication from Dr. Oppenheim, "Locum Consultant in Psychiatry" at the Charing Cross Hospital, London. Interesting is the use of methadone by injection in the course of withdrawal. His brief account follows:

> ...In this clinic, we are using methadone where possible orally, although at first only by injection, as a substitute for heroin. After a short period on a stable dose, provided the patient is doing well, we reduce this very slowly indeed, often taking months over the process. The maximum dose of methadone given may correspond to the heroin previously taken, or the minimum the patient can tolerate without getting any discomfort.
>
> All our patients are treated as out-patients on a voluntary basis. Any patient has access to the clinic. We do not serve a definite population area. Patients come from all social classes, and all levels of intelligence.
>
> We have only been working in this field for two years, and hence it is difficult to be dogmatic about the effectiveness of the programme. Out of 160 patients, approximately 30 are now off all drugs, and are on a follow-up programme to assess the outcome.

VIRGIN ISLANDS LAW ENFORCEMENT COMMISSION PROGRAM

Dr. George A. Moorehead, Research Director of the Virgin Islands Task Force on Narcotics, Dangerous Drugs and Alcoholism provided us with the following description of three methadone programs under the Department of Health:

A. Department of Health, Division of Public Health Services,

Charlotte Amalie, St. Thomas.

B. Department of Health, Charles Harwood Memorial Hospital,

Christiansted, St. Croix.

C. Knud Hansen Memorial Hospital and Medical Services,

Charlotte Amalie, St. Thomas.

All addicts are placed under the supervision of the Public Health Services. Psychiatric evaluations are the basis for recommending the plan of management, either placing the addict on methadone treatment or for psychiatric care, or both.

In these methadone programs, oral medication is administered in the form of tablets until a blockading and stabilizing dose has been established. Follow-up studies are required of all addicts in order to ascertain the effectiveness and results of the treatment. The administration of liquid methadone in Tang to replace the methadone tablets has been recommended.

Psychiatric evaluation, psychological testing, group or individual therapy, and counseling with the psychiatrist of the Department of Mental Health, Department of Health are referred to this Department if the hospital finds it necessary. The guidelines and treatment plans are the same as those of Dole and Nyswander. A short term inpatient care is available if needed.

All services are offered to the addicts on a voluntary basis unless the courts of the Virgin Islands have placed the addicts under the jurisdiction of the Commissioner of Health under the laws to provide for the Civil Commitment and Rehabilitation of Narcotic Addicts and the Civil Commitment of Persons not charged with any criminal offense.

Characteristics of patient population in the Virgin Islands are as follows:

1. Most of the patients are from St. Thomas and St. Croix.

2. In St. Croix, population 35,285, the majority of drug addicts who are treated are for heroin. The ethnic groups which are involved are mostly the native Puerto Ricans, those of Puerto Rican origin, mainland residents, and a few local residents.

3. In St. Thomas, population 36,290, the picture is a little different. The drug addicts are generally mainland residents and a few local residents.

4. In St. John, population 1,828, there are no known drug addicts who have been treated.

"... At present, there have been about 10-12 patients in St Thomas, Virgin Islands who have attended the Methadone Maintenance Treatment Program at the Public Health Clinic. All patients have high regard for the program and are very much satisfied. The results are excellent.

"In St. Croix, over 100 patients have attended the clinic at one time or another. However, those that have remained in the program are very much satisfied with it and have encouraged others to attend the clinic also."

SWEDISH PROGRAM

The Psychiatric Research Center, Ulleraker Hospital, Uppsala is the locus of methadone treatment in Sweden. The modality was introduced in Sweden by Gunne in 1966. Erikson reports that at that time, the number of patients addicted to different types of narcotic analgesics was estimated to be about 300 located in a few cities, foremost Stockholm and Gothenburg. In Stockholm, an experiment with prescription of opiates was going on; and addicts were being maintained on methadone and other drugs for *parenteral* self-administration. Heroin was practically unavailable on the black market. The main narcotic drugs abused were morphine, meperidine, ketobemedone, methadone, dextromoramide and raw opium. There was a widespread mixed addiction in this group. Amphetamine and phenmetraline i.v. in high doses were often abused together with the mentioned opiates.

Selection of Patients

From January 1967 to October 1970, 83 addicts from the whole country were admitted to the clinic for detoxification from opiates; 38 or 46% entered the methadone program. The major reasons for rejection were: too short history of opiate addiction; too heavy abuse of other drugs or alcohol; and unwillingness to participate in the program be returning to an outpatient clinic every day for medication. The criteria for selection followed those of Dole-Nyswander as did the induction procedures.

After release from the stabilization hospital the patients appeared daily for medication in a pharmacy in their home town. Two times a week, they gave urine samples to be sent to the clinic for TLC to detect use of other opiates, central simulants and hypnotics. Twenty-five pharmacies all over Sweden participated in the out-patient program. Co-operation between the pharmacists and the clinic has been very good. No ambulatory induction was used.

The patients in the Methadone Maintenance Program were well established opiate addicts with an average of ten years' use prior to admission. The age distribution has a median value at 30. There were 6 women and 32 men.

A certain degree of mixed addiction was tolerated. Abuse of central stimulants was as frequent as 63%. Only nine patients had no history of previous or present abuse beside opiates.

Nineteen of the patients had a history of alcohol abuse before they started on opiates. Twelve had opiates as their first drug of abuse, but later mixed other drugs, preferably central stimulants. All patients accepted for methadone maintenance were mainline opiate addicts at the time of admission.

As of October 31st, 1970 among the 38 patients, 16 or 45% were expelled from the treatment program. The main reason for discharge was drug abuse, preferably central stimulants and alcohol, which necessitated the detoxification of 13 patients. In addition, 3 patients asked to leave the program as they found the daily dose administration inconvenient and difficult to combine with their occupational activities.

"The increase in employment from 24 to 76% is a result achieved to a large extent through cooperation with the local social agencies which supported our patients in training and seeking jobs. The remaining 24% are on welfare or are sporadically employed. In this study, medical complications during the period of self-administration were exclusively due to innoculation—hepatitis, was a frequent complication. The only medical complication observed during MMT was transient edemas of the ankles seen in two patients.

"In four cases, it was judged necessary to increase the dose after the first out-patient period. In all these cases, the patients had previously been addicted to methadone. Three patients, now functioning and self-supporting, have recently asked for withdrawal from methadone. They have all been in the program for more than three years."

The results of the Swedish study are comparable to those reported by other methadone programs. An acceptable degree of social rehabilitation was achieved in 76% in the Swedish population as compared with 82% in a New York City study. The majority of failures in Swedish patients was accounted for by a heavy abuse of drugs besides opiates.

A special problem was encountered in patients with a history of previous addiction to methadone. Six patients had used 400–500 mg. methadone daily for parenteral administration before admission. It has been very difficult to maintain these patients on the doses mentioned in our program, and the effect of methadone has been considerably shorter than in other patients in the treatment group. These six patients experienced withdrawal symptoms as early as six hours after an oral dose of 140 mg. of methadone. A dose increase up to 240, on the other hand, made the patients drowsy and difficult to handle. These cases were later stabilized on acetyl-methadol. The results support the view expressed by Dole and co-workers that a methadone maintenance program should screen out those who have a mixed drug addiction or who are heavy users of alcohol. Local pharmacies have proved to be a useful substitute for out-patient clinics and the Swedish MMTP may serve as an example of how a small country can handle an opiate addiction problem of a moderate size.

COMMENTS

This chapter, constitutes an extension of the prior section on "Innovative Methadone Programs in the United States," and covers those programs in Canada, the Virgin Islands, England and Sweden for which data were available at the time of writing. Like the earlier chapter, it describes some of the varied programs which have been leapfrogging abroad; and attempts to indicate the specific colorations and directions assumed by them, based on the geographical and social situation prevailing, specific addict populations served, and the differing conceptualizations and rationales developed by the individual program directors. In an earlier paper, the author, and a colleague discussed the relevance of some new American treatment programs for England—one of them methadone maintenance. In Britain, for example, the usefulness of methadone treatment needed to be measured against the many potent heroin supplies so freely available until recently. (Brill & Jaffe, 1967)

While most programs have followed the Dole-Nyswander model closely, some—such as the British Columbia program-anticipated developments in the United States by first experimenting with low-dose maintenance and ambulatory detoxification techniques. While the populations seem similar, it would have been worthwhile to design comparative studies which could talk to the subject of replication, and provide parameters for cross-cultural comparisons. It is, obviously still possible to do this, and the time is probably appropriate for initiating such studies. In any case, whatever the variations on approach, all programs would concur in the belief that methadone maintenance is a major treatment modality for confirmed heroin addicts. The comments of Mr. Hammond underline the need to maintain a firm structure in methadone programming to obviate misuse of the drug and illicit diversion—which may endanger a program's reputation and effectiveness.

REFERENCES

1. Narcotic Addiction Foundation: Annual Report of Narcotic Addiction Foundation British Vancouver, Canada, 1969.
2. Milligan: Personal Communication from Director of Addiction Research Foundation, Toronto, Ontario, 1970.
3. Hammond: Personal Communication re methadone situation in Canada, 1970.
4. May: Drugs without crime, *Harper's Magazine,* July, 1971.

5. "Cure": Personal Communication from National Addiction and Research Institute, London, 1970.
6. Beckett: Personal Communication from Drug Addiction Clinic, Norwood District Hospital, London, 1970.
7. Weir: Personal Communication from Consulting Psychiatrist, St. Mary's Hospital Drug Dependence Center, Paddington, London, 1970.
8. Oppenheim: Personal Communication from Locum Consultant in Psychiatry, Charing Cross Hospital, London, 1970.
9. Moorehead: Personal Communication from Research Director, Task Force on Narcotics, Dangerous Drugs and Alcoholism, Virgin Islands Law Enforcement Commission, 1970.
10. Erikson: Methadone maintenance treatment of opiate addicts in Sweden, Proceedings Third National Methadone Maintenance Conference, New York City, 1970.

PART EIGHT

Chapter 27.

Summary and Conclusions

Carl D. Chambers
Leon Brill

CONCLUSION

The previous papers confirm that methadone substitution therapy has established itself as an important modality in the treatment of chronic opiate addiction and has become, in the opinion of some workers in the field, the treatment of choice for long-term, compulsive heroin users. It has proliferated in New York, across the country and abroad as an indispensable component in any "armamentarium" of services. It is timely, therefore, that the "State of the Art" for methadone therapy be studied more carefully in order to learn the answers to outstanding issues which have never truly been clarified. The following section reviews some of the issues in relation to methadone and indicates some of the directions future research must pursue.

Philosophic Concepts Governing the Dole-Nyswander Methadone Approach

The original Dole-Nyswander model embodied certain concepts which shaped the ensuing treatment program. Basic to this model was the feeling that there exists no proof of prior psychological or social etiological problems in confirmed addicts, and that much of the psychopathic and acting-out behavior observed is a consequence, rather than cause of the addiction. All that was needed, therefore, was to provide medication (methadone) and the person could become "normal" again. Current studies in self-perception, risk-taking, stimulus-seeking would suggest that such an approach is far too simplistic.

Metabolic - deficiency concept. Dole - Nyswander stressed, rather, the idea of prior physiological factors as etiological and embodied this in their concept of a "metabolic deficiency," using the analogy of insulin and diabetes. Once this "deficiency" was relieved, the person could function normally. Unfortunately this concept was never elaborated further, nor its many ramifications considered. For example, how was it possible for some addicts to grow out of their heroin addiction even without the help of a formal program; through an abstinence program; or by the use of narcotic antagonists? Was the metabolic deficiency a short-lived condition, or did it comprise different time spans for different individuals? Because this concept, or rather hypothesis, generated a number of embarrassments, it was in time discarded by early investigators and replaced by the idea that sustained opiate use created certain physical changes which then helped perpetuate drug-acquisitory behavior and heroin use. The "protracted abstinence" theory postulated that effects following sustained opiate use could persist up to six or seven months following detoxification.

While the "metabolic deficiency" hypothesis has thus never been adequately explained or in any way substantiated, it has nevertheless played a crucial role in shaping methadone programming. Until very recently, the role of ancillary services was underplayed and the involvement of professional personnel, apart from nurses and medical doctors, minimized. As clinical experience mounted over the years, staff began to realize that not all patients were responding uniformly and different levels of services seemed indicated. Clinically, the methadone programs are now distinguishing among three general categories of patients—one group, perhaps up to a third, respond more readily to methadone and require lesser services. A larger central group requires more intensive services; and a third group of hard-core patients needs extraordinary inputs to "make it" in the program. This latter group comprise the "dropouts" who engage in continued drug supplementation and "cheating" as well as other acting-out behavior and constitute the "failures" who mount to some 40% or 50% over a period of years. The need for a variety of methadone modalities to meet the needs of these different kinds of patients has been spelled out by the authors in their "multimodality" paper included in this volume.

The Concept of "narcotic blockade." Another concept basic to the original Dole-Nyswander model is that of "narcotic blockade," which is discussed in several of the papers in this book. Briefly stated, this concept postulates that, with stabilization, methadone occupies all "receptor sites" and thus prevents heroin and other opiates from reaching these sites. A "blockade" is thus established against illegal opiate use, and extraordinary amounts of heroin or other opiates would be needed to overcome this blockade. This concept has been sharply questioned by a number of workers in the field who prefer the idea of cross-tolerance to that of blockade. It has been suggested, for example, that not all the receptor sites become saturated, which could help explain why some addicts can feel a "buzz" even on very low doses of methadone, such as 40 or 50 mg. They can feel this "buzz" even with only one or two bags of highly diluted heroin and have therefore persisted in supplementing their methadone fairly regularly.

Because the concept of blockade has been so crucial in methadone programming, it is important that research be undertaken to determine its validity. One of the problems entailed is that of separating out physiological from subjective effects. For example, how much of the "buzz" is experienced because the heroin is actually felt; or is the satisfaction derived from using a needle? because many addicts have a "needle habit," i.e., they are conditioned to the needle and enjoy "shooting" even if the needle has no drugs? We cannot overlook the context in which drug use occurs, furthermore.

The concept of "narcotics hunger." Another basic concept of the original Dole-Nyswander repertory is that of "narcotic hunger." This corresponds to the concept of "craving," which is considered by numerous workers in the field to be the hallmark of the confirmed, compulsive heroin addict. It is contended that the narcotic hunger is fully accommodated by an adequate dose of methadone: while patients might initially "challenge" the methadone stabilization to test its effectiveness, they would relinquish their drug abuse in time when they learned that methadone did indeed blockade the heroin effects. They might then continue to act out a while longer due to their addictive life style, but this too would diminish and cease well before the end of the year.

Regrettably, this facile progress did not occur in practice, as confirmed by researchers in a variety of programs, as described in the foregoing chapters. Instead, the abuse of drugs continued for one or more years and apparently indefinitely. The "narcotic hunger" was not satiated, and supplementation with other drugs was continued by large numbers of patients. Much work, therefore, remains to be done in this area as well. It is important to learn the relationship between "drug craving" and "drug-seeking" or "drug-taking"; and whether the findings of the Philadelphia Clinic were unique or typical. There is increasing evidence that the latter is true. A number of program directors have tended to underplay this continued "cheating" by patients and to minimize the central importance of urine testing for treatment as well as research purposes. They have, further, not checked for important drugs of abuse such as cocaine and doriden which are being widely abused in numerous programs.

Still other questions relate to the concept of narcotic hunger and narcotic blockade. We know, for example, that the "blockade" is not equally stable for the 36 hours or so the methadone effect is said to persist. There is a waning of effectiveness at certain points, as Goldstein has pointed out; and it is quite possible that patients are more subject to temptation during such low points of stabilization. Obviously, this area too warrants further study. One of the answers to this problem might be the use of a-acetyl-methadol, the longer-acting form used in the Chicago program and active for 72 hours and more. It is quite likely that forms lasting up to a month could be developed and could overcome the gaps in effectiveness observed with ordinary methadone.

Another question which arises is whether there are different kinds of "hunger" for drugs. For example, once the hunger for heroin is relieved, do other kinds of hunger arise—for alcohol, amphetamines or barbiturates? Or are they all variants of a central craving? If so, why is this not fully relieved by methadone? Is the provision of more intensive ancillary services the answer? If so, why? Basic here is the need to differentiate out the physiological from the psychological and social components. As mentioned earlier, it is believed that, even if the physiological needs and craving are satisfied, there still remains the addictive life-style and long-term conditioning and other reinforcing factors for acting-out behavior, including the fears so often described in the literature of growing up, assuming responsibility and succeeding.

Some Pharmacological Questions

The foregoing papers have also pointed up the need for further research and study of such aspects as the time actions and dose-curve relationships of methadone. What are the effects of methadone generally at varying levels and time-intervals in relation to different kinds of addicts? What are the effects on maturation processes (physical and psychological) if given to adolescents? What effects do varying doses have on the ability to concentrate, on memory recall, motor coordination, etc? Is it possible that patients store up methadone and metabolites differently because of differences in metabolism; and if so, what are the implications for treatment? Why are some patients able to function on very low doses of 40 to 50 mgs, which serve primarily as tranquilizers while others need 240 mgs. and more, and even then resort to "cheating" and supplementation? What are the proper ranges for different kinds of patients? What are the short-

and long-range psychological as well as physiological effects? What are the true side effects; why and how do these vary for different patients, and how do we distinguish them from withdrawal symptoms during the low points of stabilization?

Some "philosophical" questions about methadone stabilization and maintenance

The question of "goals." The question of goals is basic since it shapes the direction of the entire program. The most frequently expressed outlook for treatment in most programs is indefinite maintenance on methadone, and this is currently stressed in the New York City intake interviews. The fact is that an experiment did occur with some 25 patients in the New York City program to learn whether patients could be withdrawn from methadone, but the results were negative and the efforts were discontinued. Some programs, such as the earlier one at the Albert Einstein College of Medicine, were geared to abstinence. An important area of research would therefore be to determine what goals are appropriate for different kinds of methadone patients; and, indeed, whether it is possible to get a number of patients off methadone in time. At present, it would seem that some patients could give up methadone; while others, possibly more fragile or fragmented, might need to be maintained indefinitely. The inputs required to help selected patients achieve abstinence would thus need to be studied. An important element, here, which has hitherto not been considered in relation to helping people get off methadone has been the question of "protracted abstinence" as discussed by Martin, *et al.* If this syndrome is indeed a factor reinforcing drug-acquisitory behavior and therefore contributing to recidivism and relapse, it would need to be compensated for by more intensive services and other measures. Unfortunately, nobody has yet related these two discrete facts as elements to be considered conjointly in helping patients achieve abstinence.

Uniform approach to treatment. A basic failing in the

original maintenance model was the assumption of a universal "addict," free of prior psychological and social problems, who therefore required a uniform solution, namely methadone maintenance at a fixed level of 80 to 120 mg., with minimal psychological and social rehabilitation inputs as adjuvant services. In a number of their writings, the authors have spelled out the idea that there is no such universal as "the addict," but rather a variety of addicts from different class and social backgrounds, of varying ethnic and geographical backgrounds and age groupings, stages of involvement in the addiction system as well as states of readiness for help. If we accept this assumption, then it should be clear that no one treatment approach will be effective for all, and that variations in methadone therapy need to be tried along the lines suggested in the multimodality paper. Different goals would need to be defined for different kinds of patients.

The structuring of treatment. Still another basic question in the treatment of all addicts is the amount of acting-out behavior and continued drug abuse which can be tolerated before a patient is dropped from a program. Most programs have generally been very tolerant of continued drug abuse. The idea has even been expressed by some workers that drug abuse is relative, i.e., that the patients are better off than before since they are using "purer," legal drugs, and a "relative" definition of success should prevail. This question, which eventually becomes a philosophical question as well, relates to the goals to be sought. Must we insist on total abstinence before we consider a patient successful? If we measure the patient against the community and social background from which he derives, where a great deal of drug abuse of various kinds may prevail, should we, or can we insist on higher goals of abstinence than exist for his contemporaries?

Another question relates to the level of functioning to be sought in the areas of work, love and interpersonal relationships generally. Is it enough to be drug abstinent if patients continue to act out in other areas, as in being sexually promiscuous, especially if married, or beating their wives and neglecting their children, or otherwise up-setting the applecart? What should we expect in the way of mature behavior from graduates? What is the actual quality of their performance and behavior on the job and elsewhere? For example, most evaluation reports play up the high percentage of employment success. Nobody, however, seems to have examined this statistic more closely to determine the level of job satisfaction achieved and the kinds of jobs the graduates are filling. The authors' experience indicates that many of the jobs are marginal and transitory; and may, in the long run, become a source of discontent and grievance and reason for relapsing to drugs or engaging in other anti-social behavior. This problem has not been anticipated suffi-ciently in terms of helping methadone patients prepare for more challenging occupations which will afford them continuing job satisfaction and, therefore, stability. In the same way, the quality of the human relationships es-tablished and their general day-to-day functioning in the community has not been scrutinized closely.

The components of methadone programming.   The role which various components play in a general methadone program has never been adequately studied and needs to be researched further. Among the areas to be examined, we would mention the following:

The role of structure—If any general categorization can be made of addicts, it is that they tend to act out their anxieties and depression, and means need to be found for structuring treatment firmly in order to hold them and deal with their testing out and manipulative behavior until they can change their addictive or "psychopathic" life style. There has been much confusion around this central point, with programs veering between extreme rigidity and great slackness, or even lack of control. Some of the newer directors of programs seem to have seized on methadone almost as if it were a plaything; un-fortunately, without having had prior experience with addicts through other modalities. It is essential that they realize that addiction is indeed a chronic relapsing illness and that treatment entails a tremendous investment of energy, patience and tolerance to stay with a patient until he can "make it" even with a metha- done assist. The appropriate kinds of structures and degrees of control required in each program for different kinds of addicts have not been studied, and it is impor- tant that this be undertaken for methadone as well. The proper structuring of treatment requires great experi- ence and skill: if we draw the lines too tight at the begin- ning of treatment before the patient has been engaged, we may drive him away. If we are too "loose," we may be fostering continued acting-out behavior, thereby "diluting" the program, and contaminating other pa- tients who are trying to do well. We need to find the optimal balances between structure and permissiveness; and these will vary in different stages of the patient's progress.

The place of "ancillary services"—The role of ancillary services has been underplayed, with professionals such as psychiatrists, psychologists and social workers not ordinarily playing a central role in the program. Much of this emanated from the concept of addiction as a physico- medical disease, which therefore required medical people primarily to deal with it—mainly medical doctors and nurses. The other people used were generally untrained for counseling such as college graduates as well as the "RA's," "research assistants," who were methadone "graduates" and were used as role models. It is only in the last year or two that the need for more intensive services became apparent and some social workers were provided to serve as "trouble shooters" for the more difficult cases, as well as a few psychiatrists and social workers to conduct group therapy in isolated clinics.

There has been talk, recently, about shifting metha- done patients to private doctors as a means of building the patient population rapidly. This approach still derives from the concept that only a "methadone assist" is required for most patients, free of ancillary services. In the opinion of the authors, this would be a most unfortu- nate occurrence since ordinary doctors are not trained to work with addicts, could easily be manipulated or would otherwise be unequipped to deal with the testing-out behavior of their patients, or provide the necessary ancillary helping services. This would undoubtedly diminish methadone treatment and generally contribute to the further illicit diversion and abuse of methadone. It should be possible to find better ways for doctors to participate in formal programs by joining the staff of existing programs and receiving further training.

Urine testing—Most programs have tended to underplay the role of urine testing and some directors have even talked of eliminating it entirely as an unnecessary expense. This too would be unfortunate since, in the opinion of the authors, the use of urinalysis is essential not only for structuring treatment, but for research as well. In treatment, for example, we can ascertain when patients are abusing other drugs and use it as a basis for counseling and discussion to help the patient relinquish his continued drug abuse and other acting-out behavior. It is a crucial component of research too since, as researchers have demonstrated, counselors are not aware of the extensive abuse underway in spite of claims to the contrary, and it is necessary to have objective verification. Urinalysis thus becomes a most important avenue for learning what is, in fact, happening with patients, and what more needs to be built into a program to help different patients progress.

A third factor to be considered is political. Because so much criticism of methadone treatment still prevails, it is important to have objective data on hand confirming the progress patients are making.

The Pharmacology of Methadone

A number of questions about methadone itself have never been resolved, and it is timely that the research get underway without further delay.

1) For example, there is much disagreement still as to what constitutes a lethal dose to individuals at different tolerance levels. There is no reference to this, to our knowledge, in all the literature.

2) Another unresearched question—what are the various excretion patterns of methadone as these relate to the interruptions, waning of effects, and other parameters?

3) What should be the proper procedure for administering supplementary narcotic drugs for people already stabilized on methadone—as in the case of accidents or surgery?

4) What are the possibilities for treating addicts on low doses of methadone as against high doses? While some work has been done in this area in Philadelphia, Chicago, California and Canada, more information is needed.

5) Inpatient versus outpatient stabilization—This question seems to have been resolved in the last two years since more than 80% of new methadone patients are being stabilized on an outpatient basis. Inpatient space is now reserved for multiple drug users and addicts as well as those with severe social or emotional problems.

6) Poly-drug users—The utility of methadone for poly-drug users has hardly been discussed in the literature. Yet this is becoming an increasingly urgent problem. In recent years, we have been witnessing the gradual disappearance or submergence of the "classical" group of heroin addicts; namely, those who used heroin as their drug of choice some 91% of the time and took other drugs only incidentally, to "boost" or potentiate the effects of their heroin. More recently a "new breed" of multiple drug users has emerged, who use drugs indiscriminately. They may thus be abusing amphetamines, barbiturates, LSD, marijuana, alcohol and heroin and may be addicted to one or more of these substances simultaneously. How helpful is methadone in relation to this new breed of drug user, or how could it be used for this group?

7) Concurrent psychotropic medication—Another area which has not been explored sufficiently, and in which great variation is noted from program to program is the utility of different psychotropic medications for methadone patients. For example, what are the effects of the phenothiazines or major tranquilizers on psychotic

patients when used in conjunction with methadone? For patients who are not psychotic, how can psychotropic drugs such as librium and valium be used? Still another problem is the use of various sleeping medications since sleeplessness is a problem for many methadone patients, especially in the earlier stages. What about the use of bulk laxatives for constipation? Still other patients have complained about the loss of libido when on methadone and this, too, needs to be researched carefully. The problem is complex since we would need to know the sex life of the patient before he began heroin use, while he was on heroin, and currently on methadone. It would also be necessary to differentiate out the physiological effects of methadone or heroin from subjective factors, including also the factor of age. For example, the patient's greater libido initially may have been related to his youth, and his diminished libido a function of the aging process rather than of methadone.

8) The question of side effects—This question too, requires further investigation. There is speculation that much of what has been considered "side effects" may actually be withdrawal effects for patients not adequately maintained on methadone or, possibly observed at a low or "waning" point of their methadone stabilization. There is still much difference of opinion about the extent of side effects, their persistence over time, and the variations noted among different patients.

9) "Inexperienced" or younger addicts—The utility of methadone for neophyte narcotic addicts needs to be clarified. In the past, the criteria for admission to a program were strict, stipulating at least five years of use (more recently reduced to two years) and a minimal age of 21, (more recently lowered to 18). Can methadone be used with inexperienced or neophyte users? This is a complex problem since the age of heroin addicts has been dropping steadily and now includes some youngsters under 10. There is much feeling still about using methadone maintenance or other drugs with youthful users. A number of program directors have experimented with low-dose methadone at the level of 40-50 mg. for younger

users and claim "success" in reaching them. More needs to be undertaken along these lines, comparing also the effectiveness of narcotics-antagonists with such youthful heroin or poly-drug users.

10) The newest issue—An important issue, with philosophical overtones and implications for treatment was recently brought into focus by the authors. The question posed was whether the methadone maintenance modality can be an appropriate regimen of choice for persons who are primarily methadone addicts? Can methadone ever be a "medicine" for those persons who have chosen to abuse it for its euphoric effects? Recent findings by Chambers in Miami, Florida indicate that as many as 50% of all new admissions to maintenance have methadone in their urines prior to receiving *any* medication; and as many as 25% are submitting intake urines positive for methadone and negative for heroin or other narcotics. Is this a form of "self-treatment" prior to acceptance in a formal treatment program, or is it primary methadone abuse? At the present time, we do not know. We do understand that, until programs begin to control the diversion of their "take-home" medications, primary methadone addiction, medicine supplementation, self-treatment and the initiation of drug-naive persons to methadone will continue.

Expansion of Methadone Programming

It has been observed that quantitative changes in a program lead to qualitative changes as well, and this has been a source of concern for methadone programmers as they envision the proliferation of methadone programs. It is feared that dilution of the program could occur and its effectiveness be reduced. The optimal size for each "satellite" clinic was originally indicated to be 75 to 100 addicts. This has expanded to 150 and, in some cases, beyond. This area therefore poses a number of questions: what changes are produced by expanding facilities beyond the capacity initially envisioned, and what staff are required to maintain firm control of each program?

No studies have been done to determine the optimal size of methadone maintenance clinics, nor the optimal staffing patterns required.

Illicit Diversion of Methadone

A growing problem has been the diversion of methadone for illicit purposes. It has been noted, for example, that a number of patients sell their methadone over the weekend, when they are not being scrutinized, to purchase heroin and experience a "high." Others may sell their methadone by accumulating portions over a period of time. Still others may feel their dose is not adequate and purchase methadone to supplement their own supply. With the "diskettes" now available, patients can gauge how much methadone they are receiving. The growing problem of illicit abuse is being documented increasingly both here and abroad and is a continuing source of anxiety to the community and to the programs. This question obviously relates, additionally, to the problem of death from methadone overdose. The reasons for such deaths, whether attributable to methadone abuse or other causes, need to be studied.

Retention Rates and "Success"*

Last, but not least, is the question of adequate evaluation of methadone programming. Apart from the numerous areas which have not been researched adequately is the problem of *effective* and *accurate* evaluation of each patient's progress in the program. There is an ever-increasing, quite understandable criticism of the evaluations conducted to date. Concerned clinicians and researchers have become aware that frequently-touted retention figures of some 80% are deliberate attempts to mislead critics of the modality. Unfortunately, *not everyone counts everyone* when compiling "retention" or "attrition" statistics to share with their

* The authors are indebted to William McGlothlin and Victor Tabbush for their obvious assistance in this section.

professional peers, with funding sources or with the less-than-informed public.

Clearly, addicts' admissions into methadone programs are not, *per se,* measures of success. Admission and retention data can be used as indicators that methadone programs may be considered successful only when combined with additional criteria. If, for example, methadone maintenance *does decrease* criminal activity and *does increase* employment, then the numbers of addicts accepted into, and retained in these programs (relative to non-addicts and other treatment modalities) represent "derived" success data. Stated somewhat differently, if this program "does some good," then the number of addicts it attracts and retains may be viewed as a measure of "the good they do."

It is entirely possible, and not entirely undesirable to keep in mind that retention in a maintenance program could be essentially attributed to the medication alone, just as heroin addiction dictates, or at least focuses drug-seeking behavior.

While it is obvious that variations do and will exist in retention figures because of the known differences in admission requirements and discharge policies, other reasons for the variations are not so obvious.

Regardless of admission or discharge policies, we believe all programs should count all patients in exactly the same way. For a variety of reasons, this has not been done. In addition, when it was not done, attempts too often were made to make it appear as if it was.

A much more subtle subterfuge occurs when terminations are reported as a simple percentage of total admissions. Clinicians and researchers, particularly when dealing with the news media, funding sources and the criminal justice system, often quote percentages of this type as a measure of the retention success of the modality. This is most misleading. Figures in this form are simply census data; they indicate only the numbers of patients admitted and the numbers terminated. Patient continuance in programs *must* be placed in a time concept, which can be correctly measured only in those terms which reflect length-of-stay. The termination percentages in most published reports include *no* information about the length-of-stay. Moreover, they are strongly biased by the timing of admissions. Admissions into most methadone programs have been increasing rapidly over time. Admissions in one program, for example, have increased at a rate sufficient to almost double the number of patients in treatment each year. The large proportion of recently-admitted patients in most of the reported study samples produce strong downward biases in termination percentages since these reports explicitly avoid accounting for patient length-of-stay.

It would appear that the following are true, but *do* require replication:

a) The "magic" retention figure for maintenance programs is probably 50-60%. Variations exist only in how quickly one arrives at that point. Programs with no selection criteria, for example, have earlier attritions than those which have them.

b) Particularly high attrition rates occur during the early months of treatment.

None of this is, of course, meant to downgrade the efficacy of methadone programming, but rather to reemphasize the need for expanding our understanding of the "State of the Art" and plan the inputs needed to upgrade and standardize the accounting systems through these elaborations.

Central Data Bank

There is need to establish a national central data bank for a variety of reasons: to avoid patients' duplication of programs and to permit the collation and comparison of data on a continuous basis, among others.

Need for Typology

The authors, in their multimodality paper attempted to draw together the varied experiences of different methadone programs under an inclusive rationale. It was hoped that a typology of the various kinds of addicts who come to methadone could, in time, be developed and differentiated approaches elaborated. The range of "modalities" outlined in the paper varied from detox to low-dose to high-dose maintenance, to the combined methadone maintenance-therapeutic community for the most recalcitrant patients and potential "dropouts."

It is possible to conjecture at this time that many of the heroin addicts admitted to methadone programs never really relinquished conventional social goals, but were troubled individuals who required a "medical assist" such as methadone to help them function. This group would therefore be not too different from patients maintained on insulin, tranquilizers or dilantin. Their apparent "deviant" behavior and frequent arrests and criminal involvement were a result of our criminal definition of the problem rather than any basic "psychopathic personality" or "character disorder."

In contrast to these "adaptive" users, we might then speculate about the truly "deviant" users who remain opposed to conventional social goals and are unable to relate themselves to a program whose primary treatment emphasis is productive social functioning. It is possible that this latter group comprises the recalcitrant "third" of methadone patients who continue to act out in a variety of ways and ultimately drop out of treatment. This dichotomy points up some of the questions we may need to confront before we can reach and help certain addicts who do not respond to our ordinary approaches.

This reinforces the need to define a typology which distinguishes among the various kinds of methadone patients in terms of characteristics; and to ascertain the kinds of structure, medications and ancillary services required to help them succeed. A striking finding in the last years has been the fact that some patients can make it on low-dose methadone stabilization, and we need to develop criteria to learn which respond best at this level. We should eventually save much time, energy and money by understanding generally which approach or services can help each kind of addict and probably head off many of the "failures" as well. We must further examine the modifications in approach required for younger heroin users and multiple drug users. Because of the numerous continued gaps in our understanding, as outlined above, it is apparent that we cannot achieve these goals or maximize methadone's potential for helping different segments of the addict population. It is urgent that this research be instituted forthwith in order to increase our scientific understanding of the proper uses of methadone, its benefits and potential dangers and its true role as a helping agent for opiate users.

Department of Health, Education, and Welfare Food and Drug Administration [21 CFR Part 130] New Drugs Proposed Special Requirements For Use of Methadone

Methadone has been under investigation for use in the maintenance treatment of narcotic addicts for approximately 9 years. For the past 2 years, interest in this use has grown steadily and intensely. In the FEDERAL REGISTER of April 2, 1971 (36 F.R. 6075), the Food and Drug Administration published § 130.44 (21 CFR 130.44) which established guidelines for investigating the use of methadone in maintenance treatment, for assuring the availability of valid data on such use, and for protecting the community from the hazards of diversion and abuse of methadone. These guidelines were developed in cooperation with the National Institute of Mental Health (NIMH) and the Bureau of Narcotics and Dangerous Drugs (BNDD), Department of Justice. To date the Food and Drug Administration and the Bureau of Narcotics and Dangerous Drugs have approved a substantial number of individual treatment units for use of methadone in treating addiction.

In addition to being used for investigational purposes, methadone has been prescribed by individual physicians and has been dispensed in medical institutions both for heroin detoxification and for maintenance therapy. It is not possible to determine how widespread the use of methadone for maintenance therapy has been outside investigational new drug plans, but there is evidence that this use is substantial.

The Food and Drug Administration, in cooperation with the National Institute of Mental Health and the Special Action Office for Drug Abuse Prevention, is undertaking an intensive inspection program to ascertain that existing programs operating under investigational new drug status (IND) meet the requirements of § 130.44. Within the immediate future, each program will be visited by an inspection team. Programs will be allowed to continue to operate if they meet the existing requirements of § 130.44. However, in addition, the proposed special requirements contained in this notice are being encompassed by the inspection in anticipation of improved requirements to be in effect in the future. To reduce the potential for diversion and misuses methadone is also being withdrawn systematically from pharmacies that are not dispensing it solely as part of approved treatment programs using methadone.

The use of methadone presents difficult and unique questions of medical judgment, law enforcement, and public policy that have not previously been encountered with other new drugs. Methadone presently represents the only drug for which there is substantial evidence of effectiveness in the treatment of heroin addiction. Although the short-term use of the drug has been shown to be relatively safe from a toxicity standpoint, more information is necessary on the toxicity of long-term use. Balancing the benefits against the risks, the Food and Drug Administration and numerous professional groups, advisory committees, and experts with whom it has consulted have concluded that the drug should be made available for all addicts who consent to use it in approved treatment programs. Retention of the drug solely on an investigational status appears to be no longer warranted.

At the same time, concern has been expressed that the usual form of NDA (new drug application) approval could lead to greater diversion or misuse of the drug, since it permits unrestricted distribution and allows physicians to use wide discretion in prescribing the drug. It has been suggested that the investigational status of the drug should be retained both to obtain additional toxicity data and as a control mechanism, at least until greater experience is obtained in reducing the potential dangers of diversion and medical misuse. The FDA recognizes these dangers and agrees that strong control must be maintained over the distribution and use of the drug. Since it is an opiod the potential for abuse is greater than for other drugs permitted for widespread medical use. The Food and Drug Administration could not conclude that it is safe if it cannot be properly controlled and would be required to disapprove its use. Some diversion and misuse will inevitably result from the availability of any drug, but it is particularly important that strong controls be available for methadone because of its known addicting potential. Finally, some have pointed out that it is premature to move completely from IND to NDA status because more information has yet to be obtained. The Commissioner concurs that unlimited approval of an NDA for methadone would not be appropriate at this time.

To provide the strongest possible control over the distribution and use of methadone, the Commissioner has concluded that both the IND and NDA control mechanisms should be utilized together with the authority granted under the Comprehensive Drug Abuse Control Act of 1970. Like an NDA, the drug will be available for treatment in all cases where there is medical justification. Like an IND controlled drug, there will be a permanent record showing the pattern of distribution of the drug because the institutions using the drug and the physicians and pharmacists operating in cooperation with the institution will be required to register all use of the drug. It will permit the Food and Drug Administration to withdraw methadone from its present unqualified approval status in pharmacies for detoxification, analgesic, and antitussive purposes. Thus, a new closed system of distribution will be established, under which any diversion or misuse can immediately be stopped at the source of supply. At the same time the drug will be available for use without all the IND restrictions for all addicts for whom it is medically justified.

The Commissioner recognizes that this is a novel form

of control designed to reflect the unique problems posed by this drug. It has not previously been necessary to utilize IND and the NDA procedures concurrently in order to assure the safe and effective use of a new drug. Because of the seriousness of the medical and social problems associated with heroin addiction and because methadone is the only drug available for the treatment of heroin addiction, the Commissioner has concluded that it is no longer feasible to retain methadone solely for investigational use. It is therefore appropriate to add the special requirements set forth in this proposal in order to permit the drug to be available wherever medical opinion concludes that it should be used in the treatment of heroin addiction.

The Commissioner feels that the mandate in section 4 of the Comprehensive Drug Abuse Prevention and Control Act of 1970 can be appropriately applied to determining the conditions under which methadone may be safely used in treating narcotic addicts. This section requires the Secretary of Health, Education and Welfare after consultation with the Attorney General and with national organizations representative of persons with knowledge and experience in the treatment of narcotic addicts, to determine the appropriate methods of professional practice in the medical treatment of narcotic addiction. . . . The Secretary has delegated the authority to make this determination to the Commissioner of Food and Drugs.

In carrying out the requirements of the Comprehensive Drug Abuse Prevention and Control Act, the Commissioner has widely consulted and maintained close communications with the medical profession regarding use of methadone. Among those associations or groups consulted are the American Medical Association's Council on Mental Health, the National Research Council's Committee on Problems of Drug Dependence, the American Psychiatric Association's Commission on Drug Abuse, a task force of the American Society of Pharmacology and Experimental Therapeutics, the Joint Food and Drug Administration/National Institutes of Mental Health Psychotomimetic Advisory Committee, the FDA Drug Abuse Advisory Committee, the Special Action Office of the White House, and the National Institute of Mental

Health. The consensus is strong among medical experts and the Food and Drug Administration that currently available evidence on the safety and effectiveness of methadone is sufficient to permit its use for the maintenance treatment of narcotic addiction as proposed in this notice.

On the basis of the above considerations, the Commissioner of Food and Drugs, after consultation with the associations and groups listed above and the Bureau of Narcotics and Dangerous Drugs, and with the endorsement of the Special Action Office of the White House, proposes that the special requirements set out in this notice be imposed upon the use of methadone. These new controls should not interfere with the availability of methadone in the treatment of severe pain or for detoxification or hospitalized addicts. Methadone for the treatment of severe pain on either an inpatient or outpatient basis will be available from hospital pharmacies.

It is proposed that patients under 18 not be admitted to a treatment program using methadone until additional study is completed to determine whether methadone may be safely and effectively used in their treatment. Such additional study must be conducted pursuant to all the requirements of the usual investigational new drug plan. This will mean that juveniles will be excluded from virtually all ongoing treatment programs using methadone except investigational programs with an IND approval. Comment is solicited as to whether the benefits of completing additional studies outweigh the risks of excluding these patients from treatment programs at this time with the likely result that they will continue to use injected heroin.

Under this proposal, the distribution of the drug is limited to treatment programs using methadone and to hospital pharmacies approved by the Food and Drug Administration. Requests for approval of programs received by FDA will be sent to BNDD for any comment it may have prior to FDA approval. BNDD may inspect any such program or may furnish FDA any relevant information from its files. FDA will give great weight to any information, comments, or recommendation received from BNDD in determining whether approval should be granted or, once granted, should be revoked. Methadone will no longer be permitted for antitussive use as the benefits of methadone for this use do not outweigh the risk involved from unsafe and ineffective use.

The Food and Drug Administration believes that State health or mental health authorities are essential to adequately controlling methadone, to assuring that the need for a methadone program exists, and to establishing criteria and guidance for rehabilitation efforts. Approval of a program by the State health or mental health authority designated under the provisions of section 314(d) of the Public Health Service Act or by his designee will be a part of approval of the treatment programs using methadone by FDA. The Food and Drug Administration will contact each State to establish the necessary channels of communication and to establish procedure for the implementation of the program, and will provide information upon request.

Section 130.44 *conditions for investigational use of methadone for maintenance programs for narcotic addicts* (21 CFR 130.44) will continue in effect until a final order is issued after consideration of the comments submitted on this proposal. To increase control over methadone and to improve patient care prior to the finalization of this proposal, however, the guidelines in § 130.44 will be enforced as a requirement for a methadone maintenance investigational program. Any IND that varies in any material respect from the protocol in § 130.44 will require justification.

The following additional provisions will be required of all methadone maintenance investigational programs during the time between the publication of this proposal and its final promulgation:

1. Only oral dosage forms of methadone formulated in such a way as to reduce its potential for parenteral abuse and accidental ingestion will be provided patients for unsupervised use under approved programs.

2. The selection of patients is to be carried out in accordance with the requirements of item V, B, of the form "Application for Approval of Treatment Program Using

Methadone" which appears in proposed section 130.48 (b) (2) (i).

3. Dosage for detoxification and maintenance is to be in accordance with the requirements of item VIII, A, of the form "Application for Approval of Treatment Program Using Methadone" which appears in proposed section 130.48 (b) (2) (i).

4. The recordkeeping requirements are to be in accordance with the information requested in the form "Annual Report for Treatment Program Using Methadone" which appears in proposed section 130.48 (b) (2) (iii).

5. All patients in the methadone investigational program are to be given careful consideration for discontinuance of methadone in accordance with item VIII, D, of the form "Application for Approval of Treatment Program Using Methadone" which appears in proposed section 130.48 (b) (2) (i).

6. Distribution of methadone will be restricted to direct shipments to approved investigational programs and hospital pharmacies, unless an alternative method of distribution is approved by FDA after consultation with BNDD.

The above stated provisions will be required of all new and ongoing methadone investigational programs within 30 days of the date of publication of this notice. An amended "Notice of Claimed Investigational Exemption for Methadone for Use in the Maintenance Treatment of Narcotic Addicts" shall be submitted by all ongoing programs and by new programs. These amended forms may be obtained from the Food and Drug Administration, 5600 Fishers Lane, Rockville, Maryland 20852.

Accordingly, purusant to provisions of the Federal Food, Drug, and Cosmetic Act (secs. 505, 701(a), 52 Stat. 1052-53 as amended, 1055; 21 U.S.C. 355, 371(a))and the Comprehensive Drug Abuse Prevention and Control Act of 1970 (sec. 4, 84 Stat. 1241; 42 USC 257a) and under authority delegated to him (21 CFR 2.120), the Commissioner of Food and Drugs proposes that § 130.48 be amended by adding a new paragraph (b), as follows:

§130.48 Drugs that are subjects of approved new drug applications and that require special studies, records, and reports.

(a) * * *

(b) *Methadone.* Methadone is an approved drug for marketing as an analgesic and for the detoxification and treatment of narcotic addicts. Methadone has been under investigation for a number of years for use as an oral substitute for heroin in the maintenance treatment of narcotic addicts. The nature of the use of methadone in maintenance treatment is such that the drug may be used for long periods of time. Further chronic toxicity studies are needed to establish the safety of long-term use. In view of the usefulness of methadone and the tremendous social problems associated with the narcotics problem, the Commissioner of Food and Drugs finds that it is not in the public interest to withhold the drug from the market until further long-term studies have been completed. In view of problems of abuse and misuse associated with the widespread availability of methadone, adequate controls are essential for the safe use of the drug. The drug should nevertheless continue to be available for treatment of severe pain in patients where no substitute therapy is suitable.

In view of these considerations, the Commissioner of Food and Drugs has concluded that it is essential to the public interest to prescribe detailed conditions for safe and effective use of methadone. Methadone maintenance treatment will be permitted under both the IND and NDA control mechanisms established in the statute and regulations. These conditions of use are intended to assure that the required studies for assessing the safety of the long-term administration are performed, to monitor records and determine that required reports are maintained, to maintain close control over distribution and availability of the drug, and to detail responsibilities for such control:

(1) The following conditions must be met in order for methadone to be used for maintenance and detoxification in connection with a treatment program using methadone:

(i) The drug is limited to oral dosage forms formulated in such a way as to reduce its potential for parenteral abuse and accidental ingestion.

(ii) The manufacturers of methadone will develop additional data from chronic animal toxicity studies in which the drug is administered orally at high doses to dogs or monkeys for 1 year and rats for 18 months or mice for 2 years. Observations will include effects on behavior, growth, food and water consumption, blood and urine chemistry, hematological systems, cardiovascular and respiratory systems. Postmortem examinations will include complete gross and histopathological examinations. Reproduction studies following the FDA 1966 guidelines will be performed.

(iii) Further chronic clinical studies with particular attention to the toxicity of methadone in the hematopoietic, cardiovascular, endocrine, hepatic, and immunological systems will be performed under Federally sponsored programs.

(iv) Reports of studies will be submitted pursuant to § 130.13.

(v) At the end of each year after the date of approval, representatives of the Food and Drug Administration, the applicant, appropriate experts, and, if necessary, the investigator(s) will meet to determine whether or not clinical studies should be continued.

(vi) Shipments of the drug are restricted to direct shipments by the holders of approved or investigational new drug applications for methadone to approved treatment programs using methadone. Alternative methods of distribution may be used if they are approved by FDA after consultation with the Bureau of Narcotics and Dangerous Drugs. These treatment programs using methadone must have been reviewed by the appropriate State health or mental health authority designated pursuant to section 314(d) of the Public Health Service Act, or his designee, and notification of the program's approval must have been received from the Food and Drug Administration. Prior to such notification, applications for treatment programs using methadone shall be reviewed by FDA and shall be sent by FDA to BNDD for any information, comments, or recommendations it may have.

(2) A treatment program using methadone shall be approved by FDA if all of the following conditions are met:

(i) The person assuming responsibility for the program

must complete, sign, and file in triplicate with the Food and Drug Administration a Form FD_____, "Application for Approval of Treatment Program Using Methadone" as follows:

FORM FD_____
APPLICATION FOR APPROVAL
OF TREATMENT PROGRAM
USING METHADONE

Name of other identification of program
Address

Commissioner
Food and Drug Administration
Bureau of Drugs (BD-22)
Rockville, Maryland 20852

Dear Sir:

As the person (program director) responsible for this program, I submit this request for approval of a treatment program using methadone to provide maintenance treatment and detoxification for narcotic addicts. I understand that failure to abide by the requirements described below are a violation of the law and may result in revocation of approval of my application, seizure of my drug supply, an injunction, and criminal prosecution.

I. Attached is evidence to indicate approval of the program by the State authority designated pursuant to section 314(d) of the Public Health Service Act (or his designee).

II. Attached is the name, complete address, and a summary of the scientific training and experience of each physician and all other professional personnel having major responsibilities for the program and rehabilitative efforts and a signed Form FD_____, "Medical Responsibility Statement for Treatment Program Using Methadone" for every licensed practitioner authorized to prescribe, dispense, or administer methadone under the program. (Copies of the required form are obtainable from this agency at the same address to which this application is mailed).

III. Attached is the name, address, and description of each hospital, institution, clinical laboratory facility or other facility available to provide the necessary services. The program must have ready access to a comprehensive range of medical and rehabilitative services. These shall be described and shall comply with any guidelines established by Federal or State authorities.

IV. Attached is a statement of the approximate number of addicts to be included in the program.

V. The following minimal treatment standards will be used:

A. Attached is a statement which will be given to the addicts to inform them about the program. Participation in the program should be voluntary.

B. Care will be exercised in the selection of patients to prevent the possibility of admitting a person who has not been dependent upon heroin or other morphine-like drugs and thereby creating de novo a state of dependence upon methadone. The mere use of an opiate, even if periodic or intermittent, cannot be equated with drug dependence. Admission to the program will be dependent upon a history of physiological dependence on one or more opiate drugs (which will be recorded in the applicant's medical record) and evidence of current physiological dependence on opiates of demonstrated by the results of urinalysis and signs of opiate withdrawal. It is highly unlikely that an individual would be currently dependent on opiates without a positive urinalysis for opiates and/or without demonstrating at least the early signs of withdrawal (lacrimation, rhinorrhea, pupillary dilatation, and piloerection) during the initial period of abstinence. Other positive evidence of use can be obtained by noting the presence of needle tracks and by obtaining additional history from relatives and friends. The withdrawal signs may be observed during an initial period of hospitalization or while the individual is an outpatient undergoing diagnostic evaluation (history, physical examination, and laboratory studies). Loss of appetite and increased body temperature, pulse rate, blood pressure, and respiratory rate are also signs of withdrawal, but their detection requires inpatient observations.

C. An exception to the requirement for evidence of current physiological dependence on opiates will be allowed under exceptional circumstances. For example, methadone treatment may be initiated for an individual with a history of opiate addiction a short time prior to or upon release from a stay of 1 month or longer in a penal or chronic care institution. In these circumstances, the reasons for this exception, appropriate descriptions of the facilities, procedures, and qualifications of the personnel of the institution or other appropriate justification will be sent to the Food and Drug Administration at the time of filing this application or with the Annual Report.

D. Additional study is necessary to determine whether methadone may be safely and effectively used in the treatment of patients under 18. No such patients will be admitted to a treatment program using methadone unless prior approval of a Form FD 1571, "Notice of Claimed Investigational Exemption for a New Drug," has been obtained. Such approval will be granted only for a controlled clinical study and not for an ongoing treatment program.

VI. I agree that an admission evaluation and record will be made and maintained for each patient upon admission to the program and will consist of the following:

A. Personal history including age, sex, educational level, employment history, criminal history, and past history of drug abuse of all types;

B. Medical history and history of psychiatric illness and current legal problems, if any; and

C. Physical examination results.

VII. I understand that there is a danger of drug dependent persons attempting to enroll in more than one methadone maintenance program in order to obtain quantities of methadone either for the purpose of self-administration or illicit marketing. To prevent such multiple enrollments, I will participate in whatever local, regional, or national patient identification system exists or is developed. Except in an emergency situation, methadone shall not be provided to a patient who is known to be currently receiving the drug from any other treatment program using methadone. Except as provided in item XV of this form, information that would identify the patient will be kept confidential pursuant to section 303 of the Public Health

Service Act and will not be divulged in any civil, criminal, administrative, legislative, or other proceedings conducted by Federal, State, or local authorities.

VIII. The following minimal procedures will be used for ongoing care:

A. Dosage and administration for detoxification and maintenance.

1. The methadone will be administered in oral form.

2. In detoxification, the patient may be placed on a substitutive methadone administration schedule when there are significant symptoms of withdrawal. The dosage schedule indicated below is recommended but should be varied depending upon clinical judgment. Initially, a single oral dose of 15-20 milligrams of methadone will often be sufficient. Additional methadone can be provided if withdrawal symptoms are not suppressed or whenever symptoms reappear. When patients are physically dependent on high doses of methadone, it may be necessary to exceed these levels. With the exception of such patients, 40 milligrams per day in single or divided doses will usually constitute an adequate stabilizing dose level. Stabilization can be continued for 2 to 3 days and then the amount of methadone can be gradually decreased. The rate at which methadone is decreased will be determined separately for each patient. The dose of methadone can be decreased on a daily basis or, at most, in 2-day intervals. However, the amount of intake must always be sufficient to keep withdrawal symptoms at a tolerable level. In hospitalized patients a daily reduction of 20 percent of the total daily dose usually will be tolerated and causes little discomfort. When the total dosage has decreased to 20 milligrams per day, the dose can be reduced by 50 percent per day without producing significant discomfort. If a patient complains of undue distress, phenothiazine may be used in lieu of increasing the methadone dose. In ambulatory patients, a somewhat slower schedule may be needed.

In any event, if methadone is administered for more than 3 weeks, the procedure will be considered to have pro-

gressed from detoxification or treatment of the acute withdrawal syndrome to that of methadone maintenance even though the goal and intent may be eventual total withdrawal.

3. In maintenance treatment the initial dosage of methadone should control the abstinence symptoms that follow withdrawal of heroin but should not be so great as to cause marked sedation or respiratory depression. It is important that the initial dosage be adjusted to the narcotic tolerance of the new patient. If such a patient has been a heavy user of heroin up to the day of admission, he may be given 20 milligrams orally for the first dose and another 20 milligrams 4 to 8 hours later or 40 milligrams in a single oral dose. If he enters treatment with little or no narcotic tolerance (e.g., if he has recently been released from jail or other confinement), the initial dosage can be one half these quantities. When there is any doubt, a smaller dose can be used initially. Then the patient should be kept under observation, and, if symptoms of abstinence are distressing, 10-milligram doses may be repeated as needed. Subsequently the dosage can be adjusted individually as tolerated and required with a maintenance level of approximately 40 to 100 milligrams daily. Occasionally, higher dosage levels may be required but must be justified in the medical record.

4. The methadone will be dispensed by a practitioner licensed by law to administer drugs and administered by him or under close supervision. For maintenance, initially (the first several weeks), the subject will receive the medication under observation daily, or at least 6 days a week. For detoxification, the drug will be administered daily under close observation. It is recognized that diversion occurs primarily when patients take medication from the clinic for self-administration. It is also recognized, however, that daily attendance at a clinic may be incompatible with gainful employment, education, and responsible home-making. Therefore, in maintenance treatment, after demonstrating satisfactory adherence to the program regulations for at least 3 months and showing substantial progress in his rehabilitation, the patient may be permitted to reduce to twice weekly the times when he

must receive the drug under observation. The rest of the time he may administer the drug himself, but no more than a 3-day supply will routinely be allowed in his possession. However, the requirement that the drug always be administered under supervision will be relaxed only in the following instances: (a) If the patient is responsibly employed on a regular and full-time basis, or (b) if the patient is a full-time student in a recognized institution of learning and is regularly in attendance and performing satisfactorily, or (c) if the patient is a part-time employee and part-time student and otherwise meets the criteria set forth in (a) and (b) above, or (d) if the patient is directly responsible, as a parent or as one in *loco parentis,* for the day-to-day welfare of one or more children under the age of 10 and customary observed medication intake would cause such a child or children to be without adequate supervision. Additional medication may also be provided in exceptional circumstances such as illness, family crises, or necessary travel when hardship would result from requiring the customary observed medication intake for such specific period as may be in question. In such circumstances the reasons for providing additional medication will be recorded.

B. In maintenance treatment, a urinalysis will be performed at least once a week for morphine and any other drug clinically indicated. Patients with take-home privileges for methadone should also be tested weekly for methadone. Urine specimens will be collected under direct observation. It is recommended but not required that patients be followed for other drug and alcohol abuse.

C. An adequate clinical record will be maintained for each patient. This record will contain the date of each visit, the results of each urinalysis, a detailed account of any adverse reactions, any significant physical or psychological disability, and other relevant aspects of the treatment program. If a patient misses appointments for 2 weeks or more without notifying the program, the episode of care will be considered terminated, and this will be noted on his clinical record. If he returns for care, he will be readmitted and his record will be reopened.

D. All patients in the maintenance program will be

given careful consideration for discontinuance of methadone after social rehabilitation has been maintained for a reasonable period of time. The patient will be given sufficient information regarding the methadone maintenance technique, so that he can elect to pursue the goal of eventually withdrawing from methadone and becoming drug-free.

IX. A report on Form FD_____, "Annual Report for Treatment Program Using Methadone" will be submitted to the Food and Drug Administration by January 30 of each year. (Copies of the form are available from this agency at the same address to which this application is mailed).

X. To prevent diversion into illicit channels, adequate security will be maintained over stocks of methadone and over the manner in which it is distributed, as required by the Bureau of Narcotics and Dangerous Drugs.

XI. Accurate records traceable to patients will be maintained showing dates, quantity, and batch or code marks of the drug used. These records should be retained for a period of 3 years.

XII. In a maintenance program, the program director may establish satellite operations for treatment and dispensing of medication but will obtain and submit to FDA a signed FD_____, "Medical Responsibility Statement for Treatment Program Using Methadone," for every such operation. Only after patients have been stabilized at their optimal dosage level may they be referred to the satellite operations for obtaining medication and other treatment including any appropriate rehabilitative services. Subsequent to such referral, the program director will retain continuing responsibility for the patient's care, and the patient must be periodically checked at the primary facility of the program. No satellite operation will provide care for more than 25 patients at any one time, unless the program director has justified an increase and obtained approval from the State authority.

XIII. All representations in this application are currently accurate, and no changes will be made in the program until they have been approved by the Food and Drug Administration.

XIV. If the program or any individual under the program is disapproved, the program director will recall the methadone from the disapproved sources and return the drug to the manufacturer.

XV. Inspections of this program may be undertaken by the State authority and the Food and Drug Administration. The identity of the patient will be kept confidential except when the patient or his legal representative consents to the release of such information, when it is necessary to make followup investigations on adverse effect information related to the drug, when the medical welfare of the patient would be threatened by a failure to reveal such information, or when it is necessary to verify records pursuant to preceedings to revoke approval of the program.

Signature:_____
Program Director

(ii) The following completed and signed form referred to in items II and XII of Form FD_____ is submitted in duplicate to the Food and Drug Administration:

Department of Health, Education, and Welfare
Food and Drug Administration
Form FD _____
Medical Responsibility
Statement For
Treatment Program For
Using Methadone

(To be completed by the individual responsible for the dispensing of medication in each facility and every physician working in an approved program, whether ultimately responsible for dispensing medication or not.)

Name of practitioner licensed by law to administer drugs

_____.

Name of program or program director _____
Program address _____.
Date _____.
The undersigned _____ agrees to assume responsibility for the prescribing and administering of

methadone under the above identified program and to abide by the standards for maintenance treatment and detoxification.

The name of each patient treated at a satellite facility and the frequency of visits will be registered with the program director. An annual report (Form FD _____) "Annual Report for Methadone Maintenance Programs" will be submitted to the program director for submission to FDA. The patient must always report to the same satellite operation unless prior approval is obtained from the program director for treatment at another satellite operation.

I. The following minimal treatment standards will be used:

A. A program statement will be given to the addicts to inform them about the program. Participation in the program should be voluntary.

B. Care will be exercised in the selection of patients to prevent the possibility of admitting a person who has not been dependent upon heroin or other morphine-like drugs and thereby creating de novo a state of dependence upon methadone. The mere use of an opiate, even if it is periodic or intermittent, cannot be equated with drug dependence. Admission to the program will depend upon a history of physiological dependence on one or more opiate drugs (which will be recorded in the applicant's medical record) and evidence of current physiological dependence on opiates as demonstrated by the results of urinalysis and signs of opiate withdrawal. It is highly unlikely that an individual would be currently dependent on opiates without a positive urinalysis for opiates and/or without demonstrating at least the early signs of withdrawal (lacrimation, rhinorrhea, pupillary dilation, and piloerection) during the initial period of abstinence. Other positive evidence of use can be obtained by noting the presence of needle tracks and by obtaining additional history from relatives and friends. The withdrawal signs may be observed during an initial period of hospitalization or while the individual is an outpatient undergoing diagnostic evaluation (history, physical examination, and laboratory studies). Loss of appetite and increased body temperature, pulse rate, blood pressure, and respiratory rate are also signs of withdrawal, but their detection requires inpatient observation.

C. An exception to the requirement for evidence of current physiological dependence on opiates will be allowed under exceptional circumstances. For example, methadone treatment may be initiated for an individual with a history of opiate addiction a short time prior to or upon release from a stay of 1 month or longer in a penal or chronic care institution. In these circumstances, the reasons for this exception, appropriate descriptions of the facilities, procedures, and qualifications of the personnel of the institution or other appropriate justification will be sent to the Food and Drug Administration at the time of filing this form or with the Annual Report.

D. Additional study is necessary to determine whether methadone may be safely and effectively used in the treatment of patients under 18. No such patients will be admitted to a treatment program using methadone unless prior approval of Form FD 1571, "Notice of Claimed Investigational Exemption for a New Drug," has been obtained. Such approval will be granted only for a controlled clinical study and not for an ongoing treatment program.

II. I agree that an admission evaluation and record will be made and maintained for each patient upon admission to the program and will consist of the following:

A. Personal history including age, sex, educational level, employment history, criminal history, and past history of drug abuse of all types;

B. Medical history and history of psychiatric illness and current legal problems, if any; and

C. Physical examination results.

III. The following minimal procedures will be used for on-going care:

A. *Dosage and administration for detoxification and maintenance*

1. The methadone will be administered in oral form.
2. In detoxification, the patient may be placed on a

substitutive methadone administration schedule when there are significant symptoms of withdrawal. The dosage schedule indicated below is recommended but should be varied depending upon clinical judgment. Initially, a single oral dose of 15-20 milligrams of methadone will often be sufficient. Additional methadone can be provided if withdrawal symptoms are not suppressed or whenever symptoms reappear. When patients are physically dependent on high doses of methadone it may be necessary to exceed these levels. With the exception of such patients, 40 milligrams per day in single or divided doses will usually constitute an adequate stabilizing dose level. Stabilization can be continued for 2 to 3 days and then the amount of methadone can be gradually decreased. The rate at which methadone is decreased will be determined separately for each patient. The dose of methadone can be decreased on a daily basis or, at most, in 2-day intervals. However, the amount of intake must always be sufficient to keep withdrawal symptoms at a tolerable level. In hospitalized patients a daily reduction of 20 percent of the total daily dose usually will be tolerated and causes little discomfort. When the total dosage has decreased to 20 milligrams per day, the dose can be reduced by 50 percent per day without producing significant discomfort. If a patient complains of undue distress, phenothiazine may be used in lieu of increasing the methadone dose. In ambulatory patients, a somewhat slower schedule may be needed.

In any event, if methadone is administered for more than 3 weeks, the procedure will be considered to have progressed from detoxification or treatment of the acute withdrawal syndrome to that of methadone maintenance even though the goal and intent may be eventual total withdrawal.

3. In maintenance treatment, the initial dosage of methadone should control the abstinence symptoms that follow withdrawal of heroin but should not be so great as to cause marked sedation or respiratory depression. It is important that the initial dosage be adjusted to the narcotic tolerance of the new patient. If such a patient has been a heavy user of heroin up to the day of admission,

he may be given 20 milligrams orally for the first dose and another 20 milligrams 4 to 8 hours later or 40 milligrams in a single oral dose. If he enters treatment with little or no narcotic tolerance (e.g., if he has recently been released from jail or other confinement), the initial dosage can be one half these quantities. When there is any doubt, a smaller dose can be used initially. Then the patient should be kept under observation, and, if symptoms of abstinence are distressing, the administration of 10-milligram doses may be repeated as needed. Subsequently the dosage can be adjusted individually as tolerated and required with a maintenance level of approximately 40 to 100 milligrams daily. Occasionally, higher dosage levels may be required but must be justified in the medical record.

4. The methadone will be dispensed by a practitioner licensed by law to administer drugs and administered by him or under close supervision. For maintenance, initially (the first several weeks) the subject will receive the medication under observation daily, or at least 6 days a week. For detoxification, the drug will be administered daily under close observation. It is recognized that diversion occurs primarily when patients take medication from the clinic for self-administration. It is also recognized, however, that daily attendance at a clinic may be incompatible with gainful employment, education, and responsible homemaking. Therefore, in maintenance treatment, after demonstrating satisfactory adherence to the program regulations for at least 3 months and showing substantial progress in his rehabilitation, the patient may be permitted to reduce to twice weekly the times when he must receive the drug under observation. The rest of the time he may administer the drug himself, but no more than a 3-day supply will routinely be allowed in his possession. However, the requirement that the drug always be administered under supervision will be relaxed only in the following instances: (a) If the patient is responsibly employed on a regular and full-time basis, or (b) if the patient is a full-time student in a recognized institution of learning and is regularly in attendance and performing satisfactorily, or (c) if the patient is a

part-time employee and/or part-time student and otherwise meets the criteria set forth in (a) and (b) above, or (d)
if the patient is directly responsible, as a parent or as one
in *loco parentis,* for the day-to-day welfare of one or more
children under the age of 10 and customary observed
medication intake would cause such a child or children to
be without adequate supervision. Additional medication
may also be provided in exceptional circumstances such
as illness, family cirsis, or necessary travel when hardship would result from requiring the customary observed
medication intake for such specific period as may be in
question. In such circumstances the reasons for providing additional medication will be recorded.

B. In maintenance treatment, a urinalysis will be performed at least once a week for morphine and any other
drug clinically indicated. Patients with take-home privileges for methadone should also be tested weekly for
methadone. Urine specimens will be collected under
direct observation. It is recommended but not required
that patients be followed for other drug and alcohol
abuse.

C. An adequate clinical record will be maintained
for each patient. This record will contain the date of each
visit, the results of each urinalysis, a detailed account of
any adverse reactions, any significant physical or
psychological disability, and other relevant aspects of
the treatment program. If a patient misses appointments
for 2 weeks or more without notifying the program, the
episode of care will be considered terminated, and this
will be noted on his clinical record. If he returns for care,
he will be readmitted and his record will be reopened.

D. All patients in the maintenance program will be
given careful consideration for discontinuance of methadone maintenance after socail rehabilitation has been
maintained for a reasonable period of time. The patient
will be given sufficient information regarding the methadone maintenance technique, so that he can elect to pursue the goal of eventually withdrawing from methadone
and becoming drug-free.

IV. To prevent diversion into illicit channels, adequate security will be maintained over stocks of metha-

done under my control and over the manner in which it is distributed, as required by the Bureau of Narcotics and Dangerous Drugs.

V. All representations in this application are currently accurate, and no changes will be made in the program until they have been approved by the program director and the Food and Drug Administration.

VI. If I am disqualified, I agree to return any remaining stock of methadone to the parent program.

VII. Inspections of this program may be undertaken by the State authority and the Food and Drug Administration. The identity of the patient will be kept confidential except when the patient or his legal representative consents to the release of such information, when it is necessary to make followup investigations on adverse effect information related to the drug, when the medical welfare of the patient would be threatened by a failure to reveal such information, or when it is necessary to verify records pursuant to proceedings to revoke approval of the program.

Signature: _____
Participating Physician

(iii) The following completed and signed form referred to in item IX of Form FD _____, "Application for Approval of Methadone Program," is submitted in duplicate in accordance with the instructions in item IX.

**Department of Health,
Education, and Welfare
Food and Drug Administration
Form FD _____
Annual Report for Treatment
Program Using Methadone**

This form is to be completed in duplicate for each calendar year. One copy is to be sent to the Food and Drug Administration and one copy to the State authority on or before January 30.

1. Name of other identification of program _____

   _____

   Address _____

   _____

   Number of satellite units _____
   (Attach a list showing address and person
   responsible for each unit)

2. Total Treatment Capacity _____

3. Drug Forms Dispensed:

   Amount of each formulation dispensed (in grams)
   during the year:

   Formulation   Amount

   a. _____   _____

   b. _____   _____

   c. _____   _____

4. Number of individuals who applied to the program
   but were not admitted or given admission evaluation
   _____.

5. Census of Patients Maintained on Methadone:

   a. Number under care at the beginning of the year
      being reported _____.
      Of those in treatment at the beginning of the year:

      (1) Number continuously under care through the
          year being reported (still under care) _____.

      (2) Number discharged or transferred to other
          types of programs and not readmitted _____.

(3) Number discharged or transferred to other types of programs and readmitted (still under care) _____.

(4) Number discharged and readmitted (no longer under care) _____.

b. Number admitted to care during year—not previously treated in this program:

(1) Number still under care at the end of the year _____.

(2) Number discharged or transferred to other types of programs and not readmitted _____.

(3) Number discharged or transferred to other types of programs and readmitted (still under care) _____.

(4) Number discharged and readmitted (no longer under care) _____.

c. Number admitted to care during the year—previously treated in this program prior to the past year:

(1) Number still under care at the end of the year _____.

(2) Number discharged or transferred to other types of programs and not readmitted _____.

(3) Number discharged and transferred to other types of programs and readmitted (still under care) _____.

(4) Number discharged and readmitted (no longer under care) _____.

6. Demographic and treatment characteristics of patients under care at the end of the year being reported:

a. Give the number of males and females in each age category:

Age	Sex	
	Male	Female
Under 18		
18-20	_____	_____
21-25	_____	_____
26-35	_____	_____
36-45	_____	_____
46+	_____	_____

b. For the year being reported, give the number of patients who have been under continuous care for the following periods of time:

Under three months	_____
3 months to one year	_____
One to two years	_____
Two to five years	_____
Over five years	_____

c. Total number of individuals treated to date _____.

d. For the year being reported, give the number of patients stabilized at each dosage level:

Daily Dosage	No. of Patients
Under 40 mgm.	
40-59 mgm.	_____
60-79 mgm.	_____
80-99 mgm.	_____
100-119 mgm.	_____
120-160 mgm.	_____
Over 160 mgm.	_____

e. For the year being reported, give the number of patients in the past 8 weeks who have fallen in the following categories:

No. of patients

No positive urinalysis for opiates
for 2 months or more   _____

Occasional positive urinalysis for
opiates (monthly or less)   _____

Frequent positive urinalysis for
opiates (more than once per month;
still dependent)   _____

7. Give the number of patients having significant adverse reactions, particularly reactions related to hematopoietic, cardiovascular, endocrine, and immunological functions (attach a completed copy of Form FD-1639 "Drug Experience Report" for each incident; forms obtainable from the Food and Drug Administration):

Type of Reaction   *No. of Patients*

_____   _____

_____   _____

_____   _____

8. Give the number of patients who have died while under methadone care (attach a completed copy of Form FD-1639 "Drug Experience Report" for each incident; forms obtainable from the Food and Drug Administration):

No. of Patients

a. Definitely methadone-related   _____

b. Not methadone-related   _____

Signature: _____
            Program Director

3. Within 60 days after receipt of an application for a treatment using methadone, the applicant will receive notification of approval or refusal.

4. Refusal or revocation of a program approval.

(i) Refusal or revocation of approval of a program may be proposed to the Commissioner of Food and Drugs by the Director of the FDA Bureau of Drugs, on his own initiative or at the request of representatives of the Bureau of Narcotics and Dangerous Drugs or the designated State authority.

(ii) Before presenting such a proposal to the Commissioner, the Director of the Bureau of Drugs or his representative will notify the program applicant of the proposed action and the reasons therefor and will offer him an opportunity to explain the matters in question in an informal conference and/or in writing. If an explanation is offered by the applicant but not accepted by the Bureau of Drugs and if the hearing is requested within 10 days after receipt of notification that the explanation is unacceptable, the Commissioner will provide the program applicant an opportunity for an informal hearing on the question of whether the applicant should be entitled to receive methadone for use in a treatment program. Representatives of the State authority and/or BNDD may participate in the conference with the Bureau official or with the Commissioner.

(iii) The Commissioner will evaluate all available information, including any explanation or assurance presented by the program applicant. If he finds that the program applicant has failed to submit adequate assurance that the conditions for receiving methadone for use in a program will be met or that the program applicant has repeatedly or deliberately failed to comply with the conditions for receiving methadone for treatment of addicts or that the applicant has deliberately submitted false information to the Food and Drug Administration, the Commissioner will notify the program applicant, the appropriate State officials, BNDD, and all other appropriate persons that the program applicant is not entitled to receive methadone for treatment of narcotic addicts.

(iv) If a program applicant has had a program application refused or revoked, such refusal or revocation may be reversed when the Commissioner determines that the applicant has presented adequate assurance that he will employ such drugs solely in compliance with the requirements for a methadone program.

5. Program directors will be allowed 3 months from the final promulgation of this paragraph in order to obtain the necessary approvals and establish procedures for adhering to these conditions. During this interim period the State authority may permit one or more hospitals in areas of the State without approved programs to dispense methadone for the detoxification and maintenance treatment of narcotic addicts. The holders of approved new drug applications will be notified by the Food and Drug Administration that methadone can be distributed to these hospital pharmacies after the state authority has so informed FDA.

6. Conditions for approving the use of methadone in analgesia and in hospitalized patients in detoxification.

(i) The drug is in oral or parenteral form.

(ii) Transportation is restricted to direct shipments to hospitals which have submitted a notification (FD _____ "Application for approval of Methadone Program,") to the Food and Drug Administration that they wish to receive the drug. The Food and Drug Administration will provide methadone manufacturers with the names of the hospitals that have submitted signed Forms FD _____, "Hospital Request for Methadone for Analgesia in Severe Pain and for Detoxification".

(iii) For a hospital to receive shipments of methadone for use as an analgesic and for detoxification, a responsible hospital official must complete, sign, and file in triplicate with the Food and Drug Administration a Form FD _____, "Hospital Request for Methadone for Analgesia in Severe Pain and for Detoxification," as follows:

Department Of Health, Education And Welfare
Food And Drug Administration
Form FD _____
Hospital Request For Methadone For Analgesia In Severe Pain And For Detoxification

Name of Hospital
Address

Commissioner
Food and Drug Administration
Bureau of Drugs (BD-22)
Rockville, Maryland 20852

Dear Sir:
I submit this notice of intent to receive supplies of methadone to be used for analgesia and detoxification. I understand that the failure to abide by the requirements described below may result in discontinuance of shipments of methadone, seizure of the drug supply on hand, injunction, and criminal prosecution.

1. The name of the individual (pharmacist) responsible for receiving and securing supplies of methadone is
_____.

2. There are _____ beds in the hospital. (Give the number).

3. A general description of the hospital and nature of patient care undertaken is attached.

4. The anticipated quantity of supply needed per year is _____.

5. Adequate security will be maintained over stocks of methadone to prevent diversion into illicit channels. All stocks will be secured in a locked cabinet or safe.

6. Methadone will be dispensed for detoxification of hospitalized patients only and for analgesia in severe pain for hospitalized and outpatients. If methadone is administered for treatment of heroin dependence for more than 3 weeks, the procedure passes from treatment of the

acute withdrawal syndrome (detoxification) to methadone maintenance. Such treatment can be undertaken only by approved methadone maintenance programs. This does not preclude the maintenance of an addict who is hospitalized for treatment for medical conditions other than addiction and whose enrollment in a specific maintenance program has been verified by the hospital.

7. Prior to filling a physician's prescription for methadone for outpatients, I will obtain from the physician a statement indicating that all such prescriptions will be limited to use for analgesia in severe pain and his agreement to maintain records to substantiate such use. These records will be available in the hospital or made available at the request of the hospital administrator. On January 30 of each year, the hospital will report to the Food and Drug Administration the names of all physicians who prescribed methadone for analgesia on an outpatient basis during the previous year.

8. Prescriptions will not be filled if they are written by a physician who has not submitted the required commitment to the hospital.

9. Accurate records are maintained showing dates, quantity, and batch or code marks of the drug used. The records are to be retained for a period of 3 years.

10. The Food and Drug Administration may inspect the supplies or use of the drug. The identity of the patient will be kept confidential except when the patient or his legal representative consents to the release of such information, when it is necessary to make followup investigations on adverse effect information related to the drug, when the medical welfare of the patient would be threatened by a failure to reveal such information, or when it is necessary to verify records pursuant to proceedings to revoke approval of the hospital.

Signature: _____
Hospital Official

Interested persons may, within 90 days after publication hereof in the FEDERAL REGISTER, file with the Hearing Clerk, Department of Health, Education, and Welfare, Room 6-88, 5600 Fishers Lane, Rockville, Md.

20852, written comments (preferably in quintuplicate) regarding this proposal. Comments may be accompanied by a memorandum or brief in support thereof. Received comments may be seen in the above office during working hours, Monday through Friday.

Dated: _____ .

_____

BIBLIOGRAPHY

Actual and Selected References

Allen, J.: New life editorials. *Journal of the New York City Addiction Rehabilitation Center,* 1970.

American Medical Association: Dependence on barbiturates and other sedative drugs. *Journal of American Medical Association,* **193,** 1965, p. 673.

American Medical Association Committee on Alcoholism and Drug Dependence. Management of narcotic-drug dependence by high-dosage methadone-HCL technique; Dole-Nyswander Program. *Journal of American Medical Association,* **201,** 1967, p. 956.

American Medical Association Council on Mental Health: Report on narcotic addiction. *Journal of American Medical Association,* **165,** 1957, pp. 1707, 1834, 1968.

Arnold, W.H.: The techniques of withdrawal of opiates and barbiturates-sedatives. Unpublished monograph from the Addiction Research Center, Lexington, Kentucky, 1961.

Ausubel, D.P.: The Dole-Nyswander treatment of heroin addiction. *Journal of American Medical Association,* **195,** 1966, p. 949.

Bailey, W.C.: Nalline control of addict-probationers. *International Journal of the Addictions,* **3,** 1968, p. 131.

Ball, J.C.: Two patterns of narcotic drug addiction in the United States. *Journal of Criminal Law, Criminology, and Police Science,* **56,** 1965, p. 203.

Batterman, R.C.: The importance of addiction to the newer synthetic analgesics in human therapy. *Annals of New York Academy of Sciences,* **51,** 1948, p. 123.

Batterman, R.C. and Oshlag, A.M.: The effectiveness and toxicity of methadone: a new analgesic agent. *Anesthesiology,* **10,** 1949, p. 214.

Beaver, W.T., *et. al.:* A clinical comparison of the analgesic effects of methadone and morphine administered intramuscularly, and of orally and parenterally administered methadone. *Clinical Pharmacology and Therapeutics,* **8,** 1967, p. 415.

Beckett, A.H., and Rowland, M.: Determination and identification of amphetamine in urine. *Journal of Pharmacy and Pharmacology,* **17,** 1965, p. 59.

Beckett, H.D.: Personal communication from drug addiction clinic, Norwood District Hospital, London, 1970.

Bellevue Hospital: New York City methadone proposal for patients with severe psychiatric problems. Mimeographed, 1970.

Berger, H.: Treatment of narcotic addicts in private practice. *Archives of Internal Medicine,* **114,** 1964, p. 59.

Berle, B. and Nyswander, M.E.: Ambulatory withdrawal treatment of heroin addicts. *New York Journal of Medicine,* **64,** 1964, p. 1846.

Bennett, J.F.: Development of a newly formulated tablet for methadone maintenance programs. Proceeding of the Third National Conference on Methadone Treatment, 1970, p. 143.

Bewley, T.H.: Drug dependence in the U.S.A.. *Bulletin on Narcotics,* **21,** 1969, p. 13.

Bewley, T.H.: The diagnosis and management of heroin addiction. *Practitioner,* **200,** 1968, p. 215.

Blachly, P.H.: Management of the opiate abstinence syndrome. *American Journal of Psychiatry,* **122,** 1966, p. 742.

Blachly, P.H.: Progress report on the methadone blockade treatment of heroin addicts in Portland. *Northwest Medicine,* **69,** 1970, p. 172.

Blachly, P.H.: Report on Oregon program. Described in *Narcotic Research Information Research Exchange Newsletter,* 1970.

Blinick, G.: Menstrual function and pregnancy in narcotics addicts treated with methadone. *Nature,* **219,** 1968, p. 180.

Blinick, G., *et. al.:* Pregnancy in narcotics addicts treated by medical withdrawal. *American Journal of Obstetrics and Gynecology,* **105,** 1969, p. 997.

Bloom, W.A. and Butcher, B.T.: Methadone side effects and related symptoms in 200 methadone maintenance patients. *Proceedings of the Third National Conference on Methadone Treatment,* 1970, p. 44.

Blumberg, H., *et. al.:* Narcotic antagonist activity of naloxone. *Federation Proceedings,* **24,** 1965, p. 676.

Blumberg, H., *et. al.:* Use of writing test for evaluating analgesic activity of narcotic antagonists. *Proceedings of the Society for Experimental Biology and Medicine,* **118,** 1965, p. 763.

Brill, H. and Larimore, G.W.: The British narcotic system—a report to Governor Rockefeller. New York State Department of Health and Mental Hygiene, 1960.

Brill, H. and Larimore, G.W.: Second on-site study of the British narcotic system—a report to Governor Rockefeller. New York State Narcotic Addiction Control Commission Reprint Series, 1967.

Brill, L. and Chambers, C.D.: A multimodality approach to methadone treatment. *Social Work,* **16,** 1971, p. 39.

Brill, L. and Jaffe, J.: The relevancy of some newer American treatment approaches for England. *British Journal of Addictions,* **62,** 1967, p. 375.

Brill, L. and Lieberman, L.: *Authority and Addiction.* Boston: Little, Brown and Company, 1969.

Brill, L., *et. al.:* Pharmacological approaches to the treatment of narcotic addiction: Patterns of response. In: *National Academy of Sciences, National Research Council Committee on Problems of Drug Dependence,* 1967, p. 5145.

Brown, T.T.: Narcotics and nalline: six years of testing. *Federal Probation,* **27,** 1963, p. 27.

California Department of Correction: Proposal for methadone program, 1970.

Chambers, C.D.: Barbiturate-sedative abuse: A study of prevalence among narcotic addicts. *International Journal of the Addictions,* **4,** 1969, p. 45.

Chambers, C.D.: Drug Abuse in Philadelphia: Current Treatment, Legislative and Research Activity. *The Yearbook of Drug Abuse,* L. Brill and E. Harms (eds.), New York: Behavioral Publications, 1972 (In Press).

Chambers, C.D.: The detoxification of narcotic addicts in out-patient clinics. *Major Modalities in the Treatment of Drug Abuse,* L. Brill and L. Lieberman (eds.), New York: Behavioral Publications, 1972.

Chambers, C.D., et. al.: Cocaine abuse during narcotic substitution therapy. Paper presented to the American Society of Clinical Pharmacology and Chemotherapy and the American Therapeutic society. Seventh Annual Meeting, Atlantic City, N.J., 1970.

Chambers, C.D., et. al.: The incidence of cocaine abuse among methadone maintenance patients. *International Journal of the Addictions,* **7,** 1972 (Forthcoming).

Chapple, P.A.L. and Gray, G.: One year's work at a centre for the treatment of addicted patients. *Lancet,* **1,** 1968, p. 908.

Chapple, P.A.L., et. al.: Treatmen of heroin addiction. *Lancet,* **1,** 1969, p. 940.

Chase, H.F., et. al.: N-allylnormorphine in treatment of dihydromorphinone and methorphinan overdosage. *Journal of American Medical Association,* **150,** 1952, p. 1103.

Cochin, J: Analysis for narcotic analgesics and barbiturates in urine by thin-layer chromatographic techniques without previous extraction and concentration. *Psychopharmacological Service Center Bulletin,* **3,** 1966, p. 53.

Cochin, J., and Daly, J.W.: Rapid identification of analgesic drugs in urine and thin-layer chromatography. *Breiv Communicazioni,* **4,** 1962, p. 294.

Coen, R.W., et. al.: Methadone substitution in neonatal narcotic withdrawal. Presented at the 79th. Annual Meeting of the American Pediatric Society, April-May, 1969.

Collins, R.J. and Weeks, J.R.: Relative potency of codeine, methadone and dihydromorphinone to morphine in self-maintained addict rats. *Archives of Experimental Pathology and Pharmacology,* **249,** 1965, p. 509.

"Cure": Personal Communication from National Addiction and Research Institute, London, 1970.

Cushman, P., et. al.: Hypothalamic-pituitary-adrenal axis in methadone-treated addicts. *Journal of Clinical Endocrinology,* **30,** 1970, p. 24.

Daly, J.R.L.: A clinical study of heroin. *Boston Medical Surgical Journal,* **142,** 1900, p. 190.

David, N.A.,, et. al.: Control of chronic pain by dl-alpha acetylmethadol. *Journal of American Medical Association,* **161,** 1956. p. 599.

DeKornfeld, T.J.: Clinical and laboratory study of hydroxydihydromorphinone (Numerphan HCL). *Federation Proceedings,* **20,** 1961, p. 309.

Devine, M.F., et. al.: The effect of simultaneously administered N-allylnoroxymorphone on the respiratory depression induced by oxymorphone. *American Journal of Medical Science,* **247,** 1964, p. 412.

Dole, V.P.: Drug maintenance as a treatment approach. *Journal of Hillside Hospital,* **16,** 1967, p. 157.

Dole, V.P.: In the course of professional practice. *New York State Journal of Medicine,* **65,** 1965, p. 927.

Dole, V.P.: Planning for the treatment of 25,000 heroin addicts. Proceedings of the Third National Conference on Methadone Treatment, New York City, 1970, p. 111.

Dole, V.P.: Thoughts on narcotics addiction. *Bulletin of the New York Academy of Sciences,* **41,** 1965, p. 211.

Dole, V.P. and Nyswander, M.E.: Heroin addiction: A metabolic disease. *Archives of Internal Medicine*, **120**, 1967, p. 19.

Dole, V.P. and Nyswander, M.E.: A medical treatment for diacetylmorphine (heroin) addiction: A clinical trail with methadone hydrochloride. *Journal of American Medical Association*, **193**, 1965, p. 646.

Dole, V.P. and Nyswander, M.E.: Methadone maintenance and its implications for theories of narcotic addiction. *Addictive States*, **46**, 1966, p. 359.

Dole, V.P. and Nyswander, M.E.: Rehabilitation of heroin addicts after blockade with methadone. *New York State Journal of Medicine*, **55**, 1966, p. 2011.

Dole, V.P. and Nyswander, M.E.: Rehabilitation of the street addict. *Archives of Environmental Health*, **14**, March 1967, p. 477.

Dole, V.P. and Nyswander, M.E.: Study of methadone as an adjunct in rehabilitation of heroin addicts. *Illinois Medical Journal*, **130**, 1966, p. 487.

Dole, V.P. and Nyswander, M.E.: The treatment of heroin addiction. *Journal of American Medical Association*, **195**, 1966, p. 972.

Dole, V.P. and Nyswander, M.E.: The use of methadone for narcotic blockade. *British Journal of Addictions*, **63**, 1968, p. 55.

Dole, V.P. and Warner, A.: Evaluation of narcotics treatment programs. *American Journal of Public Health*, **57**, 1967, p. 2000.

Dole, V.P., et. al.: Detection of narcotic drugs, tranquilizers, amphetamines, and barbiturates in urine. *Journal of American Medical Association*, **198**, 1966, p. 349.

Dole, V.P., et. al.: Methadone treatment of randomly selected criminal addicts. *New England Journal of Medicine*, **280**, 1969, p. 1372.

Dole, V.P., et. al.: Narcotic blockade: A medical technique for stopping heroin use by addicts. *Archives of Internal Medicine*, **118**, 1966, p. 304.

Dole, V.P., et. al.: Successful treatment of 750 criminal addicts. *Journal of American Medical Association*, **206**, 1968, p. 2709.

Dreser, H.: Uber die wirkung einiger derivate des morphins auf die athmung. *Archive fur Gesamte Psychologie*, **72**, 1898, p. 485.

Dupont, R.: Personal communication and program materials for Narcotic Treatment Administration of Washington, D.C., 1970.

Ebony: The methadone method. Report on Black Action Program, 1970.

Eckenhoff, J.E., et. al.: N-allylnormorphine in the treatment of morphine or Demerol narcosis. *American Journal of Medical Science*, **223**, 1952, p. 191.

Eddy, N.B.: Chemopharmacologic approach to the addiction problem. *Narcotics*, D.M. Wilner and G.G. Kassebaum (eds.), New York: McGraw-Hill, 1965, p. 57.

Eddy, N.B.: *Methadone Maintenance for the Management of Persons with Drug Dependence of Morphine Type*. Washington: Bureau of Narcotics and Dangerous Drugs, 1969.

Eddy, N.B.: The use of drugs in the management of drug dependence. *Journal of Tennessee Medical Association*, **60**, 1967, p. 269.

Eddy, N.B. and Lee, L.E., Jr.: Analgesic equivalence to morphine and relative side action liability of oxymorphone (14-hydroxydihydromorphinone). *Journal of Pharmacology and Experimental Therapeutics*, **125**, 1959, p. 116.

Eddy, N.B., et. al.: Drug dependence: its significance and characteristics. Bulletin of the World Health Organization, 32, 1965, p. 72.

Edwards, G.: Relevance of American experience of narcotic addiction to the British scene. British Medical Journal, 3, 1967, p. 425.

Edwards, G.: The British approach to the treatment of heroin addicts. Yale Law Review, 78, 1696, p. 1175.

Erickson, J.H.: Methadone maintenance treatment of opiate addicts in Sweden. Proceedings Third National Methadone Maintenance Conference, New York City, 1970.

Fink, M. and Freedman, A.M.: Antagonists in the treatment of opiate dependence. In: Modern Trends in Combatting Drug Dependence and Alcoholism, R.V. Phillipson (ed.), London: Butterworth, 1970.

Fink, M., et. al.: Methadone induced cross-tolerance to heroin. In: National Academy of Sciences, National Research Council, Committee on Problems of Drug Dependence, 1969, p. 5733.

Fink, M., et. al.: Naloxone in heroin dependence. Journal of Clinical Pharmacology and Therapeutics, 9, 1968, p. 568.

Fink, M., et. al.: Narcotic antagonists and substitutes in opiate dependence. Excerpta Medica International Cong. Series, 180, 1968.

Fiut, R.E., et. al.: Antagonism of convulsive and lethal effects induced by propoxyphine. Journal of Pharmaceutical Sciences, 55, 1966, p. 1085.

Foldes, F.F., et. al.: The respiratory, circulatory, and analgesic effects of naloxone-narcotic mixtures in anesthetized subject. Canadian Anaesthology Society Journal, 12, 1965, p. 608.

Foldes, F.F., et. al.: Studies of the specificity of narcotic antagonists. Anesthesiology, 26, 1965, p. 320.

Fraser, H.F.: Human pharmacology and clinical uses of nalorphine (N-allylnormorphine). Medical Clinics of North America, 41, 1957, p. 393.

Fraser, H.F. and Grider, J.A.: Treatment of drug addiction. American Journal of Medicine, 14, 1953, p. 571.

Fraser, H.F. and Isbell, H.: Actions and addiction liabilities of alpha-acetyl-methadols in man. Journal of Pharmacology and Experimental Therapeutics, 105, 1952, p. 458.

Fraser, H.F. and Rosenberg, D.E.: Comparative effects of (I) chronic administration of cyclazocine, (II) substitution of nalorphine for cyclazocine, and (III) chronic administration of morphine, Pilot crossover study. International Journal of the Addiction, 1, 1966, p. 86.

Fraser, H.F., et. al.: Death due to withdrawal of barbiturates. Annals of Internal Medicine, 38, 1953, P. 1319.

Fraser, H.F., et. al.: Methods for evaluating addiction liability. Journal of Pharmacology and Experimental Therapeutics, 133, 1961, p. 371.

Fraser, H.F., et. al.: Studies on N-allylnormorphine in man: Antagonism to morphine and heroin and effects of mixtures of N-allylnormorphine and morphine. American Journal of Medical Science, 231, 1956, p. 1.

Fraser, H.F., et. al.: Use of N-allynormorphine in treatment of methadone poisoning in man. Journal of American Medical Association, 148, 1952, p. 1205.

Freedman, A.M.: Drug addiction: An eclectic view. Journal of American Medical Association, 197, 1966, p. 878.

Freedman, A.M., et. al.: Clinical studies of cyclazocine in the treatment of narcotic addiction. *American Journal of Psychiatry,* **124,** 1968, p. 1499.

Freedman, A.M., *et. al.*: Cyclazocine and methadone in narcotic addiction. *Journal of American Medical Association,* **202,** 1967, p. 191.

Freymuth, H.W.: Methadone and the private practitioner. *Journal of the Medical Society of New Jersey,* **67,** 1970, p. 128.

Friend, D.G.: Accidental therapeutic drug addiction. *Clinical Pharmacology and Therapeutics,* **7,** 1966, p. 832.

Gearing, F.: Evaluation of methadone maintenance treatment program: progress report through October 3, 1968 (mimeographed).

Gearing, F.: Evaluation of methadone maintenance program: program progress report through March 31, 1969 (mimeographed).

Gearing, F.: Methadone maintenance treatment program. Progress report of evaluation through March 31, 1970 (mimeographed).

Gerwirtz, P.D.: Methadone maintenance for heroin addicts. *Yale Law Journal,* **78,** 1969, p. 1175.

Goldstein, A.: Blind controlled dosage comparisons with methadone in 200 patients. Proceedings of the Third National Conference on Methadone Treatment, 1970, p. 31.

Goldstein, A.: Uniform dosage of methadone hydrochloride. Decribed in Narcotic Research Information Exchange Newsletter, 1970.

Gordon, N.B.: Reaction time in methadone treated ex-addicts. *Psychopharmacologia,* **16,** 1970, p. 337.

Gordon, N.B., *et. al.*: Psychomotor and intellectual performance under methadone maintenance. In *National Academy of Sciences, National Research Council, Committee on Problems of Drug Dependence,* 1967, p. 5136.

Gunne, L.M.: Treatment of drug addiction with narcotic blockade. *Lakartidningen,* **63,** 1966, p. 4060.

Haertzen, C.A., and Meketon, M.J.: Opiate withdrawal as measured by the addiction research center inventory (ARCI). *Diseases of the Nervous System,* **29,** 1968, p. 450.

Hammond, R.O.: Personal Communication re methadone situation in Canada, 1970.

Hart, E.R.: N-allyl-norcodeine and N-allyl-normorphine, two antagonists to morphine. *Journal of Pharmacology and Experimental Therapeutics,* **72,** 1941, p. 19.

Hart, E.R. and McCawley, E.L.: The pharmacology of N-allylnormorphine as compared with morphine. *Journal of Pharmacology and Experimental Therapeutics,* **82,** 1944, p. 5339.

Heaton, A.M. and Blumberg, A.G.: Thin-layer chromatographic detection of barbiturates, narcotics and amphetamines in urine of patients receiving psychotropic drugs. *Journal of Chromatography,* **41,** 1969, p. 367.

Himmelsbach, C.K.: Clinical studies of drug addiction. Physical dependence, withdrawal and recovery. *Archives of Internal Medicine,* **69,** 1942, p. 766.

Himmelsbach, C.K.: Studies on the addiction of demerol (D-140). *Journal of Pharmacology and Experimental Therapeutics,* **75,** 1942, p. 64.

Himmelsbach, C.K. and Small, L.F.: Clinical studies of drug addiction II "Rossium" treatment of drug addiction. *Public Health Report,* Supplement Number **125,** 1937.

Hoffman, L.: A methadone program for addicts with chest diseases. *Journal of American Medical Association*, **211**, 1970, p. 977.

Hoogerbeets, J.: Methadone in Miami. *International Journal of the Addictions*, **5**, 1970, p. 499.

Holmes, S.J.: Paper presented at the 28th Annual Meeting of the Committee on Problems of Drug Dependence, National Research Council, National Academy of Sciences—National Academy of Engineering, Division of Medical Sciences, 1966.

Hurley, C.T.: Anti-narcotic testing: A physician's point of view. *Federal Probation*, **27**, 1963, p. 32.

Isaac, R.H. and Nyswander, M.E.: Points raised on methadone. *American Journal of Psychiatry*, **124**, 1967, p. 570.

Isbell, H.: Addiction to barbiturates and the barbiturate abstinence syndrome. *Annals of Internal Medicine*, **33**, 1950, p. 108.

Isbell, H.: Attempted addiction to nalorphine. *Federation Proceedings*, **15**, 1956, p. 442.

Isbell, H.: Nalline-a specific narcotic antagonist. Clinical and pharmacological observations. *The Merck Report*, **62**, 1953, p. 23.

Isbell, H., and Eisenman, A.J.: The addiction liability of some drugs of the methadone series. *Journal of Pharmacology and Experimental Therapeutics*, **93**, 1948, p. 305.

Isbell, H., and Eisenman, A.J.: Physical dependence liability of drugs of the methadone series and of 6-methyldihydro-morphine. *Federation Proceedings*, **7**, 1948, p. 1.

Isbell, H., and White, W.: Clinical characteristics of addictions. *American Journal of Medicine*, **16**, 1953, p. 558.

Isbell, H., *et. al.*: Chronic barbiturate intoxication: An experimental study. *Archives of Neurology*, **64**, 1950, p. 1.

Isbell, H., *et. al.*: Effect of single doses of 10820 (4-4-diphenyl-6-methyl-amino-heptanone-3) on man. *Federation Proceedings*, **6**, 1947, p. 341.

Isbell, H., *et. al.*: Experimental addiction to 10820 (4-4-diphenyl-6-dimethylamino-heptanone-3) in man. *Federation Proceedings*, **6**, 1947, p. 264.

Isbell, H., *et. al.*: Liability of addiction to 6-dimethylamino-4-4-diphenyl-heptanone-3 (methadone, amidone, or 10820). *Archives of Internal Medicine*, **82**, 1948, p. 362.

Isbell, H., *et. al.*: The effects of single doses of 6-dimethylamino-4-4-diphenyl-heptanone-3 (amidone, methadone or 10820) on human subjects. *Journal of Pharmacology and Experimental Therapeutics*, **92**, 1948, p. 83.

Isbell, H., *et. al.*: Tolerance and addiction liability of 6-dimethylamino-4-4-diphenyl-heptanone-3 (methadone). *Journal of American Medical Association*, **135**, 1947, p. 41.

Isbell, H., *et. al.*: Treatment of the morphine abstinence syndrome with 10820 (4-4 diphenyl-6-dimethylamine-heptanone-3). *Federation Proceedings*, **6**, 1947, p. 340.

Jaffe, J.H.: Methadone maintenance: variation in outcome criteria as a function of dose. Proceedings of the Third National Conference on Methadone Treatment, 1970, p. 37.

Jaffe, J.H. and Brill, L.: Cyclazocine, a long-acting narcotic antagonist: its voluntary acceptance as a treatment modality by narcotics abusers. *International Journal of the Addictions*, **1**, 1966, p. 99.

Jaffe, J.H., and Kirkpatrick, D.: The use of ion-exchange resin impregnated paper in the detection of opiate alkaloids, amphetamines, phenothiazines and barbiturates in urine *Psychopharmacological Service Center Bulletin,* **3,** 1966, p. 49.

Jaffe, J.H., *et. al.:* Comparison of acetylmethadol and methadone in the treatment of long-term heroin users: A pilot study. *Journal of American Medical Association,* **211,** 1970, p. 1834.

Jaffe, J.H., *et. al.:* Experience with the use of methadone in a multi-modality program for the treatment of narcotics users. *International Journal of the Addictions,* **4,** 1969, p. 481.

Jaffe, J.H., *et. al.:* Pharmacological approaches to the treatment of narcotics addiction; patterns of response. Paper presented at the 29th annual meeting of the Committee on Problems of Drug Dependence, National Research Council, National Academy of Sciences—National Academy of Engineering, Division of Medical Sciences, Lexington, Kentucky, 1967.

Jan, R.: Personal communication with the director of the West Side Medical Clinic, July 1970.

Jasinski, D.R. and Mansky, P.: The subjective effects of GPA-2087 and nalbuphine (EN-2234A). Bulletin, Committee on Problems of Drug Dependence, National Academy of Sciences, Washington, D.C. 1970, p. 6920.

Jasinski, D.R., *et. al.:* Antagonism of the subjective, behavioral, pupillary, and respiratory depressant effects of cyclazocine by naloxone. *Clinical Pharmacology and Therapeutics,* **9,** 1968, p. 215.

Jasinski, D.R., *et. al.:* The human pharmacology and abuse potential of N-allylnoroxymorphone (Naloxone). *Journal of Pharmacology and Experimental Therapeutics,* **157,** 1967,p. 420.

Jasinski, D.R., *et. al.:* Progress report on the assessment of the antagonists nalbuphine and GPA-2087 for abuse potential and studies of the effects of dextromethorphan in man. Paper presented at the 33rd annual meeting of the Committee on Problems of Drug Dependence, National Academy of Sciences—National Academy of Engineering, Division of Medical Sciences, Toronto, Canada, 1971.

Joseph, H.: Court services and methadone treatment. *Proceedings of the Third National Methadone Conference,* New York, 1970, p. 104.

Joseph, H.: Heroin addiction and methadone maintenance. *Probation and Parole,* **1,** 1969, p. 18.

Joseph, H. and Dole, V.P.: Methadone patients on probation and parole. *Federal Probation,* **34,** 1970, p. 42.

Keats, A.S. and Beecher, H.: Analgesic activity and toxic effects of acetyl methadol isomers in man. *Journal of Pharmacology and Experimental Therapeutics,* **105,** 1952, p. 210.

Keats, A.S. and Mithoefer, J.C.: Nature of antagonism of nalorphine to respiratory depression induced by morphine in man. *Federation Proceedings,* **14,** 1955, p. 356.

Keats, A.S. and Telford, J.: Nalorphine, a potent analgesic in man. *Journal of Pharmacology and Experimental Therapeutics,* **117,** 1956, p. 190.

Kolb, L.C.: Drug Addiction. *Bulletin of the New York Academy of Medicine,* **41,** 1965, p. 306.

Kolb, L.C.: *Drug Addiction: A Medical Problem.* Springfield: Charles C Thomas, 1962.

Kolb, L. and Himmelsbach, C.K.: Clinical studies of drug addiction. III. A critical review of the withdrawal treatments with method of evaluating abstinence syndromes. *American Journal of Psychiatry,* **94,** 1938, p. 759.

Kramer, J.C.: New directions in the management of opiate dependence. *New Physicians,* **18,** 1969, p. 205.

Kurland, A.A. and Kerman, F.: N-allyl-14-hydroxydihydronormorphinone (Naloxone) in the management of the narcotic abuser. A pilot study. Paper presented at the 33rd annual meeting of the Committee on Problems of Drug Dependence, National Research Council, National Academy of Sciences—National Academy of Engineering, Division of Medical Sciences, Toronto, Canada, 1971.

Kurland, A.A., *et. al.:* Urine detection tests in the management of the narcotic addict. *American Journal of Psychiatry,* **122,** 1966, p. 737.

Lasagna, L.: Drug interaction in the field of analgesic drugs. *Proceedings of the Royal Society of Medicine,* **58,** 1965, p. 978.

Lasagna, L.: Nalorphine (N-allylnormorphine); practical and theoretical considerations. *American Medical Association Archives of Internal Medicine,* **94,** 1954, p. 532.

Lasagna, L. and Beecher, H.K.: The analgesic effectiveness of nalorphine and nalorphine—morphine combinations in man. *Journal of Pharmacology and Experimental Therapeutics,* **112,** 1954, p. 356.

Laskowitz, D., *et. al.:* Cyclazocine intervention in the treatment of narcotic addiction: another look. *Major Modalities in the Treatment of Drug Abuse.* L. Brill and L. Lieberman (eds.), New York: Behavioral Publications, 1972 (Forthcoming).

Martin, W.P.: Commentary on the Second National Conference on Methadone Treatment. *International Journal of the Addictions,* **5,** 1971, p. 545.

Martin, W.R.: Opioid antagonists. *Pharmacological Reviews,* **19,** 1967, p. 463.

Martin, W.R.: Pharmacologic factors in relapse and the possible use of the narcotic antagonists in treatment. *Illinois Medical Journal,* **130,** 1966, p. 489.

Martin, W.R.: The basis and possible utility of opioid antagonists in the ambulatory treatment of the addict. *Association for Research in Nervous and Mental Disease,* **46,** 1968, p. 367.

Martin, W.R. and Gorodetzky, C.W.: Cyclazocine, an adjunct in the treatment of narcotic addiction. *International Journal of the Addictions,* **2,** 1967, p. 85.

Martin, W.R. and Gorodetzky, C.W.: Demonstration of tolerance to and physical dependence on N-allylnormorphine (nalorphine). *Journal of Pharmacology and Experimental Therapeutics,* **150,** 1965, p. 437.

Martin, W.R. and Jasinski, D.R.: Physiological parameters of morphine dependence in man-tolerance, early abstinence, protracted abstinence. An official memorandum to the Surgeon General of the United States from the Director of NIMH reporting on the mental health activities of the Addiction Research Center in Lexington, Kentucky, 1968.

Martin, W.R. and Sloan, J.W.: The pathophysiology of morphine dependence and its treatment with opioid antagonists. *Pharmakopsychiatric Neuropsychopharmakologie,* **1,** 1968, p. 260.

Martin, W.R., *et. al.:* An experimental study in the treatment of narcotic addicts with cyclazocine. *Clinical Pharmacology and Therapeutics,* **7,** 1966, p. 455.

Martin, W.R., *et. al.:* Tolerance to and physical dependence on morphine in rats. *Psychopharmacologia,* **4,** 1963, p. 247.

Maslansky, R.A., *et. al.*: Pregnancies in methadone maintained mothers: A Preliminary Report. Proceedings Third National Conference on Methadone Treatment, New York City, 1970, p. 56.

May, E.: Drugs without crime. *Harper's Magazine,* July, 1971, p. 60.

Medea, E.: L'impiego terapeutico dell' heroina. *Margagni,* **41,** 1899, p. 381.

Mering, J.V.: Physiological and therapeutical investigations on the action of some morphine derivatives. *Merck's Jahrest,* **1,** 1898, p. 5.

Methadone Maintenance Evaluation Committee: Progress report of methadone maintenance treatment program as of March 31, 1968. *Journal of American Medical Association,* **206,** 1968, p. 2712.

Milligan, A.: Personal Communication from Director of Addiction Research Foundation, Toronto, Ontario, 1970.

Millman, R.B. and Nyswander, M.E.: Slow detoxification of adolescent heroin addicts in New York City. Paper presented at Third National Methadone Maintenance Conference, New York City, 1970.

Moorehead, G.A.: Personal communication from Research Director, Task Force on Narcotics, Dangerous Durgs and Alcoholism, Virgin Islands Law Enforcement Commission, 1970.

Morel-Levalée, A.: La morphine remplace par l'heroine pas d'euphorie, plus de toxicomanes traitment heroique de la morphinemaie. *Rev. Med.* **20,** 1900, p. 872.

Narcotic Addiction Foundation: Narcotic Addiction Foundation of British Columbia 14th Annual Report, Treatment Supplement, Vancouver, British Columbia, 1969.

New York Academy of Medicine—Subcommittee on Drug Addiction: Report on drug addiction. *Bulletin of the New York Academy of Medicine,* **31,** Second Series. No. 8, 1955, p. 592.

New York Academy of Medicine—Subcommittee on Drug Addiction: Report on drug addiction II. *Bulletin of the New York Academy of Medicine,* **39,** Second Series No. 7, 1963, p. 417.

New York Academy of Medicine—Subcommittee on Drug Addiction: Report on drug addiction. *Bulletin of the New York Academy of Medicine,* **41,** Second Series No. 7, 1965, p. 825.

Nix, J.T.: Control programs for heroin addiction. *Journal of American Medical Association,* **211,** 1970, p. 1378.

Nix, J.T.: Methadone for narcotic addicts. *Journal of American Medical Association,* **207,** 1969, p. 2439.

Nyswander, M.E. and Dole, V.P.: The present status of methadone blockade treatment. *American Journal of Psychiatry,* **123,** 1967, p. 1141.

Ono, M., *et. al.*: Procedures for assured identification of morphine, dihydromorphinone, codeine, norcodeine, methadone, quinine, methamphetamine, etc., in human urine. *Bulletin on Narcotics,* **XXI,** No. 2, April-June, 1969, p. 31.

Oppenheim, G.P.: Personal Communication from Locum Consultant in Psychiatry, Charing Cross Hospital, London, 1970.

Paulus, I. and Halliday, R.: Rehabilitation and the narcotic addict: results of a comparative methadone withdrawal program. *Canada Medical Association Journal,* **96,** 1967, p. 655.

Perkins, M.E. and Bloch, H.I.: Methadone maintenance treatment program: a survey. *American Journal of Psychiatry,* **125,** 1970, p. 1389.

Perkins, M.E. and Bloch, H.I.: A study of some failures in methadone treatment. Presented at the 123rd Annual Meeting of the American Psychiatric Association, San Francisco, 1970.

Pohl, J.: Uber das N-allylcodein, einenatagonisten des morphins. *Atschr. Exper. Path. u Ther.,* **17,** 1915, p. 370.

Powers, B.R.: Use of methadone to combat withdrawal symptoms of "Dilaudid" addiction: a case report. *Journal of the Tennessee Medical Association,* **42,** 1949, p. 83.

Primm, B.J.: Ancillary services in methadone treatment in the Bedford-Stuyvesant experiences. Proceedings of the Third National Methadone Conference, New York, 1970, p. 66.

Prior, D.: Medical treatment of addiction. *Sciences,* **9,** 1969, p. 10.

Raskin, H.A.: Rehabilitation of the narcotic addict. *Journal of American Medical Association,* **189,** 1964, p. 180.

Rasor, R.W. and Crecraft, H.J.: Addiction to meperdine (demerol) hydrochloride. *Journal of American Medical Association,* **157,** 1955, p. 654.

Reinhold, R.: Methadone for drug addicts is gaining in popularity. *New York Times,* July 26, 1970.

Resnick, R.B., et. al.: A cyclazocine typology in opiate dependence. *American Journal of Psychiatry,* **126,** 1970, p. 9.

Resnick, R.B., et. al.: A typological approach to the therapy of opiate dependence by cyclazocine and methadone. In National Academy of Sciences, National Research Council, Committee on Problems of Drug Dependence, 1969, p. 5738.

Rice, J., and Cohen, L: Narcotic drug addiction: One year's experiences at Pilgrim State Hospital. *Psychiatric Quarterly,* **39,** 1965, p. 457.

Riordan, C.: Progress report of addiction research and treatment corporation evaluation team. Report submitted to the Department of Law Enforcement Assistance Administration. Unpublished, Mimeographed, 1970.

Roxburgh, R.C., and Munro-Faure, D.: Amidone overdosage in a child. *Lancet,* **1,** 1951, p. 174.

Sadove, M.S., et. al.: Study of a narcotic antagonist. N-allylnoroxymorphone. *Journal of American Medical Association,* **183,** 1963, p. 666.

Schur, E.M.: *Narcotic Addiction in Britain and America: The Impact of Public Policy.* Bloomington: Indiana University Press, 1962.

Scott, C.C. and Chen, K.K.: The action of I, I, diphenyl —I (dimethyl-amino-isopropyl)-butanone-3, a potent analgesic agent. *Journal of Pharmacology and Experimental Therapeutics,* **88,** 1945, p. 63.

Smits, S.E., and Takemori, A.E.: Quantiative studies on the antagonism by naloxone of some narcotic and narcotic-antagonist analgesics. *British Journal of Pharmacology,* **39,** 1970, p. 627.

Stern, R.: The Pregnant Addict, *American Journal of Obstetrics and Gynecology,* **94,** 1966, p. 253.

Strober, M.: Treatment of acute heroin intoxication with nalorphine (nalline) hydrochloride. *Journal of American Medical Association,* **154,** 1954, p. 327.

Tabor, M.C.: Capitalism plus dope equals genocide. Paper distributed by the Black Panther Party, 2026 Seventh Avenue, New York, 1970.

Telford, J., et. al.: Studies of analgesic drugs, VII. Morphine antagonists as analgesics. *Journal of Pharmacology and Experimental Therapeutics*, **133**, 1961, p. 106.

Terry, C.E. and Pellens, M.: *The Opium Problem*. New York: Bureau of Social Hygiene, 1928.

Unna, K.: Antagonistc effect of N-allyl-normorphine upon morphine. *Journal of Pharmacology and Experimental Therapeutics*, **79**, 1943, p. 27.

Wallach, R.C., et. al.: Pregnancy and menstrual function in narcotic addicts treated with methadone. *American Journal of Obstetrics and Gynecology*, **105**, 1969, p. 1226.

Weijlard, J. and Erickson, A.E.: N-allylnormorphine. *Journal of the American Chemical Society*, **64**, 1942, p. 869.

Weir, J.G.: Personal Communication from Consulting Psychiatrist, St. Mary's Hospital Drug Dependence Center, Paddington, London, 1970.

Wesley, J.F.: Program description of Harlem Hospital narcotic program. Mimeographed, 1969.

White House Conference on Narcotic and Drug Abuse. *Proceedings*. Washington, September, 1963.

Wieland, W.F.: Methadone maintenance treatment of heroin-addiction: Beginning treatment on an outpatient basis. Paper read before Annual Meeting of American Psychiatric Association, Boston, 1968.

Wieland, W.F. and Chambers, C.D.: Methadone maintenance—a comparison of two stabilization techniques. *International Journal of the Addictions*, **5**, 1970, p. 645.

Wieland, W.F. and Chambers, C.D.: Narcotic substitution therapy. *International Journal of Clinical Pharmacology Therapy and Toxicology*, (Forthcoming) 1972.

Wieland, W.F. and Chambers, C.D.: Outpatient detoxification of narcotic addiction. Proceedings 32nd Annual Meeting of Committee on Problems of Drug Dependence, World National Research Council, Washington, 1970.

Wieland, W.F. and Chambers, C.D.: Two methods of utilizing methadone in the outpatient treatment of narcotic addicts. *International Journal of Addictions*, **5**, 1970, p. 431.

Wieland, W.F. and Moffett, A.D.: Results of a low-dosage methadone treatment. Paper presented at the Third National Methadone Maintenance Conference, New York City, 1970.

Wieland, W.F. and Yunger, M.: Sexual effects and side effects of heroin and methadone. Proceedings of the Third National Conference on Methadone Treatment, 1970, p. 50.

Wikler, A.: Clinical and electroencephalographic studies on the effects of mescaline, N-allylnormorphine and morphine in man. *Journal of Nervous and Mental Diseases*, **120**, 1954, p. 157.

Wikler, A.: Conditioning factors in opiate addiction and relapse. *Narcotics*, D.M. Wilner and G.G. Kassebaum (eds.). New York: McGraw-Hill, 1965, p. 85.

Wikler, A.: Interaction of physical dependence and classical operant conditioning in the genesis of relapse. *Association for Research in Nervous and Mental Disease*, **46**, 1968, p. 280.

Wikler, A. and Frank, K.: Tolerance and physical dependence in intact and chronic spinal dogs during addiction to 10820 (4-4-diphenyl-6-dimethylamino-heptanone-3). *Federation Proceedings,* **6,** 1947, p. 384 (Abstract).

Wikler, A. and Pescor, F.T.: Factors disposing to "relapse" in rats previously addicted to morphine. *Pharmacologist,* **7,** 1965, p. 171.

Wikler, A., *et. al.:* N-allylnormorphine: Effects of single doses and precipitation of acute "abstinence syndromes" during addiction to morphine, methadone or heroin in man (post-addicts). *Journal of Pharmacology and Experimental Therapeutics,* **109,** 1953, p. 8.

Zaks, A., *et. al.:* Naloxone treatment of opiate dependence: A progress report. *Journal of American Medical Association,* **215,** 1971, p. 2106.